Stepping Stones with Children

Praise for the book

'AIDS is about social justice. We cannot achieve our goals to end AIDS by 2030 until we meet the needs of the most vulnerable in society, often children and adolescents who are living with HIV and those affected by the virus. Stepping Stones with Children provides a way that communities can support and nurture these children and build their resilience. This is what we must do first -- care for the most vulnerable.'

Michel Sidibé, Executive Director of UNAIDS

'This is a very important manual for children and caregivers. It will help support the building of closer relationships through meaningful communication that helps children and caregivers overcome barriers and build a close and supportive family unit.'

Martha Tholanah, Global Chair, International Community of Women Living with HIV/AIDS

'I wish that all children aged 5 to 14 years and their caregivers affected by HIV could have an opportunity to experience Stepping Stones with Children. I am confident that it will help them realize their dreams and overcome their challenges. It is unique because it works with peer groups separately and together and covers so many issues – psychological, physical, sexual, material and spiritual – that matter deeply to us all.'

Vincent Mwale, Minister for Youth, Sport and Child Development, Zambia

'Programmes and manuals like Stepping Stones with Children can make the difference for a human being between a healthy development and a vision of a world with possibility and, in the most extreme cases, life overshadowed by death.'

L'Orangelis Thomas, a young woman living with HIV

'Gill Gordon is to be congratulated for writing a highly readable and applied manual. Stepping Stones with Children is full of practical 'how to' tips, and most importantly, contains a rich repertoire of practical exercises. The book will make an excellent resource for any practitioner working with vulnerable children and young people.'

Morten Skovdal, Associate Professor, Department of Public Health, University of Copenhagen

'It is wonderful to see the culmination of such important thinking and practice around working with children affected by HIV. This resource provides a rich programme of training that builds on the immense success of Stepping Stones. If we can give this resource the similar time and commitment to its methodology SSWC has the potential to address key gaps in our response for children affected by HIV.'

Kate Iorpenda, Senior Advisor, Children and Adolescents, International HIV/AIDS Alliance

'At first when PASADA introduced Stepping Stones people thought they were mad. Later on they realized it was an important and powerful tool for society. If my voice can be heard all over the world, I'll tell people to use Stepping Stones with Children as it will change their life and the way they think about HIV and AIDS.'

Mrisho Mpoto, poet, actor and musician

'Gill Gordon has a great talent for writing manuals which trigger self-understanding and at the same time build confidence, assertiveness, and lots of useful life skills. She brings her wealth of experience working with young people on so many different issues. I will certainly use these exercises and adapt them for work with kids in other contexts.'

Ross Kidd, Participatory Trainer and author of several manuals, including Understanding and Challenging HIV

'We strongly recommend Stepping Stones with Children as unique in helping in the implementation of children's sexual and reproductive health and HIV and AIDS.'

Zikhalo Phiri, CEO of Young, Happy, Healthy and Safe, Zambia

Stepping Stones with Children

A transformative training for children affected by HIV and their caregivers

Gill Gordon

with Nelson Chiziza, Sue Holden,
Florence Kilonzo, Pfiriaeli Kiwia,
Willbrord Manyama, Elspeth McAdam, and Alice Welbourn

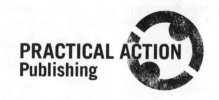

PRACTICAL ACTION
Publishing

Practical Action Publishing Ltd
The Schumacher Centre, Bourton on Dunsmore, Rugby, Warwickshire, CV23 9QZ, UK
www.practicalactionpublishing.org

A catalogue record for this book is available from the British Library.
A catalogue record for this book has been requested from the Library of Congress.

ISBN 978-1-85339-8933 Hardback
ISBN 978-1-85339-8940 Paperback
ISBN 978-1-78044-8930 Library Ebook
ISBN 978-1-78044-8947 Ebook

Citation: Gordon, G. (2015) *Stepping Stones with Children:
A transformative training for children affected by HIV and their caregivers*,
Rugby, UK: Practical Action Publishing, <http://dx.doi.org/10.3362/9781780448930>.

Since 1974, Practical Action Publishing has published and disseminated books and information in support of international development work throughout the world. Practical Action Publishing is a trading name of Practical Action Publishing Ltd (Company Reg. No. 1159018), the wholly owned publishing company of Practical Action. Practical Action Publishing trades only in support of its parent charity objectives and any profits are covenanted back to Practical Action (Charity Reg. No. 247257, Group VAT Registration No. 880 9924 76).

The views and opinions in this publication are those of the author and do not represent those of Practical Action Publishing Ltd or its parent charity Practical Action. Reasonable efforts have been made to publish reliable data and information, but the authors and publisher cannot assume responsibility for the validity of all materials or for the consequences of their use.

Cover design by Mercer Design
Typeset by Bookcraft Ltd, Stroud, Gloucestershire
Printed by Replika Press Pvt. Ltd., India

CONTENTS

ABOUT THE AUTHOR

Gill Gordon has nearly 50 years' experience of working in the development sector, and is a social development and health promotion specialist. She has particular expertise in gender, sexual, and reproductive health and rights (and its integration with HIV); community-based participatory approaches; and curriculum development. She is the author of several popular books and learning materials including Choices: a guide for young people. Working as a freelance consultant, she gained experience of using participatory methodologies for planning, health education and promotion, monitoring and evaluation; in using performing arts, including Stepping Stones, to explore choices and change; in working with young people; and in addressing issues of gender, sexuality and equity. At the International HIV/AIDS Alliance, she provided technical support to programmes working with young people in and out of schools, with a focus on Southern Africa. Gill also worked in health promotion and primary health care in rural Ghana for 10 years and with IPPF, supporting Family Planning Associations to integrate HIV into their programmes. During her career she has worked in a number of countries across Africa, Asia and The Caribbean.

DEDICATION

To all the children affected and orphaned by AIDS around the world, their mothers, their fathers and their caregivers: we dedicate this book to you all with gratitude for all you have taught us about life.

ACKNOWLEDGEMENTS

We would like to thank the numerous people who have contributed to the development of this manual; their creativity and insights bring the richness to the exercises. We particularly want to express our gratitude to:

The staff of PASADA (Pastoral Activities and Services for People with AIDS Dar Es Salaam), particularly Nelson Chiziza and his team who co-ordinate the project activities, Jovin Risiki and Simon Yohana the Executive Director.

Pfiriaeli Kiwia and Willbrord Manyama who facilitated, reviewed and translated sessions into Kiswahili and showed appreciative inquiry in practice. All the facilitators who tested the manuals with caregivers and children deserve special thanks. The caregivers and children directly affected by HIV in Dar Es Salaam and the Coastal Region who identified the issues they wanted the workshops to cover, tried out the exercises and suggested improvements.

Fiona Hale and Sue Holden for managing the project and Nigel Padfield for finance and accounting. Nell Osborne for managing www.steppingstonesfeedback.org and the community of practice and supporting the development of the manuals and films.

The international Advisory Group and particularly Dieudonne Bassonnon, Amandine Bollinger, Kate Iorpenda, Jill Lewis, Luisa Orza and Silvia Petretti. The monitoring and evaluation team, Sue Holden, Christine Nabiryo, Kato Nkimba, and Luisa Orzo. Fabienne Hejoaka whose participatory research with caregivers and children with HIV in Burkina Faso was an inspiration for the development of this package.

Kate Durrant, Martha Hardy and Petra Rohr-Rouendaal for their lively illustrations. Kate Durrant (Sessions 1, 2; and pages 87, 101 and 131) Martha Hardy (Sessions 5, 10, 11, 12, 13, 14, 15, 16, 17, 18, 21, 24, 26, 27, 28 and 29; and pages 80, 81, 108, 244, 245, 268, 301, 302, 306, 312 and 337) Petra Rohr-Rouendaal (sessions 3, 4, 22; and pages 82, 89, 98, 155, 241, 247, 251, 265, 271, 275, 309, and 333).

Alison and Glen Williams of 'Strategies for Hope' for their support in developing the concept of *Stepping Stones with Children*.

We are grateful to Comic Relief and UNAIDS for funding the development of *Stepping Stones with Children.*

We wish to acknowledge the huge range and diversity of ideas and creativity of the many practitioners who have been developing these areas of work over many years and in many countries. The key documents that we have used in developing the manuals are listed below and indicated with superscripts through the manual linked with References p.410.

Materials used with the kind permission of the authors and copyright holders

Exercise numbers	Adapted from following sources
1.4, 1.6, 1.7, 1.8, 1.9	Brakarsh, J. (2005) *The Journey of Life: A community workshop to support children.* Section 3 'The Journey of Life for Children REPSSI (Regional Psychosocial Support Initiative) and CIIT (Community Information and Inspiration team), pp. 59-66, 73-80. Under Creative Commons licence
5.1, 5.2, 5.3, 10.4	Georgia, Jovia, Kenny, Lucy and Sandra (2009) 'The "Tree of Life" in a Community Context' *CONTEXT* (2009), Number 105, pp. 50-54
11.4	REPSSI (2005) *The Journey of Life: A community workshop to support children.* 'Action Workshop 2: Helping our children to understand Death' REPSSI, pp.38-42 Under Creative Commons licence
1.7, 13.7, 27.4	McAdam, Elspeth; Welbourn, Alice; Steinberg, Charles; Oljemark, Kicki and McAdam, Keith (2011) 'NAMWEZA - Friends' Intervention Programme', pp.29, 36, 73, 79; 146; personal communication
2.3, 2.4, 2.5, 2.6, 2.7, 2.8, 2.9, 2.10, 8.1, 15.7	Siegel, D. and Payne Bryson, T. (2012) *The Whole-Brain Child: 12 Proven Strategies to Nurture Your Child's Developing Mind*, Robinson UK pp.10-13, 62-63, 88-89, 105, 114-116, 110-112, 135-137, 140-142, 129, Copyright ©2012 by Mind Your Brain, Inc. and Bryson Creative Productions, Inc.
2.1, 9.3, 9.4	Siegel, D. and Payne Bryson, T. (2014) *No-Drama Discipline: The Whole-Brain Way to Calm the Chaos and Nurture Your Child's Developing Mind,* Bantam Books, New York, pp.34-52, 57-59, 20-23, 226-227 Copyright ©2014 by Mind Your Brain, Inc. and Bryson Creative Productions, Inc.
8.5, 8.6, 9.5	Moyo, F. L. (2011) *Parenting – A Journey of Love: Called to Care, No.10,* Strategies For Hope, Oxford, pp.26-28, 38-39, 45-46
10.1, 11.5, 13.5, 29.8	Carnegie, R.; Kato-Kabunga, P. and CCATH partners. (2006) *'River of Hope: Child-centred approaches to HIV and AIDS. A resource manual for working with children and their communities.'* HealthLink Worldwide, pp.74,75,57 and 65-67
2.11	Gilbert, P. (2009) *The Compassionate Mind,* London, Constable and Robinson, p.24
9.1, 9.6	Neff, Kristin (2015) 'Self-compassion guided meditations and exercises', Exercise 4, www.selfcompassion.org/category/exercises
10.2, 10.3, 11.1, 11.3, 27.1	Brakarsh, J. with Project Concern International (2009) *'Say and Play: A Tool for young children and those who care for them'*, Project Concern International, pp.31,32,33-34,35, 22-24
3.4, 4.2, 6.1, 7.1, 7.2, 7.3, 7.4, 7.5, 7.6, 7.7, 8.2, 9.1, 16.1, 16.5, 28.3 Virtues picture	Popov, Kavelin Linda (2000) *The Virtues Project, Educator's Guide* Jalmar Press, Torrance, California, pp.151-152, 191-192, 135, 3, 16, 5, 8, 9, 18, 97, 195, 171-172, 161-162 132 and 134
10.5, 11.2, 11.6	Crossley, D. and Sheppard, K. *(2000) Muddles, Puddles and Sunshine: Your activity book to help when someone has died,* Hawthorn Press and Winston's Wish, pp.21, 18-19, 26

Exercise numbers	Adapted from following sources
Introduction. How can we safeguard and protect children? 1.3	International HIV/AIDS Alliance (2014) *Safeguarding the rights of children and young people*: *A guide to facilitating a workshop with Alliance Linking Organisations and partners working with vulnerable children and young people.* International HIV/AIDS Alliance, pp.21, 35
3.3, 6.1, 6.3, 6.4, 12.4, 16.1, 23.4	International HIV/AIDS Alliance (2008) *Sexuality and life-skills Participatory activities on sexual and reproductive health with young people*, International HIV/AIDS Alliance, pp.37, 48-50, 51, 52-53, 137, 46, 65,
3.1, 4.3, 19.2, 25.2	International HIV / AIDS Alliance (2006) *Our Future: Sexuality and Life Skills education for young people, Grades 4 – 5,* International HIV / AIDS Alliance, pp.73, 19-21, 62, 39-44, 89,
16.2, 26.2	International HIV/AIDS Alliance (2004) *A Parrot on your Shoulder A guide for people starting to work with orphans and vulnerable children*, International HIV/AIDS Alliance, pp.32-33, 34-35
17.2	Harrison, K. (2009) *'Building Hope, Supporting work with children affected by HIV and AIDS'* International HIV/AIDS Alliance, Macmillan, pp.51-63
29.2	Bolles, R. (2013) *What Color is Your Parachute*? 2013 Edition, pp.56-57 Adapted, with permission, from Richard Bolles' *What Color Is Your Parachute? 2015 edition*, 10,000,000 copies in print, used in 26 countries

ACRONYMS

AIDS   acquired immune deficiency syndrome

ARV   anti-retroviral

FGC   female genital cutting

HIV   human immunodeficiency virus

NGO   non-governmental organization

PASADA   Pastoral Activities and Services for People with AIDS Dar Es Salaam

SIFT   sensations, images, feelings and thoughts

STI   sexually transmitted infections

INTRODUCTION

Welcome to *Stepping Stones with Children*. This introduction sets out what you need to know about the programme and running workshops. You can also check www.steppingstonesfeedback. org for updates about using this manual, based on users' experiences.

WHY and HOW did we develop *Stepping Stones with Children*?

Children living with HIV can live normal, healthy lives if they have love, care, and treatment when they need it. Yet they and their caregivers face many challenges, including stigma and self-stigma, discrimination, violence and abuse, and services that may not serve children well. While we would all prefer to experience relationships of love, appreciation, and compassion, challenges including grief, bereavement, stress, and poverty can get in the way. The result is that children suffer in many ways, and some die because they have not received treatment, and the care and support needed to take it, in time.

The *Stepping Stones* training process has been used for over 20 years around the world.[1] Community members who go through its process – taking time to explore issues in peer groups, and to find ways forward together – are able to make important and lasting changes. This version of *Stepping Stones* is our response to the scarcity of materials which fully address the needs of children who are growing up either with HIV, or directly affected by HIV. It combines new exercises with adapted existing materials to create a comprehensive process for both younger and older children and their caregivers.

The workshop sessions were developed by Salamander Trust and Pastoral Activities and Services for people with AIDS Dar es Salaam Archdiocese (PASADA), working with children and caregivers in Tanzania. In December 2013 three communities went through the whole process. Using their feedback we revised the sessions; the revised versions are the ones in this manual.

WHO are the participants of the workshops?

Stepping Stones with Children workshops are for *children and caregivers from households directly affected by HIV*. This means that someone in their household has HIV or AIDS, or has died with AIDS-related illness. They are not open meetings: the people who agree to take part at the beginning are the same ones who come to each session. You may need to describe the workshop to community members as a workshop for some children and their caregivers, without mentioning HIV at all.

In the workshop sessions the participants usually work in their peer groups:
- girls and boys aged 5–8 years;
- girls and boys aged 9–14 years;
- female and male caregivers of these children.

For the children's peer groups, the ideal number of participants in each group is between 10 and 15. For the caregivers, up to around 25 will work.

WHAT does *Stepping Stones with Children* contain?

Content of the sessions

A loving and appreciative relationship between children and their caregivers is crucial for children's development. HIV often disrupts this at a time when the child and caregivers are grieving and under great stress. The relationship can rapidly go downhill as children act out their feelings, and caregivers try to cope with their own grief, anger, and anxiety about meeting the basic needs of their bigger family. *Stepping Stones with Children* enables caregivers and children to reflect on their own issues with their peers, and then come together to share across the generations in a safe way.

The *Stepping Stones with Children* manual is split into two parts, which jointly contain 29 workshop sessions, each with full instructions and information.

Part 1. This contains 15 sessions, to be used in sequence, like a journey. The process of following all these sessions enables participants to develop group trust and cooperation, knowledge, virtues, and skills, and to build on these as they reflect on key issues in their lives.
- In Sessions 1 to 11, the caregivers and children learn about virtues such as love and self-compassion, how our brains work, gender and rights, how to cope with loss and death, and positive ways of bringing out the best in one another.
- Children and caregivers have many concerns about HIV. These include how to protect each other from HIV, talking about having HIV, living positively with HIV, using HIV services, and taking treatment. Sessions 12 to 15 address these issues.

Part 2. This contains 14 sessions on specific issues. *Stepping Stones* groups may choose to use them in the suggested sequence, or select priority issues.
- Having friends and going to school are hugely important for social wellbeing in the lives of children, both now and to prepare them for the future. The use of alcohol and drugs is related to friendship groups and ways of coping with stress. Sessions 16 to 18 explore these issues.
- Supporting children in protecting themselves and others from sexually transmitted HIV, other sexually transmitted infections, and early pregnancy is made more difficult by reluctance to accept the reality of (even young) children's sexual lives. Sexual abuse, pornography, and sexual exchange for money or goods are some of these realities. Sessions 19 to 25 explore sexual wellbeing, while sexual abuse of children is addressed in Sessions 26 and 27.
- Poverty is a root cause of many of the problems faced by children and caregivers. Sessions 28 and 29 address the value of work and build caregivers' and children's visions for safe and meaningful work in the future.

Throughout the workshops, we take a holistic approach which combines the psycho-social, physical, sexual, and material issues facing children, embedded in a spiritual appreciation of the importance of love, respect, care, and support for children.

Learning methods

We use a variety of participatory methods and activities which enable learning by doing. Throughout the process we practise life skills and virtues such as listening, questioning, critical thinking, assertiveness, love, compassion, diligence, and courage.

We all learn in different ways. Some people learn best by listening, others by seeing, others by saying, and yet others by doing. Throughout this manual we use a variety of methods in order to build on and reinforce different learning patterns for everyone. Please use them too. They include songs and dancing, as well as the methods listed in Table 0.1. For all of the methods, symbols or drawings can be used in place of text, so that no one is excluded by lack of literacy.

Table 0.1 Learning methods used in *Stepping Stones with Children*

Method	Why we use this method	How to use this method
Drawing	• Enables people to express themselves, including less literate participants • Helps participants create powerful images to take home and remind them of what they did in the sessions	• Encourage people to express themselves without any concern for whether it 'looks right'
Role play	• Gives us a powerful way of practising new behaviours • Enables people to explore the effects of different behaviours • Improves empathy by asking people to put themselves in others' shoes through acting	• Encourage people to have fun pretending to be someone else • You can ask actors to stay in role while the audience asks them about their feelings, and ask actors to reflect on how they felt in the role once they are back out of it
Mind maps[1]	• Enables a group discussion to be captured – this improves the group's understanding and analysis • Provides a quick way of sharing a group discussion with others • Can also be used by individuals to clarify thinking and analysis	• Put a single theme or question in the middle of a piece of paper • Add key thoughts, then add more thoughts, using lines to join related ideas • Use different-coloured pens for different aspects: for example, to add possible solutions to challenges
Ability spotting[2]	• Increases participants' awareness of the abilities they already have, and how they might use them further • Helps raise self-esteem • Provides participants with a positive way of looking at a situation and finding ways forward, rather than focussing on negatives	• In pairs, one person interviews the other about something they have done well, and looks for the abilities the interviewee showed • The interviewer names the other person's abilities and affirms them • The interviewer then writes each ability on a small bit of paper and threads it onto the other person's ability necklace
Visioning and 'backlighting'	• Provides a creative way of thinking about the future, free from the constraints of real life • Creates memorable dream images and identifies practical steps towards the dream • Enables positive planning for the future	• Encourage people to dream about an ideal situation in the future • Ask them to look back from the vision to their situation now, to identify practical steps required to achieve their dream (this is backlighting)

Method	Why we use this method	How to use this method
Storytelling	• Gives participants a joint basis from which to widen their discussion • Enables participants to discuss relevant issues through the characters, rather than having to reveal their own stories	• Read the story, or ask someone else to read it • You may want to tell the story again, with participants acting it out • Ask questions to explore the story and its relevance to participants' lives
Using virtues[3]	• Recognizing and using virtues helps participants develop the best aspects of their characters and interact well with people • By getting into the habit of naming and acknowledging each other's virtues and their own, participants feel good about themselves and are better able to improve their lives	• Invite people to choose a different virtue for each session • Draw or write the virtue in the middle of a flipchart, and invite people to write or draw behaviours that show this virtue around it • Ask people to spot participants who use the virtue during the session, and add their names to the flipchart

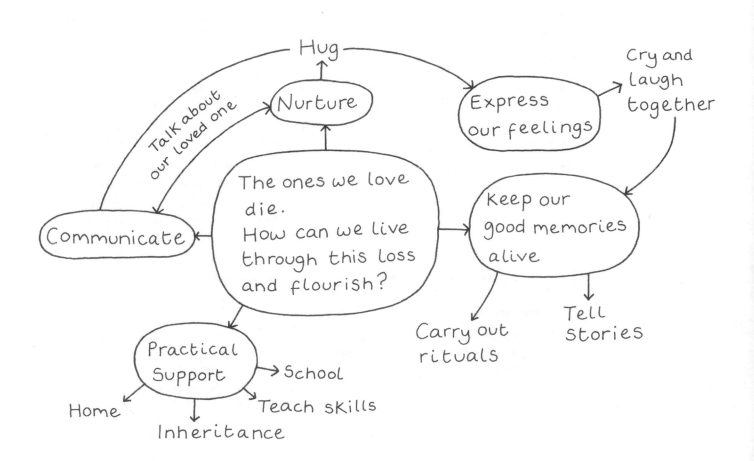

An example of a mind map

We encourage facilitators to adapt exercises using methods to suit their different age groups. For example, the youngest children may find drawing and storytelling easier, while older groups may also like role plays. In general, we have found younger children far more capable of all these methods than adults have imagined.

WHO is this manual for?

This manual is written for organizations or community groups that are working with households, caregivers, and children with HIV or affected by HIV. It sets out all the information that facilitators need to facilitate the *Stepping Stones with Children* programme.

To run workshops with all three peer groups at the same time you need a team as follows:
- Three facilitators, one for each peer group;
- Three assistants, one for each peer group;
- ideally, the facilitator team (comprising one facilitator and one assistant) for each peer group should be made up of one man and one woman;
- if possible, one volunteer counsellor or trusted community member who can support any participants who are ill or upset.

Facilitators need to be skilled people who already work with local groups in their communities. They might be volunteers or paid staff, and could be community leaders, health workers, educators, members of an HIV support group, religious leaders, or simply members of the community concerned by the issues covered in the workshop. Encourage people with HIV to consider becoming facilitators or facilitator's assistants. They will bring their understanding of living with HIV to the workshop. If they are open about having HIV and comfortable talking to others about it, they can help the group feel comforted that they can live a 'normal', good life with HIV.

Box 0.a Recommendation to potential facilitators

We strongly recommend that all potential facilitators attend a training course to familiarize themselves with the content of the manual and enable them to practise using the tools.

Use the quiz in Table 0.2 to see whether you have the experience and skills needed to facilitate the workshops straight away, or if you need some training first. For information about how to be trained and recognized as a *Stepping Stones with Children* trainer, please visit our website (www.steppingstonesfeedback.org) or send an email to: enquiries@steppingstonesfeedback.org.

Table 0.2 Facilitators' quiz (tick your answer)

Are you motivated to work with children and caregivers?	Yes	Quite	No
Are you able to read and understand this text easily?	Yes	Quite	No
Are you able to speak the community's first language fluently?	Yes	Quite	No
Are you able to make notes when needed?	Yes	Quite	No

Do you have experience of working with:
   children aged 5–8 years?
   children aged 9–14 years?
   caregivers of children affected by HIV?
	
	Yes
	Yes
	Yes
		
		A little
		A little
		A little
			
			No
			No
			No

Do you have good communication skills, e.g. listening, questioning, empathy, and compassion?	Yes	A little	No
Do you have experience of facilitating active learning, using role play, drawing, and storytelling?	Yes	A little	No
Are you a fast learner, creative, and flexible?	Yes	Quite	No
Are you able to say 'I don't know but I will find out', and 'I'm sorry', and to learn from your mistakes?	Yes	Quite	No
Do you have a positive attitude towards challenges?	Yes	Quite	No
Are you able to keep what you learn from workshop participants private?	Yes		No
Are you willing to share what you learn from workshop participants if a child is at risk, in order to protect the child?	Yes		No
Can you relate well to adults and children from all backgrounds in an understanding, positive, and non-judgemental way?	Yes	Quite	No
Are you in good mental health?	Yes	Quite	No
Are you willing to explore issues concerning gender and sexuality, including your own feelings and behaviours?	Yes	Quite	No
Are you willing to explore the basic facts of HIV transmission, prevention, and treatment?	Yes	Quite	No
Are you able to discuss sexual matters with people, including children, clearly and sensitively?	Yes	Quite	No

 Anyone who has been convicted of sexual, physical, or emotional abuse against children, or neglect, is not an appropriate person for this work. See 'HOW can we safeguard and protect children?' (p.10).

How did you get on?

If you have ticked 15 or more of the boxes in the first column, then it seems that you have the skills and experience needed to run the sessions.

If you ticked fewer than 15 of the boxes in the first column, but more than 15 boxes in the first and second columns, then it seems you would make a great assistant.

If you have ticked four or more of the boxes in the last column, it seems that you will need some training to gain the skills and experience needed to run these sessions well. Alternatively, perhaps you can find someone else to take on the role of facilitator. You will find it very difficult to run a workshop if you do not have training or assistance in the areas mentioned in the table.

Recommendation. Whatever your score, we recommend that you attend a 'Training of Facilitators' to enable you to:

- gain familiarity with the material in the package;
- anticipate and explore likely areas of particular interest or difficulty relevant to your own communities;
- gain confidence in handling the subject matter and methods, in large and small groups;
- increase your own understanding of the topics;
- increase your empathy and solidarity with different community groups by understanding that it is not only them who face these issues, but all of us together;
- develop an ongoing support group structure with other facilitators in your area.

You can find guidance on training for facilitators on the *Stepping Stones* website, where we will also provide information on the accredited training that we intend to provide in the future.

If you think you already have the skills and experience to facilitate *Stepping Stones with Children*, we strongly recommend that you:

- read through the whole manual – either by yourself or with the other facilitators. You will need at least two full days for this.
- as a form of practice, run some sessions and exercises with friends or colleagues with whom you plan to use the package for training others.

WHY organize the participants into peer groups?

We use peer groups because people share and learn best from talking first with those who are most similar to themselves. It also enables children to find a voice and gain confidence and self-compassion; they can talk more easily with their peers, without the fear or shyness they may feel if caregivers are present. Children can often feel lonely, and isolated, and feel that they are somehow to blame for these feelings. Bringing them together with others of their own age who have had similar experiences soon helps them to feel less lonely, and happier. The same applies to their caregivers. Sometimes the peer group also splits into males and females and they work separately.

The peer groups come together to share their learning at key points. When caregivers and children do activities together and have fun, it strengthens their relationships and respect for each other. They are encouraged to talk about the workshop at home and, sometimes, to do homework.

The manual explains when to work in peer groups and when to come together. You may want to change things to suit your participants. For example, if the girls are shy of speaking in front of the boys, you will need to split the group initially, even though the instruction is for them all to work together. You need to be aware of this possibility all the time. Or, when asking caregivers to do small group work, you might ask younger and older caregivers to form different groups, as they will have more in common with people of their own age.

In general, caregivers gain knowledge and practise skills related to themselves and how to support their children, while children gain knowledge and practise skills related to themselves and how to support their families and friends. The facilitator working with the caregivers generally asks them to talk about the children in their care, while the facilitators working with the children's peer groups focus on the children talking about themselves.

How can young children and adults work on the same issues?

The themes, sessions, and aims are all relevant to children aged 5–14 years and their caregivers, with adaptations. The peer group activities allow children and adults to reflect on the topics from their own perspectives using their preferred activities, level, and language. There are opportunities for them to share their learning across peer groups in safe ways.

The children, particularly the younger children, sometimes do fewer exercises than the caregivers, or do the exercises in less detail. They typically need more energizing activities and more play time.

Every session includes aims, approximate timing, activities, and examples appropriate for the three age groups. Facilitators may adapt activities as necessary – see our 'Tips on working with children' (p.16–17).

Must the sessions be run with all three peer groups?

The programme is designed so that all three peer groups work on the same issues at the same time, and come together to share their learning. This means that both children and caregivers are exposed to new ideas and new ways of doing things, can share and remind each other what they have learned, and practise together. They travel on the same journey. However, there are two other ways to use the programme:

1. If it is not practical for all three groups to work at the same time, the peer groups could have their sessions at different times and meet at home and at training halls for everyone to share ideas. For example, if there is only one suitable meeting space in the community, you would need to run the sessions at different times. Or if there is only one facilitator and assistant able to work with the children's peer groups, their sessions would need to be at different times.

2. You might opt to use the sessions with just one peer group, for example, with children in schools or with adults in an HIV support group. We would expect the sessions to be beneficial, but not nearly as much as when working with all three age groups.

HOW to organize the sessions

Making contact with potential participants

It is very important to introduce *Stepping Stones with Children* to the community and potential participants in a way that encourages people directly affected by HIV to take part, but also ensures that confidentiality about HIV in families is maintained. This is difficult to do: if you describe the programme too generally (for example, saying that it is about raising happy, healthy children), then people who are not affected by HIV may want to participate; if you are too specific, you risk informing the community that all the participants are affected. Here are some suggestions:
*   Meet with any HIV support groups or HIV service providers to explain fully the content and purpose of the workshops, and talk about the best way of meeting with and encouraging caregivers and children directly affected by HIV to participate. You may also wish to meet with one or two trusted and discreet stakeholders from religious, women's, youth, or other groups, and invite them to suggest ways of meeting people who would benefit from the workshop.
*   Very soon afterwards, meet with local government and community leaders to explain the programme, perhaps in more general terms, and gain their support for the workshops.

If they are motivated by the workshops they will encourage others to participate and support changes that result. *Be careful not to disclose the status of anyone with HIV without that person's permission.*

- Decide on a geographic zone from which to seek participants, so that they share a common language, can support each other in their communities, and are able to travel to the workshops.

- Within your chosen zone, make contact with caregivers and their children aged 5–14 years who are directly affected by HIV, and invite them to participate in the workshop. *Do not say to the children that the workshop is linked to there being HIV in their household, without first gaining permission from their caregivers.* Explain the *general* content and purpose of the workshops and invite them to ask questions. Ask them to suggest or invite other people, like themselves, who would benefit from the workshops, and to suggest a convenient time and place for a meeting involving all possible participants. Ask them whether that meeting should be just for potential participants, or should include other relevant people too.

- Identify trusted service providers, such as health workers and teachers, who will be able to provide support to the workshops and participate in Session 15 'Partners in health care' and Session 17 'Going to school'.

- Hold a meeting for all the people invited to attend the workshops and, if agreed with them, other relevant people. Use the meeting to set out what the workshops involve, to answer questions, and to agree when and where to hold them. Talk about what you will do and what participants will do, including what you can and cannot offer participants. For example, clarify whether you will provide refreshments or if participants will be responsible for them, and whether transport costs or attendance allowances (to replace lost earnings) can be covered.

Where might you hold the workshops?

- Discuss possible venues for the workshop with the caregivers and children; if anyone is worried about revealing their HIV status, it may need to be somewhere where people can arrive without being seen by neighbours.

- Ideally the venue needs to have three private spaces, so that the three peer groups can work, talk, and play separately and freely. It also needs a big enough space for everyone to come together to share their ideas and have fun.

- You need enough privacy so that people who aren't participants aren't able to listen in to the sessions.

- You may be able to incorporate *Stepping Stones with Children* sessions into an existing regular event. For example, if children already come together for a kids club, perhaps there is space for the caregivers to come too. Or if adults already meet as an HIV support group, perhaps the children could attend that.

When might you hold the workshops?

This will depend on where you will be running the sessions and who will be attending. You need to consider the time of year, key festivals and religious events, the day of the week, and the time of day. Be sure to find out from the participants – adults and children – when would best suit them, and find a compromise that is OK for most of them and for the facilitators.

You might end up running sessions intensively, for example, covering four sessions on the first weekend of every month. Or you might run single sessions at a regular time, such as after school every Wednesday. What's important is that the schedule suits people, so they are more likely to attend, and so they have the chance to use and develop their skills between sessions or clusters of sessions.

Involving people who are living with HIV

People living with HIV are at the heart of the *Stepping Stones with Children* process, as the participants are all people directly affected by HIV, and the participatory methodology supports them in sharing their experiences if they wish to. The process can be strengthened further by having suitably skilled facilitators and assistants who are living with HIV, particularly if they are willing to be open about their HIV status.

We recognize, however, that participants and facilitators may not want to share their status, so activities in Sessions 12, 13, 24, and 25 involve inviting people who are open about living with HIV to join those sessions and share their experiences.

HOW can we safeguard and protect children?

The aim of child safeguarding is to prevent and respond to violence towards, exploitation of, and abuse against children, and to provide a safe and healthy environment in which children can grow and develop. The *Stepping Stones with Children* process aims to reduce abuse and violence against children, including:
- *neglect*: failure to provide food, clothing, shelter, medical care, and supervision to the extent that the household can afford to do so;
- *physical violence*: aggression which may be used as punishment or to control the child through fear; this may include beating, burning, cutting, or the use of harmful substances; it may also be used against others, causing fear and trauma in observers;
- *emotional abuse*: this might be excessive criticism, name-calling, ridicule, destruction of personal belongings, humiliation, and withholding of communication and love;
- *sexual abuse*: this might be indecent exposure of genitals, showing pornography to a child, creating pornography involving a child, sexual touching, sexual intercourse, and selling the sexual services of children;
- *female genital cutting*: a form of physical, sexual, and emotional violence against girls and women;
- *early marriage*: if before the age of consent, this is, in law, child sexual abuse; if, at any age, the girl or boy does not consent, forced marriage violates their human and child rights;
- *harmful work*: this may include sexual, physical, or emotional abuse, and deprive children of the right to go to school.

The process also aims to promote the safe and healthy environment which children need to thrive, by enabling children and caregivers to increase their awareness of their rights and find a voice. We can be sure that some of the children participating have faced or are facing abuse and violence, and we have a duty of care to prevent or protect them from further abuse and violence.

Before beginning *Stepping Stones with Children* workshops

It is essential to prepare for the workshops as follows:
- Ensure that you have a Child Protection Policy for your organization and all the people you work with (there are examples on the Stepping Stones website). This should include: 1) the

written policy; 2) who is responsible for implementing it; 3) the procedures to follow, such as how to respond to reports of abuse; and 4) how you will ensure that the policy is being implemented by reporting and monitoring accountability.[4]

- Ensure that you have a child-friendly version of your policy to share in Exercise 1.3 'Making our ground rules'.[5]

- Ensure that everyone in your organization knows their role with regard to child protection and safeguarding, and is able to fulfil their role. Provide training if necessary.

- Carry out a child risk assessment with regard to the workshop. Look at issues which could put children at risk during the workshop, between sessions, and in the community. For example, there may be a risk of child sexual abuse by adults or other children during workshops, particularly if the workshop is residential, or of children experiencing violence at home after a session, as a result of breaking confidentiality about having HIV. Assess levels of risk and identify strategies to keep children safe.

- Find out what human, legal, and institutional resources exist locally to protect children and respond if they are being abused or harmed (for example, child protection workers, law courts, and home counsellors).

- Identify possible ethical dilemmas and develop strategies to safeguard children in these situations; for example, a child reports sexual violence but asks you to keep it secret because they fear more violence, and the abuser earns most of the income for the family.[6]

Safeguarding children during the workshop sessions

Children and caregivers may feel ill, upset, or angry during a session. We need to: attend to each child's physical, emotional, and social wellbeing; be ready for the possibility of a child disclosing physical, sexual, or emotional violence, having HIV or being sexually active; and foster supportive relationships between children and their caregivers, other participants, and the facilitators.

- Teach participants about your child-friendly Child Protection Policy in Exercise 1.3 'Making our ground rules'.

- Attend to individuals' wellbeing by being aware of their body language and energy levels, and listening actively to what they say. Provide snacks, toilet breaks, and opportunities to play at regular intervals, as well as rest and sleep breaks if needed.

- Encourage children and caregivers to talk about 'people like them' in the sessions, rather than talking about themselves, and invite them to come to you privately after the session to share any worries.

- Support children and caregivers in strengthening their relationships with communication and love, so that they are able to talk about issues safely when they feel ready.

- Encourage participants to empathize and support each other with compassion, so that the sessions are safe and supportive, especially when discussing difficult topics which may upset people.

- Be prepared to respond to strong emotions. Encourage people to use the tools that they learn to stay balanced, open, and calm, and to support others in doing so too.

- Have a support person available (this might be a trusted community member or volunteer counsellor) in case a child or caregiver is ill or upset during the session. Other supporters may include facilitators and assistant facilitators, caregivers and siblings, guardian angels (see Exercise 1.10 'Guardian angels'), and friends from the peer group.

- Organize a quiet space where participants can go to be calm or relax, or to have private counselling and comfort.

- Remind participants what they have agreed about confidentiality, and stay alert so that you and your facilitators do not put a child in danger by accidentally breaking confidentiality.

How can we support a child who reports abuse?

Safeguarding children who report abuse, or whom you suspect of being abused, demands great sensitivity and cooperation from all the facilitators and supervisors. Please discuss this issue thoroughly as a team, before the workshop begins and between each session as the workshop progresses.

Follow the procedures in your Child Protection Policy. Here are some actions you might take:
- Support the child in talking with a trusted person or counsellor about the abuse. If the child agrees, and if appropriate, support the child and caregiver in talking together.
- Talk through Exercise 27.5 'Protecting children from further abuse', and see how the caregiver can protect the child from further abuse.
- Ask the child how they feel and what they would like to happen to keep them safe.
- If a child or caregiver has confided in a member of their peer group about the abuse, they may wish to continue supporting each other back in the community. Encourage members of the peer groups to think of ways of supporting each other.
- Arrange for home visits by facilitators, counsellors, or child protection workers.
- Work with relevant local services and support groups dealing with child protection.
- Refer the child for follow-up care such as counselling, health services, or spiritual help.
- Support the *Stepping Stones* groups, if they are interested, in mobilizing the community to protect children from violence.

HOW to use the manual

Deciding which sessions to use

All the sessions in *Part 1* are essential and work best if done in the order they are written.

For *Part 2* you may want to assess with the participants which themes are most important to them, or which they would like to do first. Be careful of picking out a single session. For example, you need to do Sessions 12 ('All about HIV'), 21 ('Sexual feelings and sexual safety'), and 23 ('Delaying, starting, and stopping having sex') before doing Session 24 ('All about condoms'). We have noted at the start of each session if it is important to do other sessions first.

We recommend that you always do the sessions 1–9 before using certain sessions as stand-alone modules with peer groups facing specific challenges, for example: losing parents, having HIV, or being sexually abused. Doing this ensures that participants benefit from the process of building skills which happens when working through sessions 1–9. This increases the impact of the sessions.

Preparing for each session

- Do prepare thoroughly for each session with the rest of your team so that you all understand how the aims and exercises for caregivers and children link up.

- Read through the session and use the aims to help you work out what you want the participants to know and feel by the end of the session.
- If appropriate, in *Part 2*, decide which exercises you will use and consider any adaptations you may need to make to suit your peer group and the context in which you are working.
- Be aware that you may need to split longer sessions into two.
- Make sure you understand and can remember any 'information for facilitators' (this appears in boxes in each session).
- Pay attention to these small pictures:

This picture indicates the special importance of safeguarding and protecting children in this session or exercise

This picture indicates information on how to monitor and evaluate the workshop.

- Do any preparation needed, as listed at the beginning of each exercise.
- Have a list of local games, songs, dances, or stories that you can use to liven any session up, if needed.
- Gather whatever materials you need, as listed at the beginning of each session.

We have listed only any special materials needed for each exercise, such as a piece of rope. You should always carry basic workshop materials of chalk, flipchart paper, other paper, a way of attaching paper to the wall, a watch, and different-coloured pens or crayons.

How to run the sessions

Be a good role model

Do take care to model the behaviours you would like to see from participants and to follow the ground rules which you jointly create in Exercise 1.3 'Making our ground rules'. For example, be on time for sessions, have your mobile phone turned off during sessions, listen carefully, and use the language of virtues.

Opening circle

Every session begins with an opening circle, usually with just your peer group, but sometimes with the whole group. We have not listed the steps in each session as they are the same each time, as follows.

1. *Attendance record.* As participants arrive, tick them off in your Facilitator's Journal (available from http://www.steppingstonesfeedback.org/index.php/page/Resources/gb?resourceid=80).

2. *Welcome.* Welcome participants and enquire about anyone who is missing.

3. *One good thing.* Invite participants, in pairs, to: 'Tell each other one good thing that has happened to you that you feel grateful for since the last session.' Invite one or two people to share their experience.

4. *Using our learning.* From Session 2 onwards:
   - Ask the three volunteers who evaluated the previous session (see 'Closing circle', below) to share if they have used their learning from the previous session and, if so, what happened. Record their feedback in your journal.
   - If you have time invite one or two other participants to share how they have used their learning from the last session and record their feedback in your journal.

5. *Questions.* Ask: 'Do you have any questions about the last session?'

6. *Last session's virtue.* Put up the virtue flipchart from the previous session. Ask two people: 'Tell us one way you have used this virtue since the last session, and how it made you feel.'

7. *This session's virtue.*
   - Invite someone to choose a virtue or, for sessions linked to a certain virtue, tell the group today's virtue.
   - Put up a flipchart with the virtue in the middle, and say: 'Let's write or draw a few ideas which show that someone is practising this virtue.'
   - Ask everyone to look out for participants using this virtue during the session, and to add their names to the flipchart.

Closing circle

 As with the opening circle, the steps are the same for each session.

1. *Pause.* Invite participants to sit up in a relaxed and alert way and to take 10 soothing breaths.

2. *Session evaluation.*
   - Ask for three volunteers to stay behind to review today's session (see 'Monitoring using the Facilitator's Journal' on p.18).
   - Ask each of them to say one thing they have learned in this session and why it is important. Record them in your journal. Ask them to try to use this learning before the next session, to share at the next opening circle.

3. *Using our learning.* Ask everyone to think, to themselves, of one way they will make use of their learning before the next session.

4. *This session's virtue.*
   - Ask: 'How did what we have done today connect with the virtue for this session?' Add the ideas to the virtue flipchart.
   - Say: 'After the session, agree with your child or caregiver on one thing you will do this week to bring today's virtue into your house or community.'

5. *Questions*. Ask: 'Do you have any more questions about the session?'

6. *Guardian angels*. Remind everyone of their role as guardian angel.

Box 0.b Recommendation to facilitators: opening and closing circles

We suggest that you write the opening and closing circle steps on a flipchart and display them at each session as a reminder.

Using pictures

The manual uses pictures and diagrams to help participants learn, remember, and analyse. Often participants will draw pictures to represent ideas or objects, which are called 'symbols'. In keeping with adult literacy programmes, it is good to write the word for what the symbol represents by the symbol.

We have provided images in the Annex. You can photocopy these onto bigger pieces of paper to use in the sessions. If you aren't able to do this, invite participants who like to draw to make the pictures on flipchart paper instead.

It's also good to have key images pinned up in every session, to remind participants (and facilitators) about earlier sessions. This helps everyone link up their learning and create permanent pictures in their brains. For example, a picture of a bug on the hub of a bicycle can remind everyone to stay on their hubs and not get overwhelmed by feelings.

Using the anonymous question box

Participants may have questions that they feel shy to ask. Make a box into which they can 'post' these questions on slips of paper, anonymously. If a person is not able to write, invite them to tell you their question privately so you can write and post it for them.

Using 'Information for facilitators'

Many sessions contain information for you to read and know before facilitating the exercise; this is contained in boxes headed 'Information for facilitators'. You can then contribute new information to the discussions with the participants as they need it. This works better and is much more interesting for them than lecturing, or reading it out to them from the manual. So – learn from the information boxes, but don't read out directly from the manual unless asked to do so in the instructions.

Managing time during the session

Some sessions take a whole day to run; you may prefer to split those ones into shorter sessions. Each exercise says how long it should take, roughly. However, the time it actually takes can vary a lot! You will probably find that you take less time to run the sessions after the first time, as you become familiar with the material and how the exercises fit together. And as the participants get more skilled with the participatory activities and more confident speaking up in the group, they may also speed up.

In general, you need to keep an eye on the time taken in order to fit all the exercises into a session. However, it is also important not to rush people without giving them time to feel and think, just to get the exercises finished. People do not learn well in this way and some people take longer than others to grasp new ideas or to feel able to express themselves.

Here are some ideas to save time and to manage time in a session:

- Turn up in good time and praise participants who are on time. Do not delay the start of a session for a few people who are late. Discuss the importance of time-keeping while explaining that you appreciate transport difficulties and how busy everyone is. If someone is consistently late, ask them how the whole group can support them in arriving on time.

- Be clear about how much time you have for each activity, or each step of an activity, and try to stick to it. If the participants know they have just 10 minutes to discuss they will be quite focussed. If they know that '10 minutes' usually means closer to 20 minutes, they may not focus on the task so well.

- Divide the peer group into smaller groups rather than discussing as one big group. You can stop these small group discussions before all the groups have finished; when the groups come together and share ideas they will cover all the points.

- When small groups give their feedback, ask them to say points only if they have not yet been said. This stops people repeating points.

- Define how participants give their feedback. For example, inviting them to 'say three words to describe how you feel' may be an appropriate way to get their input and to keep it brief.

- If running out of time during a session:

  Adapt. Modify exercises to save time.

  Split the group. Get half the group to do one exercise and half to do another, then ask them to give their feedback briefly.

  Give homework. Ask participants to continue their discussions outside the workshop and to feed back the next time you meet.

  Focus on the essentials. If an exercise is not essential, miss it out, but describe what you would have done had you spent more time together. Be careful though: you don't want to spend a long time on something that could have been done more quickly, and so miss an exercise which is important.

Managing workshop products

The workshop participants will create a lot of items during the sessions. Encourage them to keep the items which are personal to them, such as their necklaces (made in Session 1 'Getting started') and their trees of life (Session 5 'The tree of life').

You will need to find a way of managing other group items, such as the reminder pictures you put up on the wall in each session, and things which participants create jointly, such as mind maps. Perhaps participants can look after them, or maybe you can store them at the workshop venue. Participants in Tanzania found it particularly valuable to pin up the drawings from Session 2 'Using our brains' in later sessions.

Tips on working with children

- Make sure the facilitators for the children's groups have relevant training, skills, attitudes, and experience (see Table 0.2 'Facilitators' quiz', p.6).

- Have between 10 and 15 children in the peer group. It is hard to manage more than this.

- If possible, always have an assistant present who is able to: support the facilitator; support children who are ill or upset; work with small groups; monitor how things are going; feed back on time-keeping; or contribute to any gaps. The assistant will gain facilitation skills through this apprenticeship and can work towards becoming a facilitator.

- All sit on mats (or chairs or stools) in a close circle, including the adults.

- Use *Stepping Stones* names (see Exercise 1.2 'Introducing ourselves') and give a lot of praise for participation.

- Use simple language. Ask the children to help you choose the right words to explain something. Probe to make sure that children have understood.

- Divide the group into smaller groups of younger and older children, or boys and girls, as this helps children feel confident and talk about issues relevant to their lives. Move around the groups to support the children. If they find it difficult to manage without a facilitator, you may need to bring them back together into the larger group.

- In pair work, put talkative and less talkative children together, or fast and slow learners, or literate and less literate children, or younger and older children, so that they can all learn to support one another.

- Don't allow exercises to run over time too much.

- Break up the activity and discussion with movement and playing.

- Be sensitive to the need for energizing activities to give everyone some fun, and for calming activities such as meditation.

- Let all the children go to the toilet together every hour. Supervise them and escort them there and back.

- Use local games, songs, and dances chosen by children. Adapt these to fit the exercise topic if appropriate. If the children choose songs, dances, or games related to courtship or sexuality, you can take the opportunity to explore their meaning and what we can learn from them.

- Have toys such as cars, aeroplanes, balls, skipping ropes, soft toys, dolls, and puppets available for children to play with at the end of the session. The children may finish their activities before the caregivers, so it's good to have things to play with as well as some organized games.

- When doing an activity which they may find difficult, begin by demonstrating it yourself with one child or with the assistant, using the relevant skills, while the group watches. Then invite older children to do parts or all of the activity while the younger ones watch; and then invite the younger ones to join in.

How can we manage confidentiality in peer groups?

You will discuss this with the participants, and make an agreement, in Session 1 'Getting started'. In general these are our recommendations:

- Encourage participants to talk about 'people like us', to make up stories or pictures, or to use stories from the manual, rather than giving personal, sensitive information to the group. This is because people have a tendency to share new information about each other with others – to gossip. If participants find that their personal information has been told to the other peer group, they may be upset or harmed by it, and the person who gossiped may be punished.

- Encourage participants *not* to tell the group that they, their caregiver, or any other person, has HIV, unless they have thought about it carefully and agreed it with the relevant person.

Children and caregivers will share information, thoughts and feelings in their peer groups which may not be known to their caregiver or child. You should only share that information with the other party *with their consent*. In general it is better to encourage them to speak directly to each other; this becomes easier as the exercises help build bridges between caregivers and children, enabling them to repair damaged relationships.

If you are involved in communication between caregivers and children and do not have consent to share information, or you need more time to share it safely, you can:

- give general reassurance: for example, telling an upset child that caregivers usually want the best for their children, but don't always know how to do it;
- generalize what you have learned until after the session, when you can handle the situation using your Child Protection Policy: for example, if a children's peer group reports sexual violence, the facilitator for the caregivers' group might say to the group that the children are concerned about children they know who are being sexually abused, and follow up later with caregiver concerned.

Agreeing how to work with your team

You and the other facilitators need to agree how you will work together and support each other as you go along. We recommend that you choose one of your team as a 'workshop coordinator'. You could rotate this role between you for each community you run the programme with.

You need to discuss and agree:

- who will be your workshop coordinator and point of contact for the community leader, in case of any questions;
- a timetable for the workshop;
- having a facilitators' meeting before each session to prepare;
- how to advise, support, and cooperate with each other well;
- having a meeting after each session to give feedback and share ideas;
- how your team will get any extra support you need;
- how you will provide additional support to the participants;
- how you will link up and work with other services such as clinics, counsellors, and schools;
- how you will manage confidentiality between yourselves regarding specific information about the participants;
- how you will record what has happened at each session; we have provided a Facilitator's Journal for this purpose, which you can download from http://www.steppingstonesfeedback. org/index.php/page/Resources/gb?resourceid=80

HOW can we monitor and evaluate the process?

We have provided a number of tools to help you track how the sessions are going and try to find out what effect they have had.

Monitoring using the Facilitator's Journal

You can download the Facilitator's Journal from our website or make your own. It contains the following monitoring tools:

An attendance record. This tracks who attended each session and who was absent. Use this to enquire after missing participants, perhaps requesting other peer group members to follow up with them. You can also use it at the end of the workshop to total up the proportion of sessions attended by males and females for each peer group, as an indicator of how much people valued the sessions.

A progress record. This records a score out of 5 for each participant's engagement and active learning in each session, as observed by the facilitators. Use this to identify and support people who are not engaged; perhaps there are things you can do to improve their experience and learning.

A participants' review for each session. After each session, ask three participants to review and score the session. Ask each person to use the fingers and thumb on one hand to show their score out of 5 (where 1 is very poor and 5 is very good) for each activity, against three categories:

- how relevant and useful they found the *content*;
- how much they enjoyed the *activity*;
- how they rated the *timing*.

Fill in their scores and get their feedback on how to improve low scores. Also record one thing that each of them learned and how they intend to use it.

A facilitator's review for each session. This is where you add your own observations and thoughts. This will build a useful reference when you next facilitate *Stepping Stones with Children* workshops. You can also use your notes to shape your evaluation: for example, to follow up with a person who said how something they had learned had helped them.

Evaluating the effects of the workshops

These are the tools we have provided to try and measure change as a result of participating in the workshop sessions:

A questionnaire for each peer group. This is to be used before the first session, after Part 1, and after completing Part 2 (available from http://www.steppingstonesfeedback.org/index.php/page/Resources/gb?resourceid=80). We suggest participants use blindfolds and show their responses with their fingers, to make it easier for everyone to do, rather than completing a written questionnaire.

'Fingers up' questions. These are included in the sessions, to gather data about something relevant to that session. For example, in Exercise 9.3 'Problems with violent punishment', participants discuss what punishment is, and are then asked to close their eyes, bow their heads, and use their fingers to show how many times they have been punished by their caregiver in the past week, or how many times they have punished their child. You record all the finger-scores for the males and females in your Facilitator's Journal and will repeat the questions later in the process to see if there is any change.

Focus groups and interviews. Focus groups are used to explore themes with peer group members, and interviews to enable individuals to explore their experiences: guidance and topic guides are available from http://www.steppingstonesfeedback.org/index.php/page/Resources/gb?resourceid=80

Other tools are likely to be added to the *Stepping Stones* website as they are suggested by users.

Share what you learn!

We very much hope you will be able to use *Stepping Stones with Children* for the benefit of children affected by HIV and their caregivers.

If you have access to the internet, please go to www.steppingstonesfeedback.org and see how to join our International Community of Practice, so that you can share your experiences and learn from other people's use of *Stepping Stones with Children*. We will be adding information about using the materials on our website, and will also be offering formally accredited training courses for facilitators and trainers in the future.

Purpose: To start the workshop in a fun way; to help peers get to know each other; and to introduce skills, virtues, and tools which participants will use later in the workshop.[7]

Contents	Materials required	Time required
Opening circle		15 mins
1.1 Getting to know each other		20 mins
1.2 Introducing ourselves		30 mins
1.3 Making our ground rules	Child Protection Policy	20 mins
1.4 The road of life		30 mins
1.5 Our dreams		30 mins
1.6 Our feelings		30 mins
1.7 Discovering our strengths	String, coloured paper, scissors	45 mins
1.8 Supporting each other in being strong		60 mins
1.9 Our happy moments		40 mins
1.10 Guardian angels		15 mins
Closing circle (see p.14–15)		15 mins

About 6 hrs

Preparation

Exercise 1.3. You need to prepare a Child Protection Policy in language that children can understand. An example is given in Box 1.a.

Opening circle

1. Sit everybody together in a circle. Everyone, including you, should be at the same level, whether on chairs, benches, or mats.

2. Introduce the facilitators and thank everyone for coming. Explain that if they want to join the workshop, you ask them to make a real commitment to coming to every meeting. This is because we will discuss new things at every meeting, which build on what we have discussed before. When members attend all the meetings, it builds trust and continuity.

3. Add that you would particularly like to welcome anyone who may have HIV or is living with another health condition. Reassure everyone that you don't know who may have HIV or any other problem, and that no one has to share this information with anyone in the group unless they want to.

4. Explain the purpose of the workshop, the topics that we will discuss, how the peer groups are going to work separately and together, and the timing of the sessions.

5. Explain the topics we are going to cover in the first session.

6. Ask if anyone has any questions.

7. Say 'If anyone feels unable to commit to the workshop at this time, please feel free to leave before we begin Session 1.' Encourage people who are unsure to attend this session and see how they feel. Suggest that people who are not able to attend might want to keep in touch with their peers.

 ## EXERCISE 1.1 GETTING TO KNOW EACH OTHER

AIMS: To welcome children and caregivers to *Stepping Stones with Children*. To get to know one other. To have fun.

DESCRIPTION: Participants play games to get to know each other.

Directions

1. Explain to participants that you will say:

'Find someone who [...]', and that people should get into the relevant pairs or groups as fast as they can.

You might say, for example:
- 'Find someone who is wearing the same colour shirt as you and tell them your name.'
- 'Find someone who is as tall as you and tell them your name.'
- 'Find someone who has the same size foot as you and tell them your name.'

2. Now ask participants to split into peer groups of children aged 5–8 years, children aged 9–14 years, and caregivers. They will work in these separate groups (ideally in different rooms) for the rest of the session.

3. In each peer group, ask participants to divide into groups of three. Invite one person in each group to sing a favourite song, and ask the others to sing along.

4. Ask the groups of three to come together into groups of six. Invite a different person in each group to show their favourite dance, and ask the others to join in.

5. Ask the groups of six to come together into groups of 12. Ask one person (who has not led a song or a dance so far) to demonstrate their favourite exercise, and ask the others to copy them.

 ## EXERCISE 1.2 INTRODUCING OURSELVES

AIM: To create a safe place in which participants can talk and listen to one other.

DESCRIPTION: The facilitator explains the Story Circle to participants, and participants then interview and introduce each other.

Directions

1. Ask your peer group to sit in a circle. Explain that this is the Story Circle, where we gather to share our experiences. In the circle we can talk about important issues and say things we might not say outside the circle. What we say in the circle stays in the circle. We won't share it with anyone outside the circle.

2. Invite participants to pair up with the person sitting next to them. Ask them to interview each other using the questions below. Answer the questions yourself first to get things going.
- What is your name?
- What information about yourself would you like to share with the group?
- What are you looking forward to in this workshop? Tell me something you are good at (for example, kindness, humour, singing, hard work).
- Tell me one fear you have about the workshop (for example, not being enough refreshments).

3. When everyone has interviewed each other, ask each person in turn to introduce their partner, saying their name, what they are looking forward to, the thing they are good at, and their fear if they have one. The group welcomes and appreciates them. Try to address the fear straight away, if you can; if you can't, say you will ask someone about it.

 4. Record the hopes and fears as people say them in your Facilitator's Journal.

5. Invite each person to tell the group the name they want to be called by, and to choose an adjective to go with their name. This adjective should describe one of their strengths or abilities. Some people may like to choose a word that starts with the same letter or sound as their name: for example, Compassionate Clare, Loyal Leonard, Happy Hamiss, or Friendly Fatuma. If they cannot think of an adjective that begins with the same letter as their name, they can choose any adjective they like, for example, Thoughtful Andile. Explain that this will be their 'Stepping Stones name'.

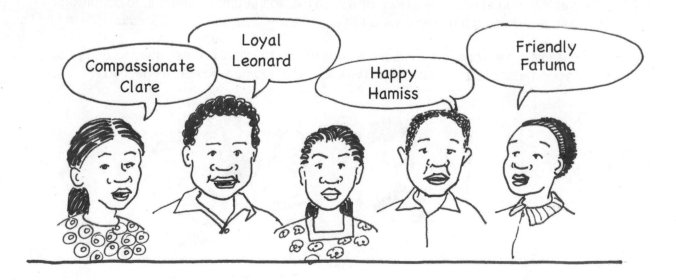

EXERCISE 1.3 MAKING OUR GROUND RULES

AIMS: To agree on how we want to work together and behave towards each other during the workshop.

DESCRIPTION: Participants agree on ground rules for the workshop, using positive language, and are familiarized with the Child Protection Policy.

Directions

1. Sitting in a circle, explain that we are now going to look at how we want to work together and behave towards one other during the workshop. We will decide on our ground rules and write them up on a poster, to remind ourselves of what we have agreed. We can add more as we go along.

2. Say: 'Let's give our ideas about what we want to *do*, using positive action language.'
Ask: 'Who can give us an example?' Participants might say:
- '*be on time* for sessions' (rather than saying *do not be late* for sessions);
- '*respect* each other';
- '*turn mobiles off*'.

3. Place a piece of flipchart paper in the middle of your circle and encourage participants to make suggestions. If everyone else agrees to a suggestion, ask the participant who made it to draw something to represent that behaviour. For example, they could draw an ear to represent listening to each other. If someone suggests an action using negative language – for example, 'no quarrelling' – turn this into a *positive* action verb by saying, for example, 'cooperate with each other' or 'listen and talk to each other in a peaceful way'. Do encourage participants to use drawings to express ideas. Explain that it doesn't matter if the drawing is not perfect, as long as everyone knows what the drawing means. We are not trying to become fine artists. Our goal is to become fine communicators.

4. Once all the ground rules have been drawn on the flipchart, ask the group to go through them again together, so that everyone is clear.

5. If appropriate, ask someone to take responsibility for the flipchart. Ask them to bring it to each of your meetings, so you can refer back to it and add new actions as needed.

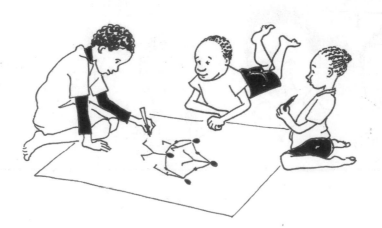

6. Explain that all children have the right to be protected, and not to be hurt or harmed in any way. Say: 'Let's talk about how we expect adults to behave, and about what to do if you feel scared or frightened, or if you feel that people are not treating you in the right way.' Put up a child-friendly version of your Child Protection Policy on flipchart paper and explain the points to the participants. See Box 1.a for an example.

Box 1.a Child Protection Policy, as written for children

The adults in this programme are expected to behave well and to protect you at all times. They must not hurt you, bully you, or make you feel frightened or scared. If you feel uncomfortable, tell someone. They will listen to you!

Speak to a caregiver or facilitator, a person in our clinic or office (tell them a name), or someone else you trust. They will help you decide what to do next. You have the right to be listened to, and the right to tell people what you think in your own words and in your own way.

Taking part. Before any activity, someone should explain clearly what they want you to do. Remember, you do not have to take part in activities in this project if you don't want to. You can stop at any time.

Nobody should take photos of you without explaining what they will use them for, and without asking permission from you and your caregiver.

Bullying. If someone is bullying you, you must tell a caregiver or trusted adult as soon as you can.

Hitting, punching, or smacking you. No one should hurt you. If a member of the group or an adult hits, punches, or smacks you, or hurts you in any way, or if you see someone else being hurt, you must tell a caregiver or trusted adult as soon as you can.

Saying strange things to you. If a member of the group or an adult says something to you or you hear something that you do not like or that upsets you, and/or if they threaten you or say you must not tell anyone, you must tell a caregiver or trusted adult as soon as you can. Do not keep it a secret.

Touching you. If someone touches your body in a way you do not like, you must tell a caregiver or trusted adult as soon as you can. Do not be scared of telling someone straight away. Their job is to listen to you. If you don't think they are listening, tell someone else.

 EXERCISE 1.4 THE ROAD OF LIFE

AIMS: To think about our lives as a journey. To create an imaginary road in the workshop space.

DESCRIPTION: Participants tell stories and make a Road of Life.

Directions

1. Explain that we can see our lives as a journey on the Road of Life. Invite participants to imagine their lives as a journey, with a road in front of them. Ask them to imagine that they are standing at the beginning of the road. Ask one or all of them to act out their journey along the road of life: first crawling as babies, then toddlers walking, then getting older until they reach the present day.

2. Ask participants to pair up and tell each other one thing about their road so far.

3. Ask them to come back together as a group. Then say: 'Work with your group to make an imaginary road in your work space or outside. Make the road in any way or any shape that you want, using local materials, chalk, or crayons. Mark the beginning and end of the road.'

4. Explain that we will be using this road throughout this session.

 EXERCISE 1.5 OUR DREAMS

AIMS: To introduce the idea of dreaming and describing our vision for the future. To find out what peers need now to achieve their dream.

DESCRIPTION: Participants imagine their vision of the future and one action that will help them get there.

Directions

1. Say: 'Roads always go somewhere. This imaginary road is going to our dream future.'

2. Ask participants to call out examples of the sort of things we dream of, or want to do, for example: becoming adults, being safe and loved, our sick relative getting better, passing school exams, becoming a good dancer, setting up a business, having enough income, having a loving partner, having children, living in peace with other people and countries.

3. Ask participants to close their eyes for three minutes. Direct the relevant peer groups as follows:

Caregivers. Ask them to picture their dreams for when their child grows up.

Children. Ask them to think of how their lives will be when they are grown up.
All peer groups. Ask them to open their eyes and to pair up. Invite them to draw a picture of their dreams, to act out one of their dreams, or to interview each other about their dreams.

4. Ask everyone to think of one action they need to practise now which will enable them to continue along the road and reach their dreams. For example, working hard at school, being kind to other people, or learning how to keep chickens. Go around the circle inviting each participant to share their action.

5. Explain that we will do more exercises using dreaming later in the workshops.

EXERCISE 1.6 OUR FEELINGS

AIM: To introduce work on feelings.

DESCRIPTION: Peers identify feelings and express them through walking and facial expressions.

Directions

1. Explain: 'Sometimes our way along the road is easy and we feel happy.' Ask everyone to walk in a happy way.

Next, say: 'Sometimes things are difficult and we feel sad.' Ask everyone to walk in a sad way.

Then say: 'Sometimes things happen which make us feel angry or afraid. The road is confusing and twisty.' Ask people to pair up and stand back-to-back holding onto each other's arms, and then walk about looking angry, or looking out for danger. Ask: 'Does life ever feel this way?'

2. Explain that every day we have feelings. Say: 'Let's show each other a *happy* face – what makes us happy?'

Next, say: 'Now make an *angry* face – what makes us angry?'

Then say: 'What about making a *sad* face – what makes us sad?'

Finally, say: 'Let's do *laughing* faces – what makes us laugh? Who can tell us a joke?'

3. When people have stopped laughing, ask: 'Did you know that *moving our bodies* can help us feel better when we have a strong feeling of sadness or anger? Let's try it out. First, imagine you are feeling sad. Smile. What happens?''Now imagine you are feeling angry. Jump, stamp your feet, or shout a bit.''Now imagine you are feeling afraid. Breathe slowly and deeply, and focus on the movement of your belly.''Now imagine you are feeling stressed. Sing a song, or dance.'

4. Ask participants to share what they found helpful. Say: 'Sometimes just moving our bodies can make us feel that things are going to be OK.'

5. Explain that our feelings come and go. We are not the same as our feelings. So instead of saying, 'I am sad', we should really say, 'I feel sad at the moment.' For example, in the morning we might feel angry with our friend, but in the afternoon we feel loving and peaceful towards them.

Say that we will learn more about feelings during the workshops.

EXERCISE 1.7 DISCOVERING OUR STRENGTHS

AIMS: To enable us to discover the abilities which help us to walk along the road to our future dream.

DESCRIPTION: Participants create a space on the Road of Life to describe different types of strength people have, and play games to explore each other's strengths. They create a necklace to represent their heart strengths.

Directions

1. Ask a participant to choose a number between one and 10. He or she walks that number of steps to come to a place called the Strengths Space along their imaginary road. Explain that we will use this space to show our strengths. We all have great strengths. We can also receive strength from others, and share our strength with others.

2. Ask participants to decorate their space with drawings, or with any available materials such as flowers, leaves, sticks, or stones, so we know it is their Strengths Space.

3. Say: 'There are three main ways we can be strong. Let's explore them in pairs. First, we can be strong in our *muscles*. Show your partner a way that you have been strong in your muscles.'

4. Say: 'Second, we can be strong in our *hearts*. We can use virtues in our behaviour; for example, by being kind, courageous, respectful, or hard-working.'

5. Ask participants to sit in pairs, and explain that we are going to make necklaces to show our heart strengths. Invite them to find out about each other's strengths: 'One of you tells the other about a time when you were strong in your heart. The other asks questions starting with "what, when, how, where, with whom", to learn more about the story. As you talk, they spot the good things you did, and write or draw them on small pieces of paper. Then you make a necklace, by threading the pieces of paper on a piece of string or wool. Then you swap roles and, when you have finished, congratulate each other on your heart strengths.'

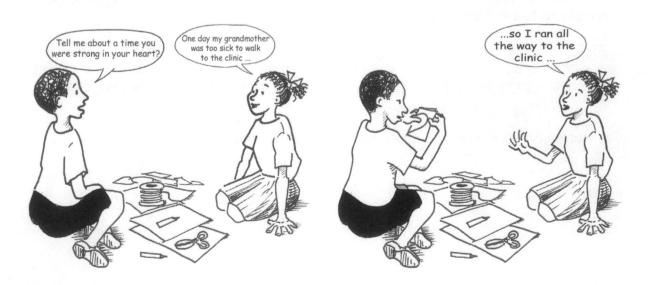

6. When the pairs have interviewed each other, say: 'The last type of strength is in our *minds*. We use mind strength by using our brains to think and make good decisions, to communicate with another person, or to cope with problems. Tell each other a story about when you used your brains. What skills did you use? Congratulate each other on your mind skills.'

7. Explain the Strength Game.

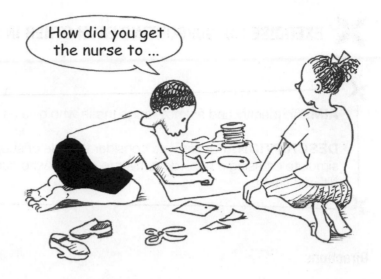

Say: 'Repeat after me: I am strong in my muscles (touch muscle of arm or leg); I am strong in my heart (touch heart); I am strong in my mind (touch head). Now let's do it as quickly as possible, 10 times.'

Invite participants to do this again 10 times, but this time touching their partner as they say: 'You are strong in your muscles, heart, and mind.' Last, ask everyone to walk around the room, pointing to each other as they say, 10 times: 'We are strong in our muscles, heart, and mind.'

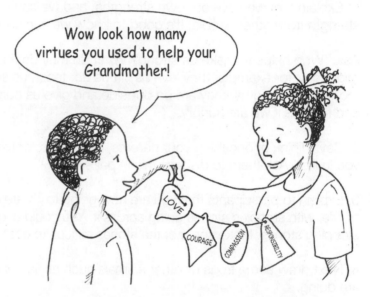

8. Ask: 'How does it make us feel to name our strengths and acknowledge one another's strengths?'
'How does it feel to be with a group of friends and recognize our collective strengths?'

9. Summarize by saying that recognizing and acknowledging our strengths lifts us up and makes us feel good about ourselves. Say: 'Shall we add it to our ground rules? Let's act in a way that lifts us up rather than puts us down.'

10. Invite participants to quickly sketch a picture of themselves as strong, drawing their muscles, heart, and mind. Suggest that they keep the picture to remind them of their strength whenever they feel weak.

11. Explain that in other workshop sessions we will use 'ability-spotting', where we look for one another's strengths. Say: 'You will be able to collect more abilities on your necklace, so remember to bring it along to each session.'

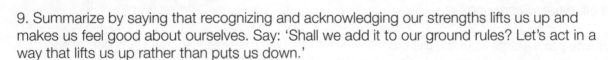

EXERCISE 1.8 SUPPORTING EACH OTHER IN BEING STRONG

AIM: To identify and acknowledge those who give us strength in our lives.

DESCRIPTION: Participants consider the role of supporters in their lives and simulate crossing a hazardous river to explore who can support them and how at difficult times.

Directions

1. Explain that we have our own strengths, and we can use them to help others. We also get strength from other people. It's good to know we can support each other in different ways.

Ask: 'Who helps to make us strong? What do they do that makes us strong?' Participants might say, for example: they love us; lift us up; teach us so we grow our abilities; act as role models of strengths; they are on our side and give us confidence; they help us if we are sick and feed us if we are hungry.

2. Say: 'Think of one thing your parents, caregivers, or teachers have taught you which helps you in life.' Ask them to discuss this in pairs.

3. Explain to participants that you are now going to create a wide, imaginary river across the Road of Life, with stepping stones going across it. You could use chalk to draw the river, banks, and stepping stones. Make some of the stones difficult to get to, some small, and some far apart.

4. Next draw some frogs or other animals such as fish or birds in the river, explaining what you are doing.

5. Now ask participants to imagine they are crossing this river using the stepping stones. If they fall off, what will happen?

6. Invite participants to cross the stones in whatever way they like. (Secretly, ask one or two participants to fall in the river.) When someone falls in, ask what happens to them.

7. Explain that sometimes we face difficult situations in life, and at these times we need to find new strengths that we didn't know we had. This is also when we call on our supporters, people who can share their strengths with us.

8. Ask people to call out some difficulties that they might need support with. Turn these into questions, like the ones in Box 1.b. Invent five questions, which must be relevant to the group.

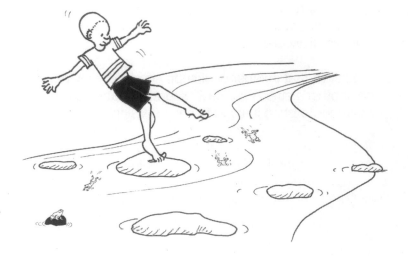

Box 1.b Sample questions for situations requiring support

- Who could comfort and love us if one of our caregivers were to die?
- Who could help us if we were to fall sick?
- Who could help us if someone were bullying us?
- Who could help us if someone were sexually abusing us?
- Who could help us if we had no money for school fees?
- Who could help us if we were to fall pregnant and didn't know what to do?
- Who could help us if we were hungry?
- Who could help us with our homework?

---

9. Write or draw a symbol for each question in the middle of a piece of paper, and place the pieces of paper apart from each other 'in the river', on the floor.

10. Divide into small groups, so that there is one group to consider each question. Ask each group to sit by a question and talk about who *could* support them with this problem. Tell them they have just three minutes to do this. Encourage them not to use the support person's name, but to describe their role; what heart, mind, and physical strengths do they have that make them a suitable person to help with this problem? Add the person to the piece of paper, using words or a drawing.

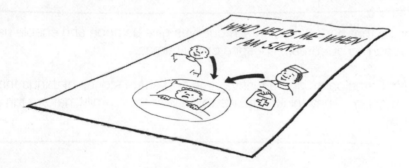

11. After three minutes, ask everyone to move to the next question on their right, and add more supporters to that piece of paper if they want to. Continue until each group has been around all the questions, and is back sitting next to the first question they considered.

As the groups are working, write the questions that they chose, and the supporters they identify, in your Facilitator's Journal. When everyone has considered all the questions, explain that we would like to learn how many of these supporters they have actually used themselves for support with these problems. Ask them to shut their eyes and, as you read out each supporter listed for each problem, to raise their hand if they have turned to this supporter for help with this problem. Record in your Facilitator's Journal how many people raise their hand for each supporter.

12. Ask each group in turn to choose one supporter from their paper, for example, a nurse or a friend, and then to invite one of their members to act as this supporter. Write the supporter's role on a piece of paper and pin it to the actor, so everyone remembers who they are. When every group has chosen a supporter, ask the supporters to form a circle surrounding the rest of their peers.

13. Ask the peers inside the circle how it feels to know these people are ready to support them.

14. Ask each small group to think of one way in which they could support a friend or family member with their problem.

15. Now invite participants to cross the river again, this time with a supporter holding each hand, and see what happens. Explain that if there were more and bigger stones, and if we crossed the river carefully, we would get across ourselves without help. But sometimes we need extra strength and guidance.

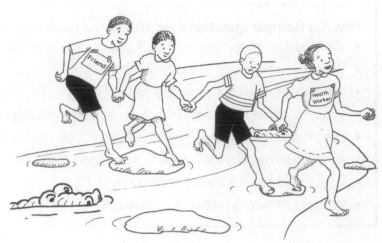

16. When everyone has crossed the river, ask:
'What was it like crossing the river now, compared to the first time?'
'What did you learn about your strengths?'

17. Ask participants to summarize what they have learned.

 EXERCISE 1.9 OUR HAPPY MOMENTS

AIM: To recognize that happy moments in our lives give us hope and enable us to move towards reaching our dreams despite difficult times.

DESCRIPTION: Participants play a funny game and share stories of things that have made them happy. They think of things to do with their family that are fun and make them happy.

Directions

1. Explain that we are now going to find a Happy Space on our Road of Life. Ask participants to say the word 'happy' as many times as possible in only one breath, and to walk in a funny way. As soon as they run out of breath, they must stop.

2. Ask participants to join the person who has gone the furthest along the road at their Happy Space, which represents moments in their lives when they have been happy.

3. Ask people to pair up. One person is the 'chicken'. Explain the game: 'Crow or cluck at your partner. Your partner tries not to laugh. Your partner rubs your hair saying "sweet chicken, sweet chicken", and tries not to laugh. If your partner laughs, they become the "chicken".'

4. Explain that playful parenting, and having fun in the family, is one of the best ways to prepare children for relationships and encourage them to connect with others. The more they enjoy the time they spend with their caregivers and the rest of the family, the more they'll value relationships and desire positive and healthy relationships in future.

5. Ask everyone to sit in a Story Circle. Direct the relevant peer groups as follows.

Caregivers. Invite them to discuss:

- Why is happiness important in our children's lives?
- How do we have fun with our children?
- What opportunities do we give our children for having fun together? What about our children and their friends?
- What more would we like to do? (for example, playing games, being silly, playing sport, cooking together, working together on a project, dancing, singing)

Children. Invite them to discuss:

- How does happiness help us in our lives?
- Show what things you do to make yourself happy, for example, acting silly, talking to your friend, or singing a happy song.
- What do you do with your caregiver that makes you happy? What would you like to do?
- What do you and your caregiver and siblings do to have fun at home? What would you like to do?

6. Invite participants to sing a happy song with you, such as *If you're happy and you know it clap your hands*.

 ## EXERCISE 1.10 GUARDIAN ANGELS

AIM: To give each person support during all the workshops.

DESCRIPTION: Each person is given the role of looking after someone else in their peer group.

Directions

1. Ask everyone to stand up in a circle and join hands. Stand yourself in the middle of the circle.

2. Then ask everyone to drop their hands and to turn to their right. This will mean that each person in the circle is facing the back of someone else.

3. Next, explain that in this kind of workshop, it is always a good idea for participants to 'look after' one another. You would like to suggest that each participant becomes the 'guardian angel' of the person standing in front of them. Ask each person to put their hand on the shoulder of the person in front and say their name out loud. Each person will be 'looking after' somebody, and each person will have somebody 'looking after' them.

4. Now ask everyone to turn back to the centre of the circle. Explain that as a guardian angel, they will regularly ask the person they are 'looking after' how they are, and whether the workshop is going OK for them. If people need to talk to the facilitator about an issue, or need more support, the guardian angel can support them.

5. Ask if anyone has any questions about this.

Purpose: To understand how our brain develops and works, and how we can use this knowledge; to learn mindsight tools to help children both survive and thrive as they grow up, and to help all of us to stay balanced in the river of wellbeing; to build loving relationships between caretakers and children.[8]

Contents	Materials required	Time required
Opening circle (see p.13–14)		15 mins
2.1 Our changing brains	Picture from p35 and in annex	30 mins
2.2 The singing game		15 mins
2.3 The river of wellbeing	Chalk or other available materials	20 mins
2.4 Helping our lower and upper brain work together		30 mins
2.5 Using the brain-in-hand model		30 mins
2.6 Memory for growth and healing	Picture from p43 and in annex (William being butted)	30 mins
2.7 SIFT: paying attention to what's going on inside us		40 mins
2.8 Our wheel of awareness	Ideally, a bicycle!	50 mins
2.9 Getting back on our hub		30 mins
2.10 The me–we connection		40 mins
2.11 The three circles of the brain		45 mins
Closing circle (see p.14–15)		15 mins

About 6.5 hrs

Preparation

By the end of this session. Please make sure you have each of the following images – either photocopied from this manual before this session or drawn by participants:

1. upper and lower brain;

2. river of wellbeing, with rapids on right and rocks on left;

3. brain-in-hand model of upper and lower parts of the brain, open and closed;

4. bicycle wheel with insect sitting on hub;

5. three circles of the brain.

We suggest that you photocopy the pictures before the session but also encourage interested participants to draw them when they have time. Put the images on the walls in future sessions, so that participants can refer back to them.

Exercise 2.6. Make a puzzle for each peer group by photocopying the picture of the boy being butted by the goat, from the Annex. Stick it on a piece of card and cut it into pieces.

EXERCISE 2.1 OUR CHANGING BRAINS[9]

AIMS: To understand how the brain changes as it grows and that it is changeable. To understand that we can use this knowledge to help our brains develop well for good mental wellbeing.

DESCRIPTION: Participants engage in a question and answer session about the brain.

Directions[9]

1. Explain that we are first going to learn about how our brains develop and change over our lives, and what we can do to strengthen our brains to enjoy mental wellbeing throughout our lives.

2. Ask: 'Who can tell us something about what the brain looks like? What different parts does the brain have?'

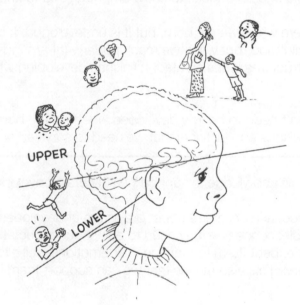

3. Show the picture above and, as needed, contribute the information in Box 2.a in your own words.

Box 2.a Our complex brains

The brain is made up of many parts, all of which have different jobs to do, for example: memory, language, empathy, responding to threats. There is the upper brain and the lower brain, the right side and the left side. When they work together as a coordinated team, they accomplish more and are more effective than if they were working on their own.

If we understand how the different parts of our brains work, we can respond to situations in ways that help them work as a team. We will learn some tools which help us do this later in the session.

---

4. Ask: 'When we are born, are our brains fully developed?'

As needed, contribute information from Box 2.b in your own words.

Box 2.b Our developing brains

When we are children, our brain is still under construction.

Lower brain. The lower part of the brain is well developed at birth and is responsible for:
- regulating basic body functions such as breathing, sleep, and digestion;
- strong emotions, such as fear and anger, and related actions such as crying and hitting without thinking about it;
- instincts such as staying close to our mothers, and responding to danger quickly, such as running away or fighting.

All of these things need to be there from the moment we are born, so that we can survive.

Upper brain. The upper part of the brain is responsible for thinking, and the emotional skills which allow us to live balanced, meaningful lives and enjoy healthy relationships. It enables us to make sound decisions and plan; to regulate our emotions and body; to understand ourselves; to be flexible and adaptable; to show empathy; and to know right from wrong.

This upper brain is there when we are born, but it is undeveloped. It begins to grow during infancy and childhood, but when we reach puberty (at around 12 years) the brain starts changing the structures it has created. It finishes developing when we are in our mid-twenties.

The upper brain doesn't need to be fully developed when we are born, as the lower brain tackles all the key functions and instincts that we need to survive.

Ask: 'How can we use this knowledge to support healthy brain development?'

If needed, explain that because children's upper brains are undeveloped, and because they change again during adolescence, we may need to adjust our expectations of our children's behaviour. We shouldn't expect them to manage their emotions well all the time; we need to be patient and empathetic. This also means that we can support them in helping their brains develop well.

5. Ask: 'Who can tell us something about what influences how well the brain develops?'

As needed, contribute information from Box 2.c in your own words.

Box 2.c Our changeable brains

The brain does not only change as we grow up, it remains *changeable*. Even as adults, we can all physically change our brains through what we experience repeatedly. For example, we change our brains in a good way by paying attention to what is going on in our minds and bodies, being loved, communicating, and learning new things such as how to play a musical instrument or ride a bicycle. It therefore makes sense that the brains of children who are nurtured and cared for are different from those of children who are abused. This means that children who are cared for are less likely to suffer from depression, drug use, and relationship difficulties. But the changeable nature of our brains means it is also possible to undo damage caused by lack of care or abuse.

---

6. *Caregivers* Ask: 'What are we doing to support our brains / our children's brains in developing well? What more can we do?'

Explain that, as repeated experiences change the structure of our brains, the experiences that children have as they grow up are important. We can try to give our children experiences that will help their brains develop well, and enable them to have better skills and mental health, now and in the future.

Explain that in the *Stepping Stones* sessions we will be thinking about issues such as:
- How do we interact positively with our children?
- How do we help them reflect on their actions and behaviour?
- What do we teach them about relationships – respect, trust, and effort?
- How do we help our children make sense of negative and challenging experiences as learning experiences, not as trauma that may limit them in future?

 EXERCISE 2.2 THE SINGING GAME

AIM: To understand the contrast between rigidity, chaos, and harmony, and the need for harmony.

DESCRIPTION: Participants form a choir and sing as instructed, followed by questions.

Directions

1. Ask the group to pretend to be a choir.

2. Sing a note, and ask everyone to sing the same note in a simple 'da-da' rhythm for 30 seconds. They must do as you say: sing just that note, in that rhythm.
Ask: 'How did you feel?' and 'What words would you use to describe this singing?'

3. Ask each person to think of a song they like. When everyone has thought of one, ask them to put their hands over their ears and sing it. After 30 seconds, ask: 'What happened, and how did it feel?' and 'What words would you use to describe this singing?'

4. Ask the group to choose a song which they all know and would like to sing. Ask them to sing it together, but encourage people to add their own ideas, such as singing harmonies, or clapping or dancing.

Ask: 'What happened? How did that feel?' and 'What words would you use to describe this singing?'

5. Ask: 'Which singing did you enjoy most, and why?' and 'How might this apply to our lives?' If necessary, explain that our brains work best when all the parts work together in a creative way.

 ## EXERCISE 2.3 THE RIVER OF WELLBEING

AIM: To understand the concept of mental wellbeing, using the idea of a river.

DESCRIPTION: The facilitator uses chalk or other materials to draw or create a river scene on the floor. Participants are invited to travel along the river and see what happens if they run into the bank of chaos or bank of rigidity, or keep going in the middle.

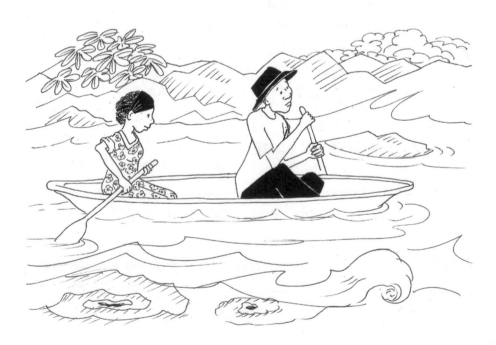

Directions

1. Draw or create a 'river' on the floor. Show whirlpool-like 'chaos' on the right side, and rocky lines of 'rigidity' on the left. Explain that this is our river of wellbeing.

2. Ask everyone to stand in the middle of the river. Then say: 'Imagine you are in a canoe on the river. You feel stable and peaceful, and in a good relationship with the world around you.

You have a clear understanding of yourself, other people, and your life. You can be flexible and change when situations change. All the parts of your brain are working together well.'
Explain that *mental health* is our ability to remain in the middle of the river of wellbeing.

3. Now ask everyone to imagine that their canoe is going too close to the right-hand bank – the *chaos* bank where they feel out of control. Say: 'You are caught up in rapids and whirlpools, causing confusion and turmoil. You are not in control of your emotions, and may be angry, loud, or rude.'

Invite everyone to move about in a chaotic way alongside the chaos bank.

4. Now ask everyone to move towards the left-hand bank. Explain: 'This is the *rigidity* bank, where we insist on our own way, and impose control on everyone and everything around us. We are unwilling to adapt, compromise, or negotiate. We may not listen to our or other people's emotions.'

Invite everyone to move about in a stiff way.

5. Explain that we all tend to move between the banks. If we find ourselves going towards the left or right bank, there are things we can do to get back to the middle. We will learn about these in this session. Being in the middle is best for our wellbeing. As with our singing in Exercise 2.2, it is not good to be too rigid or too chaotic; having all parts of our brain working harmoniously is best.

 ## EXERCISE 2.4 HELPING OUR LOWER AND UPPER BRAIN WORK TOGETHER

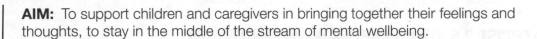

AIM: To support children and caregivers in bringing together their feelings and thoughts, to stay in the middle of the stream of mental wellbeing.

DESCRIPTION: Participants explore what happens when we are overwhelmed by our feelings, and learn how we can help ourselves or our children to calm down and get back to the middle of the river of wellbeing.

Directions

1. Explain that we are now going to learn more about how the lower and upper parts of our brain can work together. This will help us support one another in keeping calm and happy, rather than sad, scared, or angry. Show 'the picture of the brain' again and ask: 'Who can tell us what the lower and upper parts of the brain do?'

As needed, remind participants that, as we learned in Exercise 2.1, the lower part of our brain produces big feelings such as anger, fear, and frustration. These feelings can become overwhelming. It is important to use our upper brains to pay attention to these feelings, and to talk and think about them.

2. Ask participants to pair up. Say: 'Tell each other about a time when you felt really sad, scared, frustrated, or angry, but managed to control it without harm to yourself or someone else. Explain how you did that and, if someone helped you, what they did.'

Additional question for caregivers only. 'Talk about a time when your child got very angry or upset. How did you help calm them down, so they didn't do something that would make them feel bad or put them in danger?'

All peer groups. Bring the pairs back together into one big group and invite participants to share one or two of the stories about how people managed to control their feelings or support their children in doing so. Relate the stories to how the upper brain can soothe the big emotions produced by the lower brain.

3. Divide into two groups. Each person in group 1 acts as the lower brain having a big feeling. Each person in group 2 acts as the upper brain, whose job is to soothe the lower brain.

4. Ask the lower-brain people to move around the space acting out their big feelings. Now ask the upper-brain people to mill around and each find a lower-brain partner.

5. Ask each upper-brain person to connect with their lower-brain partner, and soothe and calm them down. For example, they might hold their hand or hug them, or ask them what they are feeling and empathize with them by saying 'I can see that you are really upset.'

6. As the lower brain calms down, invite the upper brain to bring in thoughts and feelings about the situation. For example, 'Let's talk about what has made you feel so [...].'

7. Ask: 'What have we learned from this activity?'

Summarize by saying that the upper and lower parts of our brain, when working together, can help put our feelings into thoughts and words, and enable us to calm down. Then we are able to use the upper part of our brains to think, understand our feelings, and make good decisions. You can say that we will learn more about a tool called Connect and Redirect in Sessions 9 and 15.

 ## EXERCISE 2.5 USING THE BRAIN-IN-HAND MODEL

AIMS: To understand the importance of keeping the upper and lower parts of the brain connected. To learn and practise a tool which helps us calm down, pause, and think before acting in emotional situations.

DESCRIPTION: Participants learn how to make the hand model of the brain, and use it to calm down, pause, and think before acting on strong emotions.

Directions

1. Ask everyone to make a fist with their hand, with the thumb tucked in between the palm and the fingers. Ask them to hold it up, so that the nails are facing outwards towards others in the circle. Explain that we are going to use this 'brain-in-hand' model to learn about the importance of keeping the upper and lower parts of our brain connected.

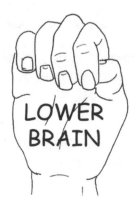
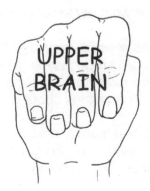

2. Explain that the upper part of the brain is where we can choose how we react to a situation, and where we can make good decisions and do the right thing even when we are feeling really upset, or really want something.

3. Say: 'Now lift your fingers a little bit. See your thumb? That's part of the lower brain, which is where our really big feelings come from.'

4. Say: 'There's nothing wrong with feeling upset. It's normal. The upper part of our brain helps us calm down. Close your fingers again. See how the upper, thinking part of your brain is touching your thumb? When the upper and lower parts of our brain are connected, as when our fingers cover our thumb, our lower brain can use our upper brain to support us in expressing our feelings calmly. If the connection is in place and everything is touching, we can act more calmly and wisely.

5. Say: 'Sometimes when we get really upset, we lose control of our emotions. Stretch your fingers up, and see how the upper brain is no longer touching the lower brain. Our upper brain can't help our lower brain to stay calm. In certain situations this may be good for our survival. But sometimes we lose control of our emotions when it is not appropriate, in ways that harm ourselves or others.'

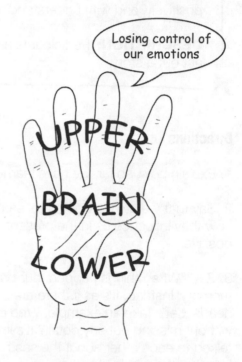

Losing control of our emotions

6. Explain that children lose control of their emotions more often than adults because their upper brain is not yet fully developed, and the connection between the upper and lower brain is not always strong. Caregivers and older children can support them in calming down again, and this helps develop their brains.

Say that adults also lose control of their emotions sometimes! We can all support each other in reconnecting our upper brains with our lower brains.

7. Explain that we can use the brain-in-hand model to help us calm down when we have big feelings. Invite three people to act out the story of Amina (see Box 2.d), or use one of your own that shows the person using their brain-in-hand model to calm down.

Box 2.d The story of Amina

Amina was doing her homework when her brother spilled his drink all over her picture, which she had spent a long time perfecting. She felt very angry and wanted to yell at him and hit him. But she remembered to make a model of the upper and lower brain with her hand. She raised her fingers straight out from her hand, and then lowered them slowly, one by one, so that they were hugging her thumb. This reminded her to use her upper brain to help her to calm those big feelings from her lower brain.

Amina was still angry, but instead of shouting at and hitting her brother, she told him that she was angry, and asked her caregiver to take him out of the room.

---

8. Ask participants to form groups of four, and to think of situations which make people like them so angry or frustrated that they lose control of their emotions. *Caregivers* should think of situations when they lose control of their emotions which involve their children. Ask the groups

to role play some of these situations within their groups, and to try using the brain-in-hand technique to calm down.

9. Invite two participants who like drawing to make a picture of the brain-in-hand model.

 EXERCISE 2.6 MEMORY FOR GROWTH AND HEALING

AIMS: To support children and caregivers in taking troubling experiences which are influencing them without their knowledge – the scattered puzzle pieces of their mind – and turning those experiences into a whole picture which they can see clearly, positively, and with understanding of how it influences them now and in the future.

DESCRIPTION: Participants are given an explanation of how memory works, and act out a story.

Directions

1. Explain how, so far, we have learned about connecting our lower and upper brains together.

2. Say that we are now going to learn why our memories are important, how they work, and how they influence us in the present. We will learn how to make our memories clear and positive.

3. Say: 'When things happen, our brain remembers them, but not always as a whole, joined-up memory. Instead, it's as if there are little puzzle pieces of what happened floating around in our heads. Let's take an example. Who can tell us, exactly, everything that happened in Session 1, without missing out any detail? It's impossible for any of us to remember every detail. But if we talked to each other about the session, we could share our different memories of it and piece together the whole story.'

4. Explain that the way we help our brain put the puzzle pieces of our memories in order is by telling the story of what happened.

5. Say: 'Telling the story is great when we do something fun, like having a Christmas or Eid party. Just by talking about it, we get to remember how much fun we had.'

Ask: 'What good stories come into your minds?' Encourage participants to name a few examples.

6. Then say: 'But sometimes something upsetting happens to us, and we might not want to remember. And when we don't think about it, those puzzle pieces never get put in order, and we might feel scared, sad, or angry, without knowing why.'

Ask: 'What upsetting stories come into your mind?' For instance, an adult may fear the sea because he nearly drowned as a child. A child might fear all dogs because one bit her when she was small.

7. Explain that when we tell a story to a trusted caregiver or friend about what has happened, they can help us put the puzzle pieces together, and to add the missing pieces. Then we feel less scared, sad, or angry. We feel braver, calmer, and happier.

8. Invite four participants to act out a story you will tell, each playing one of the following roles: a goat, William as a five-year-old, William as a 10-year-old, and William's caregiver. Read out the story in Box 2.e scene by scene, with the four participants acting out each scene.

Box 2.e The story of William and the goat

When William was five he was asked, for the first time, to look after some goats. He was proud and excited, but one of them butted him. It hurt and frightened him, and he cried. He didn't tell anyone what had happened because he thought he might get in trouble. He thought the goat had attacked him because he was doing something wrong.

Later in life, William would sometimes feel worried and anxious, especially when he was asked to take responsibility for something he hadn't done before. He didn't know why. He avoided doing new things. His auntie said he was lazy.

One day, William's uncle asked him to take care of his goats. He noticed that William looked really anxious. He talked kindly, to find out what the problem was. Gradually William told the tale of when he had been butted by a goat. With his uncle's help, he was able to remember the whole story.

Now William understood that he had not done anything wrong when the goat butted him, he had just been inexperienced. His memories of being hurt, and of feeling guilty, were only part of the story: he had also looked after the goats, when he was only five! And he had shown courage by not abandoning them after being butted.

He felt much better, and asked his uncle to show him how to take care of the goats well – and how to avoid getting butted!

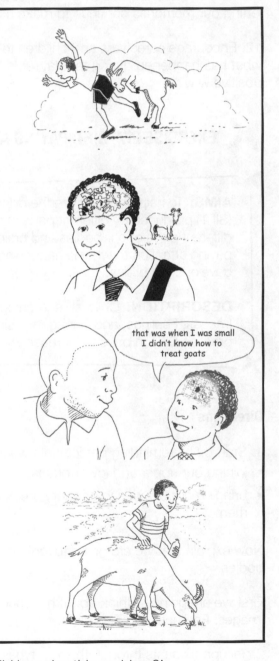

that was when I was small I didn't know how to treat goats

---

9. Ask: 'What had happened in William's brain? How did he solve this problem?'

10. Show the mixed-up jigsaw pieces you have prepared; then ask a couple of volunteers to join them together so that everyone can see the whole picture.

Explain: 'This is what we need to do to support each other in dealing with bits of memory that make us angry, sad, or scared. We can bring the pieces together to create a whole picture, so our minds can make sense of the memories and feel less angry, sad, or upset by them.'

With *caregivers*, add: 'It's important to support our children in doing this too.'

11. Explain: 'It is important for caregivers and children to tell the upsetting story to a person whom they trust. This person can help make sense of the story, empathize with our feelings, point out how we used our abilities to cope with the situation, and show us how it either ended well at the time or how things have improved since. This allows us to develop a more positive story in our mind, which does not make us feel sad, fearful, or angry. This helps us have a *whole* memory of the event, which gives us strength as we move forward with our life, rather than letting our memories continue to make us feel sad, upset, or angry.'

12. Encourage caregivers and children to talk together regularly when they get home about what has happened during the day, or in the past. This will help our memories develop in a positive way.

 EXERCISE 2.7 SIFT: PAYING ATTENTION TO WHAT'S GOING ON INSIDE US

AIMS: To help us recognize the different Sensations, Images, Feelings, and Thoughts (SIFT) produced by different parts of our bodies and brains. To understand how the different parts of our bodies and brains are integrated. To use the SIFT tool to practise paying attention to what is happening in our bodies and minds, and talk about it; this develops our brains.

DESCRIPTION: Children and caregivers learn to be aware of their Sensations, Images, Feelings, and Thoughts, using movements, examples, and a game. They practise SIFT in pairs to increase their understanding of each other.

Directions

1. Start off by reminding participants what we have learned already about:
• joining our upper and lower brains;
• bringing our bits of sad or angry memories back together, to make a more complete, positive memory.

Now explain that we are going to look at how our brains are also connected to the rest of our bodies.

First we are going to think about how our bodies experience things: through Sensations, Images, Feelings, and Thoughts.

2. Talk participants through the four types of experience as follows.

Sensations. Physical sensations in different parts of our bodies can help us recognize how we are feeling.

For example:

- The sensation of feeling a bit sick can be a symptom of anxiety. Ask: 'Who can suggest something that might make us feel anxious?' Once participants answer, ask: 'What can we do to feel better? Let's take deep, calm breaths.'
- The sensation of soreness in our shoulders and neck muscles can be a symptom of stress. Ask: 'What might make us feel stressed?' Once participants answer, ask: 'What can we do to feel better? Let's stand and turn to massage the shoulders of the person on our right, and relax our necks.'

Now say: 'Let's stretch our arms downwards and use all our fingers and thumbs to feel our feet, legs, tummy, chest, shoulders, arms, neck, and head. As we move up our bodies, what sensations do you feel? Does anywhere feel tense, painful, or relaxed, or can you feel any other sensations?'

Images. Images in our minds may be memories or imaginary pictures, or they might come from a film or book. Once we recognize them, we can enjoy them, or change them and/or control them. For example:

> Mary is very good at singing. She has been asked to sing a solo in the church choir, but she has an image in her mind of being unable to sing a note, and people laughing at her. She is feeling very nervous. Her caregiver listens to her worries and helps her to change the image to a lovely one, in which she sings beautifully and everyone claps and appreciates her.

Say: 'Let's make some glasses for ourselves to see our images better.' Ask everyone to make circles with both their first fingers and thumbs, and hold them up to their eyes, so that they can pretend to look through the 'glasses'.

Feelings. We may feel, for example, fear or happiness in different parts of our bodies, but they mostly arise in our lower brain, and are mostly transmitted into the right upper side of the brain.

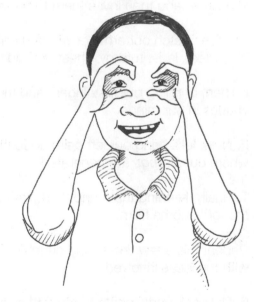

Say: 'Put your left hand on the back of your head, so your fingers point to the right to show where our feelings are generated.' Explain that it's good to recognize and talk about our feelings. We can learn to describe feelings in detail, and accurately, so we understand the richness of our feelings, like moving from a black and white photo to a colour one.

Say: 'Let's show each other how we are feeling using our faces. Pair up and, in turn, show each other how you are feeling right now. Tell your partner what you think they are feeling, before they say as clearly as they can how they are feeling. If your partner's feeling is very general, ask questions about it. For example, "I feel bad" might mean "I feel disappointed", or "jealous", or "anxious" or "sick".

'Show that you have seen and heard your partner, and empathize with their feeling. You might say, for example, "I see that you are feeling disappointed. What has made you feel that way?"'

Remind participants that we can communicate our feelings through our face and body language, and through words. It is good to do both. Invite them to choose and show one feeling, and ask their partner to 'read' the feeling. Feelings they might express include: nervousness, surprise, disgust, tiredness, excitement, shyness, guiltiness.

Thoughts. These are the things we think about, what we tell ourselves, and how we tell the story of our lives, using words.

Say: 'Let's put our left hand on the top of our heads, where our thoughts are made.'

Ask for examples of thoughts. Once participants have given their ideas, explain that thoughts are just thoughts, they are not facts. We can enjoy helpful thoughts, but we can also argue with thoughts that aren't helpful, healthy, or even true. We can listen to our thoughts, and direct our attention away from thoughts we don't like and instead think of happier thoughts or of ways to solve problems. For example, from thinking: 'I'm so stupid to forget to take my medicine', we can redirect our thoughts to think: 'Come on, I'm not stupid – that's just a thought, it's not a fact. It's normal to forget things sometimes. What can I do to make it easier to remember?'

Invite people to give examples of thoughts that are helpful. Then ask for some examples of thoughts that are not helpful, and invite people to turn them into more positive, helpful thoughts.

3. Say: 'Now put your right hand on top of your head, and your left hand on the back of your head with fingers on the upper right part of the brain.' Ask: 'What does this tell us about how different parts of our brain are working together?'

The SIFT game

4. Explain that we are now going to play the SIFT game, which we can play at any time with our friends, family, or teachers. Ask someone to say what SIFT stands for.

5. Remind everyone, using the hand actions, what SIFT means. Ask everyone to stand together in a circle, and then invite them to do each action in turn as you describe it:

S: Let's stretch our arms downwards and use all our fingers and thumbs to feel the *sensations* in our feet, legs, tummy, chest, shoulders, arms, neck, and head.

I: Then, bringing our first fingers and thumbs together to make two circles, let's look for the *images* in our minds.

F: Now, let's bring our left palm up to the back of our head, and right upper part of the brain, where our *feelings* are generated.

T: Finally, keeping that hand there, let's bring our right palm up to the top of our head, where our *thoughts* come from.

Repeat this a few times, and encourage everyone to do so, so they are associating the actions with the ideas involved.

6. Now ask participants to repeat the sequence in pairs. They should take it in turns to do the SIFT actions, this time telling their partner what their own sensations, images, feelings, and thoughts are as they do so.

7. Bring the group back together and ask: 'What did you like about the game, and what did you find difficult? What did you learn about yourselves from the game?'

8. Ask: 'Would you like to play it at home or with your friends?' Invite them to try it and report on how it went.

EXERCISE 2.8 OUR WHEEL OF AWARENESS

AIMS: To give children and caregivers a tool to help them:
- survive big emotions and fears, and thrive;
- learn more about which parts of themselves they want to develop;
- learn how to find deep peacefulness within their hub.

DESCRIPTION: Participants are given an explanation of our wheel of awareness and act out a story. They draw their own wheels of awareness and interview each other in pairs.

Box 2.f Information for facilitators

In this exercise, encourage participants to think about a manageable negative feeling or thought. Some participants may have big problems going on in their lives, and may get upset. Interact with each pair, so you can support any participant who is so worried about their problem that they can't avoid thinking about it. Respect this anxiety, and follow up after the session. If appropriate, say that later on in the workshop we will explore how we can address their concerns together. It may be more appropriate to stop the exercise after the story of Habiba, and have participants draw and use their own wheels of awareness in a later session.

Directions

1. Recap quickly on what participants have done so far in this session. We have looked at:
- getting our lower and upper brains to work together;
- joining together bits of our memories;
- paying attention to our bodily sensations, images, feelings, and thoughts.

Explain that we are now going to look at how we can *choose* what our brains think about. We are going to learn about something called 'mindsight'. This means seeing with our mind. We use our eyes for eyesight, to see actual things and people. We can use our minds for mindsight, to see what's happening in our minds.

MINDSIGHT IS SEEING WITH YOUR MIND

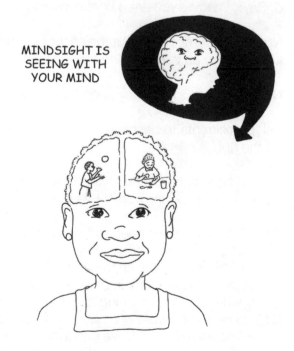

Mindsight lets us pay attention to the pictures in our head, the thoughts in our mind, the emotions we experience, and the feelings in our body. It helps connect them all together. It helps us know ourselves better. Just as we can make our shoulders relax if they are feeling tense, we can also choose to make our minds relax.

2. Explain that in this exercise we are going to use a tool which helps us see what's going on in our minds.

3. Say: 'We can picture our mind as a bicycle wheel, with a hub at the centre and spokes radiating towards the outer rim.'

Either show a picture of a bicycle wheel, or bring a bicycle into the room and wheel it around.

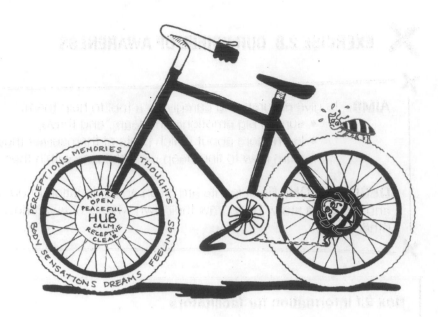

Say: 'The *rim* represents anything we can pay attention to, or become aware of: the SIFT elements, our dreams and desires, our memories, and our perceptions of the outside world. The *hub* is the inner place of the mind: our awareness. From here, we can focus calmly on everything that is happening in our lives. It helps us make good decisions and allows us to connect deeply to the wisdom within others and within ourselves. Do you see how the wheel is connected to the bicycle by the hub, so that it is well balanced and can move smoothly? In the same way, if we connect with the hub of our minds, we can be balanced in all that we feel, say, and do.'

4. Ask: 'Do you ever get stuck on a feeling or thought? Maybe an unhappy one, that's so powerful that it makes you forget about other, nicer feelings and thoughts?'

5. Say: 'The good news is that we don't have to stay stuck all the time on feelings that upset us. Of course we will still feel them at times, and that is good, but we can also learn to focus on other parts of ourselves and move away from that sad or angry feeling. How can we do this? We are going to use the "wheel of awareness".'

6. Say: 'Imagine you are a beetle, having a ride on the bicycle's wheel.'

Now invite someone to put their finger (representing the beetle) on the rim of the bicycle, and to keep it there as you wheel the bicycle.

Now ask them to put their finger on the hub, and wheel the bike again.

Ask participants to describe the beetle's two different journeys: the one on the rim, and the one on the hub.

Explain how, if the beetle settles on the rim, it goes round and round in a bumpy way and may feel sick. If it is on the hub, it has a much smoother and calmer ride along a straight line.

Say: 'This is what we need to try to achieve with our minds. If we stay on the hub, and don't allow all our thoughts and emotions to take over, we can just be aware of them, and feel much calmer about dealing with them. If instead we focus on just one or two points on the rim of the wheel, we can get stuck in a negative state of mind. But we can choose not be bossed about by negative feelings or thoughts which demand all our attention. If we get on the hub, and use SIFT to become aware of what's happening on the rim, we can achieve a more peaceful and accepting state of mind. We can focus on positive thoughts and feelings, not just problems. So the trick is: remember the beetle – hold on to the hub!'

7. Say: 'Now we are going to hear the story of Habiba and how she used this tool to help her. Who would like to act it out for us as I read it?' Invite two participants to act out Habiba's story (see Box 2.g).

Box 2.g The story of Habiba and her hub

Habiba cannot stop thinking about the spelling test coming up. She even has stomach ache. She doesn't feel like eating her lunch, or playing at break time. All she can imagine is disappointing her mother in the spelling test. She is nervous.

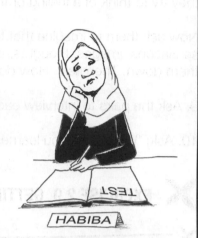

Then Habiba's teacher reminds her about the wheel of awareness. She explains that our minds are like a bicycle wheel. The centre of the wheel, called the hub, is our safe place, where our mind can relax and choose what to think about.

On the rim of the wheel are all the things Habiba could think about and feel, for example: how she likes playing netball with her friends at break; how she enjoys eating the chicken and chapati in her lunch bag; and of course, her nervousness about the spelling test. But she has left her hub, and has forgotten about the nice thoughts and feelings. She is only focussing on the nervousness point on the rim, and ignoring other, more positive points.

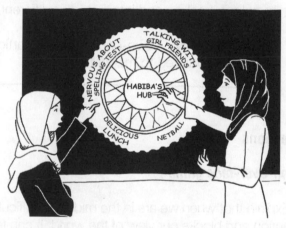

Habiba's teacher asks her to close her eyes and take three deep breaths. She says: 'You've been focussing on your worries about spelling. Now I want you to sit back on your hub, and think about the other parts of your wheel: you can focus on the part of your wheel that has fun, or imagine your lunch.' Habiba smiles, and her stomach starts to grumble. When she opens her eyes she feels better. She has used her wheel of awareness to remember to stay on her hub, so that she can focus on more positive feelings and thoughts than the spelling test. In this way, she has changed how she feels. She is still a little nervous, but she isn't stuck feeling nothing but nervousness.

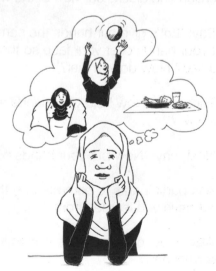

Habiba learns that she doesn't have to think only about nervous feelings, and that she can use her mind to remember to sit on her hub. She can think about other things that might help her have fun and feel less worried. Her teacher says, 'What could you do to do well in the test?' Now Habiba feels able to think about her options, and revises her spellings with her friend as they eat their lunch.

You may think it is more appropriate to finish the exercise here and have participants drawing their own wheels of awareness in a later session on a suitable topic. If not, continue with step 8.

8. Ask participants to pair up and draw their own wheels of awareness. Ask: 'Where do we focus our own minds most of the time?' Invite them to start on the rim, by drawing any negative feelings or thoughts that are in their minds a lot of the time, that they feel stuck on. Suggest that they try to think of a feeling or thought that is not too overwhelming.

Now ask them to imagine that they are sitting on their hub, breathing calmly. Ask: 'What other sensations, images, thoughts, and feelings can you see on the rim?' Ask them to draw or write them down. Then ask: 'How do you feel now?'

9. Ask the pairs to interview each other about their wheel of awareness.

10. Ask: 'What have you learned from your wheel of awareness? How does it help you?'

 ## EXERCISE 2.9 GETTING BACK ON OUR HUB

AIM: To learn how to focus our attention back to our hub, using mindsight exercises to calm ourselves and integrate our different feelings and desires.

DESCRIPTION: A two-part exercise: participants play the hand-over-face game; and are introduced to meditation.

Directions

Hand-over-face game

1. Explain that when we are in the middle of difficulty it can feel as if our problem takes up all of our attention and blocks our view of the world. It can feel all too close, like hands covering our face.

2. Say: 'Let's give our hands the name of a negative feeling, for example, fear or sadness. Now put your hands over your face so they cover it. Imagine that the hands are the feeling. What can you see? How do you feel?'

3. Then say: 'Now hold your hands away from your face. What can you see now? How do you feel now?'

4. Next, say: 'Now put your hands over your heart. What do you feel now?'

5. Ask participants to comment on the activity. For example, ask: 'What does this activity show? What have you learned from it?'

6. Ask: 'How could you use this activity to get a broader perspective on life when you feel overwhelmed?'

7. Summarize the learning and, if necessary, add: 'Observing how we feel can help us gain perspective. If we can step back a little, we can stop being overwhelmed and instead understand our experience rather than react to it. It is as if we can pull the hand (our suffering,

our reactions) away from our face. The size of our hand doesn't change (our experience doesn't disappear) but it gains a proper place, as one part of a bigger picture. Putting our hands on our heart reminds us to be kind to ourselves.'

Meditation to get back on our hub

Younger children can easily do this exercise. It's good to put a toy on their bellies so they can watch it go up and down with each breath.

1. Ask participants to make themselves comfortable in their chairs, or sitting on a mat or lying on their backs, and to follow the guidance you give. They don't have to say anything.

2. Give them the following guidance:

'Move your eyes around the room without moving your head. Look at the things I mention (for example, me, the door). Do you see how you have the power to choose where you focus your attention, all over this room? That's what I want to teach you about. We're going to learn how you can also choose to focus your attention on what's going on inside your mind and body. Close your eyes, and let's focus on what is in your thoughts, feelings, and senses. Let's start with what you can hear. I'm going to be quiet for a minute, while you pay attention to the sounds around us.'

After 30 seconds, say:

'What do you hear? You're aware of the sounds because you became still and listened on purpose.'

'Now I want you to notice your breathing. First, notice the air coming in and out of your nose and mouth (keep your mouth open). Now feel your chest going up and down. Now notice the way your stomach moves each time you breathe in and out.'

Now say:

'I'm going to be quiet for a minute. During this time, stay focussed on your breath. Other thoughts and feelings will come into your head. That's fine. Once you notice that your mind is wandering, and you're thinking about something else or starting to worry, just go back to focussing on your breath. Follow the wave of the in-breath and out-breath.'

After a minute, ask people to gently open their eyes and sit up.

3. Explain: 'This exercise is a powerful way to calm the mind and body. We can use it at any time. You may find it particularly useful when you feel anxious, confused, or worried. We can use it during our everyday lives, even with our eyes open, and sitting or standing up. This exercise helps us choose to return to our hub, so we can notice our thoughts, feelings, and sensations. This moves us into a different, calm state of mind. Remember, the bug will feel calmer if it rides on the hub!'

If you have time, ask participants to draw a picture of the bug on the hub, breathing away and looking happy.

EXERCISE 2.10 THE ME–WE CONNECTION: JOINING OURSELVES TO OTHER PEOPLE

AIM: To support each other in joining ourselves to other people, and in moving from being 'me' to being 'we'.

DESCRIPTION: Participants practise using mindsight to see things from someone else's perspective.

Directions

1. Ask: 'Who can remind us what "mindsight" means?' If necessary, remind participants that it means seeing with your mind.

Say: 'We have already learned that it means looking *inside your own mind* to see what's going on in there. Mindsight lets you pay attention to SIFT: the feelings in your body, the images or pictures in your head, the feelings or emotions you experience, and also the thoughts in your mind. It helps you know yourself better, and stay on your hub, in the middle of the river of wellbeing.'

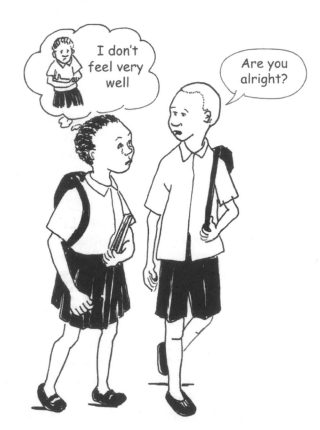

2. Say: 'Now we are going to look at using mindsight to try and see *someone else's mind*: to try to look at things from their point of view; how they are thinking and feeling.'

Show the picture opposite as an example of empathy, and invite a participant to draw it for later sessions.

3. Ask participants to pair up and sit together. Say: 'Take it in turns to tell each other about something that happened yesterday. The person listening should pay attention to what the person speaking is feeling about what happened. When the speaker stops, the listener tells him what she thinks they were feeling. The speaker then tells them how they were actually feeling, and the pair talk about how well the listener's perception matched the reality.'

4. After both partners have taken turns at speaking and listening, invite participants to share what they have learned.

5. Invite five people to act out the story of Kwame and Kofi (see Box 2.h).

Box 2.h The story of Kwame and Kofi

Kwame and Kofi are good friends and sit next to each other in school. The teacher asks Kofi to read out a poem he has written. When he sits down he sees that Kwame has drawn a silly picture of it, and his neighbour is laughing. Kofi calls Kwame 'stupid' in a loud voice, and everybody laughs.

Instead of walking home together, the two boys leave separately without speaking. Both boys look upset when they get home.

At the end of the drama, ask the actors playing Kwame and Kofi to stay in character.

6. Divide participants into four groups and direct them as follows.

Group 1. Ask this group to sit with Kofi and take it in turns to ask him these questions:
- Why is he upset?
- What did he feel when the incident happened?
- How might he feel if he did something to make friends with Kwame again?
- How might he become friends again with Kwame?

Group 2. Ask this group to use mindsight to try to answer the same questions from Kofi's perspective.

Group 3. Ask this group to sit with Kwame and ask him the same questions as Group 1 are asking, but in relation to his friendship with Kofi.

Group 4. Ask this group to use mindsight to try to answer the same questions from Kwame's perspective.

7. Come together and share the answers to the questions. Ask: 'How closely did the answers of the actors match the mindsight answers of groups 2 and 4? What can we learn from this?'

8. Ask participants to pair up and talk about a time when they used mindsight to think about how someone else was feeling and it worked out well. What abilities did they use?

9. Bring the activity to a close and say: 'The next time you're upset with someone, use your own mindsight to see how the other person feels. It can make you both feel a lot happier.'

 EXERCISE 2.11 THE THREE CIRCLES OF THE BRAIN

We suggest that children aged 5–8 years do not do this exercise.

AIM: To understand the 'protection', 'drive', and 'soothe' systems of our brains, and the importance of having them in balance for us to stay in our harmonious river of wellbeing.

DESCRIPTION: Participants are given an explanation of the three systems of the brain, draw circles to represent them and think about how they interact.

Directions[10]

1. Divide your peer group into males and females. Explain that in this exercise we are going to learn more about how our brains work, so that we can support ourselves in staying in our river of wellbeing.

Ask: 'Who can remind us about what we have learned about helping our brains to work in a coordinated way between the upper and lower brain?' Ask one or two participants to tell a story about how they stayed on their hub, or kept themselves calm.

2. Briefly explain that we have three systems in our brains, each having different functions. The three systems have to stay in balance to help us stay on our hubs. Invite one or two participants to draw a version of the picture below, showing the three brain systems – the *drive and achievement, safeness and kindness,* and *protection and safety-seeking* systems – with a star in the middle to show the hub where all three systems are balanced.

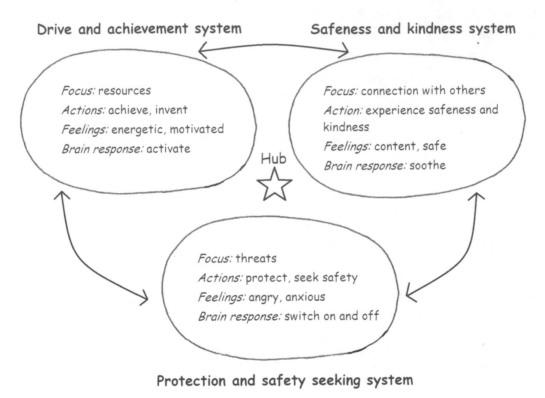

Drive and achievement system

Focus: resources
Actions: achieve, invent
Feelings: energetic, motivated
Brain response: activate

Safeness and kindness system

Focus: connection with others
Action: experience safeness and kindness
Feelings: content, safe
Brain response: soothe

Hub

Focus: threats
Actions: protect, seek safety
Feelings: angry, anxious
Brain response: switch on and off

Protection and safety seeking system

3. Read out the following, which is what we imagine the three systems might say if they could speak:

'When faced with the pain of life:
- the *protection and safety-seeking* system says, "This is bad – I need to fight or run away!";
- the *drive and achievement* system says, "Things will be better when I pass my exams!";
- compassion, intimately related to our *safeness and kindness* system, says, "Ah, pain. I recognize you. This is how life sometimes is. I will work out what needs to be done to work with this, and I will bear it in the meantime".'

4. Invite participants to draw the three circles for their own brain, including the star for the hub.

5. Explain that you will now talk to them about each circle. As you speak, they can think about what is happening in their own brain, and write or draw their ideas in the relevant circle.

Protection and safety-seeking system. This is housed in the lower brain.

As we learned in Exercise 2.1 'Our changing brains', it is from this part of the brain that we react automatically to protect ourselves from danger or threats.

Ask: 'Who can tell us some ways that we behave in response to danger or threat, and give us an example?' Invite participants to act them out. For example:

- Fight: Someone tries to take our bag and we fight them to get it back.
- Flight: We can see fire burning in the forest behind our house. We run away and report it.
- Freeze: A stranger comes into the house when we are alone. We stay completely still behind the curtain.
- Appease: A trader is angry that we owe him money. We promise to bring it immediately to calm him down, so he does not hit us – and then we think about how we can pay him.

Use the information in Box 2.i to explain the words in and around the *protection and safety-seeking* system in the picture.

Box 2.i Protection and safety-seeking system characteristics

Explain the words on the three brain systems picture:

Focus: threat;
Actions: seeking protection and safety;
Feelings: anger, anxiety, disgust;
Brain response: activating to turn it on; inhibiting to switch it off.

Ask: 'What benefits does this system give us?'

Explain that this system is very important for protecting us from harm. For example, if we touch something hot, this system makes us take our hand off the source of heat instantly without thinking about it.

Invite participants to think about the protection and safety system in their own brains. When have they used it recently, and how did it help them? How often do they feel angry, afraid, or disgusted, and seek safety and protection?

Drive and achievement system. This is housed in the upper brain. It has helped us to invent many things since the beginning of humankind.

Ask: 'Who can think of some of these ideas or inventions?'

Examples include: herding animals for milk and meat; growing crops to eat and for other uses; making clothes; using tools and weapons; wearing jewellery; learning to read and write; designing mobile phones; designing and riding bicycles, cars, planes, and spaceships.

Say: 'None of these would have been possible without the "drive" part of our brains, which is full of drive and enquiry and wants to achieve something new or different.'

Ask: 'What benefits does this system give us?'

Explain that our drive motivates us to take action to achieve a good life for ourselves and our families.

Invite participants to think about this circle in their own brains. What motivates them to take action to achieve a good life? What examples can they suggest that show this part of our brain in action? How big do they think this part of their brain is compared to the 'protection' circle?

Safeness and kindness system. This is also in the upper brain. It calms, soothes, and comforts us. It encourages us to connect with others and use our virtues to keep our relationships harmonious.

Ask: 'What examples can we suggest that show this part of our brain in action?'

Explain that this is the part of our brain that enables us to make and love friends, families, and children. It leads us to find activities that help us relax, such as singing and dancing.

Ask: 'What benefits does the safeness and kindness part of our brain give us?'

Explain that using this part of the brain, we become 'we' instead of 'I'. We use our virtues, such as compassion and kindness, to soothe ourselves and others.

Invite participants to think about this circle in their own brains. What ways do they use to soothe themselves and to stay connected with other people? What examples can they suggest that show this part of our brain in action? How big do they think this circle is in their brains compared to the 'protection' and 'drive' circles?

6. Explain that all three systems are important, and need to be *in balance and connected* to each other, so that we remain in our river of wellbeing.

7. Explain that sometimes the three systems get *out of balance*: then one or two systems become too dominating, and we no longer live in our river of wellbeing.

8. If there is time, ask participants to draw how big they think the three circles are in their own brains.

Ask participants: 'How do we keep the balance?'

Remind them of any of the tools they don't mention. Explain that we will be learning lots of ways of keeping the balance as we go through the workshop.

Closing circle

Purpose: To support participants in: understanding the difference between gender and sex; realizing that gender roles can change; and questioning the 'naturalness' of gender roles.

Contents of session	Materials required	Time required
Opening circle (see p.13)		15 mins
3.1 The difference between sex and gender	Prepared flipchart and pictures on page 60 and in Annex	45 mins
3.2 Being a female, being a male		30 mins
3.3 Checking our beliefs		60 mins
3.4 Using courage to change gender norms		45 mins
Closing circle (see p.14)		15 mins

About 3.5 hrs

EXERCISE 3.1 THE DIFFERENCE BETWEEN SEX AND GENDER

AIMS: To understand the difference between 'sex' and 'gender'. To understand that gender characteristics and roles are created by culture, and that they can and do change over time.

DESCRIPTION: Participants explore the difference between sex and gender roles.

Box 3.a Information for facilitators

You should read and understand this information before you lead the exercise, so that you feel comfortable explaining it in your own words to participants as appropriate.

You may find a lot of new ideas and information in this session. Practise it with other facilitators so that you are comfortable talking about sex and gender, and ready to explore challenging issues by questioning participants about them or responding to their questions.

Explain this information to participants as needed and appropriate:

The word 'sex' tells us about the differences between male and female bodies. Most of us get classified as a boy or a girl when we are born. Only females can have periods, get pregnant, give birth to children, and breastfeed. Only males can produce sperm, which is needed to make pregnancy happen. These differences are the work of nature and we cannot change them except by surgery and medication. A few people are born with a mixture of male and female organs. People who are born with this mixture are called *intersex*.

The word 'sex' is also used to mean sexual intercourse, for example, 'she is not old enough to have sex'.

'Gender' describes differences in the way that men and boys, and women and girls, are expected to behave: our dress, the work we do, the way that we speak, and our status in society. These differences are created by our culture rather than nature, and we can change them.

'Gender roles' describe what men and boys, and women and girls, are supposed to do in their culture. For example, in Tanzania, a man is traditionally expected to cut down trees, and a woman is expected to cook. Since people create gender roles, people can also change them. Cultures adapt them all the time.

'Gender identity' refers to one's internal personal sense of being a girl or a boy, a man or a woman. Some people feel that they have been born in the wrong body; for example, they are biologically a man but feel like a woman. They are called *transgender people* and can, if they wish, have surgery or take medication to make them feel comfortable as a male or female in their bodies and minds.

 Intersex and transgender people are often stigmatized by others. It is important that we accept and include people with different sexual and gender attributes in our work and our community. Share this information as appropriate with participants, and be aware that your group may include people with different sexual and gender characteristics.

'Gender' and 'sex' are often used interchangeably, or 'gender' is used for all references to male and female, with 'sex' only used for 'sexual intercourse'. We think that it is helpful to use 'sex' and 'gender' in this manual in the way we have defined them above. So, for example, we use 'sex' when we are dividing groups into males and females. We use 'gender' when we are talking about social attitudes and behaviours. If any participant has a gender identity that does not match their sex, they might, when you split the peer group by sex, prefer to join the half they feel comfortable in. Support them in negotiating this with the other participants.

Directions[11]

1. Explain that today we are going to talk about the differences between boys and girls, and men and women.

Ask: 'Who can tell us the difference between a person's "sex" and their "gender"?' If necessary, use information from Box 3.a to help explain these terms.

2. Show participants the pictures on the next page, and Annex, one by one, or others that your community will relate to.

Ask: 'Which pictures show the "sex" of a person?' and 'Which pictures show "gender" roles?'

3. Invite two volunteers to come forward: a girl or woman to act out something that only a female can do; and a boy or man to act out something that only a male can do.

Ask: 'What is the person doing?'

'Is it to do with their gender or their sex?' and 'Is it true that only a male or a female can do this?'

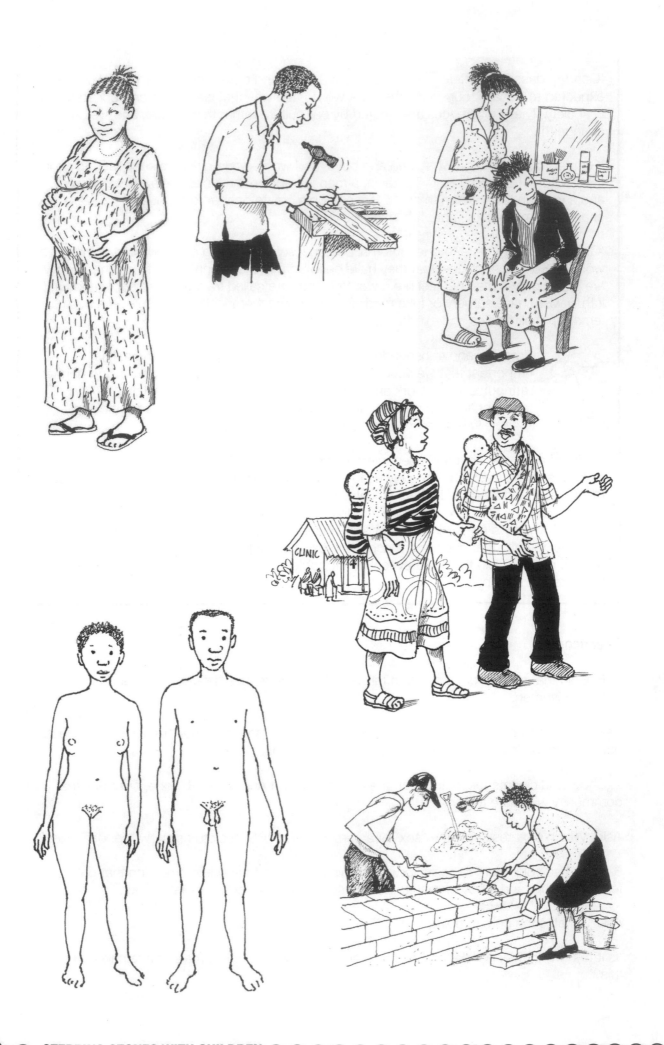

4. Put up the flipchart that you have prepared (see Table 3.1).

Table 3.1 Flipchart headings

Male-only gender roles	Female-only gender roles	Male and female gender roles	Male sex roles	Female sex roles

5. Invite participants to enter the following words into one or more columns in your flipchart.

Doctor – Secretary – Truck driver – Giving birth – Sweeping – Cooking – Nurse – Mother – Herding – Weeding – Priest – Soldier – Father – Teacher – Pregnancy – Politician – Knitting – Menstruation – Producing sperm – Clearing land – Building roofs – Breastfeeding – Making a woman pregnant – Looking after children – Carrying firewood – Labourer – Washing plates

Younger and older children. Introduce each role and say: 'Stand up if you think that a boy or girl like you could do this role, either now or when you grow up.' Discuss the answers each time, and add the role to the appropriate column.

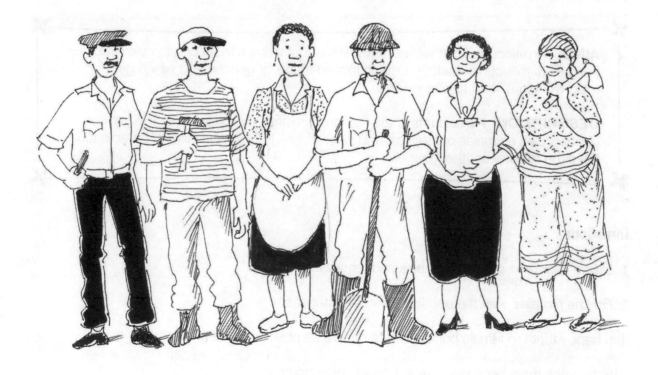

6. Ask the participants to look again at the first two columns. Ask: 'Could any of these roles be done by either a male or a female?'

If some participants disagree, ask them to explain why. Move the role into the middle column if it can be done by both males and females.

7. *Caregivers only.* Ask 'Who can think of any gender roles that have changed since you or your grandparents were children?'

You might ask:

- 'Did girls go to school then?'
- 'Did boys fetch water?'
- 'What other roles have changed over the years?'
- 'Are there any negative things about these changes?'
- 'What is negative and why?'
- 'What are the good things about these changes? Why are they good?'
- 'What do you think we as caregivers could do to support our boys and girls with these changing roles?'

8. *Younger and older children.* Explain that gender roles have changed in the past, and continue to change now. For example, girls did not go to school.

Explain that you will now call out a *new role* and ask them to stand up if they think a person like them could do this role, now or when they are older (as in point 5). Include new roles that are relevant to your country, e.g. being a member of parliament, wearing trousers, riding a bicycle, cooking for the family, being president.

 ## EXERCISE 3.2 BEING A MALE, BEING A FEMALE

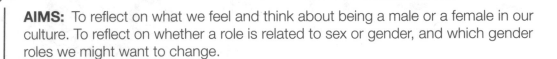

AIMS: To reflect on what we feel and think about being a male or a female in our culture. To reflect on whether a role is related to sex or gender, and which gender roles we might want to change.

DESCRIPTION: Participants share reasons why they feel happy with their sex or gender roles as males or females, and ways in which they would like to be able to have the roles of another gender.

Directions

1. Divide your peer group into males and females.

2. *For the females.* Ask them to finish these sentences:

'I'm happy that I'm female because … (e.g. I will be able to give birth).'

'I wish I were male because … (e.g. I could come home late).'

For the males. Ask them to finish these sentences:

'I'm happy that I'm male because … (e.g. I don't have to look after babies).'

'I wish I were female because … (e.g. I wouldn't have to labour hard to earn money).'

3. Bring the peer group back together. Invite participants to share their ideas, and write or draw symbols for them on the flipchart or chalkboard.

Discuss: 'Which of the roles can you change if you wish, and which can you not change?'

We can change gender roles but not sex roles. For example:

'I wish I were a boy because I could move freely at night' (gender role)

'I wish I were a girl so I could breastfeed my baby' (sex role)

4. With the group, underline those ideas that can change. Ask: 'How would you change them?'

5. Ask: 'Did you find anyone's comments surprising or interesting?'

'Is there any difference between how easily males can wish to be females, and how easily females can wish to be males?'

If participants answer 'yes', ask: 'Why do you think this is?'

 EXERCISE 3.3 CHECKING OUR BELIEFS

AIMS: To find out how we think boys and girls should behave. To discover which of these ideas promote our health and wellbeing, and which ones threaten it. To practise listening skills.

DESCRIPTION: Participants respond to a series of statements, explain their choices, and potentially change their views.

Box 3.b Information for facilitators

This exercise causes a lot of discussion, as people may feel quite strongly about gender roles. Let the participants discuss and challenge each other. Be ready to question harmful attitudes or beliefs if needed. For example, in one workshop, women said it was right for a man to beat his wife if she did not cook for him. The facilitator asked: 'If our children see their fathers beating their mothers, what does this tell our children?' This led to a good discussion; in the end everyone agreed that men beating women was a bad idea.

Directions[12]

1. Use words or symbols to label one corner of the room 'agree' and another 'disagree'. Label the middle of the room 'not sure'.

Explain: 'We are going to look at what we believe about gender, and what we believe are the correct and good ways for males and females to behave. I'm going to read out some statements. If you agree with the statement, stand in the "agree" corner; if you disagree, stand in the "disagree" corner; and if you're not sure, stand in the middle.'

2. Read out a statement (using Box 3.c and your ideas from Exercise 3.1).

3. Once everyone has moved, invite people in the same corner to share their reasons for being there with each other for two minutes.

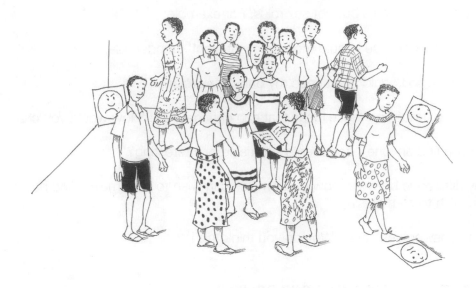

4. Invite one or two people in each corner to explain why they agree, disagree, or are not sure.

5. Ask 'Does anyone want to change corners?' If any people move, ask one or two of them to explain why.

6. Ask what consequences the statement would have for boys and girls, men and women, if everyone were to obey it.

7. Repeat the exercise with a different statement. You can also ask participants to add their own statements.

Box 3.c Possible statements for use in Exercise 3.3

Use statements that fit your peer group and context.

Girls and boys aged 5–8 years
- Boys should be asked to spend as much time as girls on household tasks.
- Women should raise children because they are more caring than men.
- Girls and women should show respect to men by keeping quiet unless asked to speak.

Girls and boys aged 9–14 years
- Girls should obey boys because boys are stronger in decision-making than girls.
- Sexually active boys should protect their sexual partners by using condoms.
- It's fine for a boy or man to beat a girl or woman because she needs to know who is in charge.

Caregivers
- When money is scarce, boys should go to school rather than girls because girls will marry and bring in dowry.
- As caregivers we should teach boys and girls their different roles in society.
- Men should make the decisions about how money is spent in the home.

---

8. Invite participants to say what they have learned about gender beliefs from this activity.

If necessary, add:

'Our gender beliefs affect our self-compassion, our relationships with others and our behaviour. They may stop girls and boys, women and men, from doing and being everything they could do and be in their lives.

'Some gender beliefs put everyone at risk of HIV, other sexually transmitted infections (STIs), unwanted pregnancy, and infertility. For example, if girls and women are expected to be quiet and obedient, they may find it difficult to say "no" to unsafe sex.'

 ## EXERCISE 3.4 USING COURAGE TO CHANGE GENDER NORMS

AIMS: To learn about the virtue of courage and how we can practise it to promote fairer gender roles and norms.

DESCRIPTION: Agreeing on what we mean by the virtue of courage; role plays to show how we can practise courage to make gender roles fairer.

Directions

1. Explain that in this exercise, we are going to talk about using courage to change unhelpful gender norms. Invite participants to say what 'courage' means to them and to give examples. Add any further information from Box 3.d as needed.

Box 3.d Information for facilitators

You may wish to share some of this information with participants in your own words.

Courage is personal bravery in the face of fear. It is doing what needs to be done, even if it is hard and makes us afraid. Courage is going ahead when you feel like giving up. Courage is needed in trying new things, for example, changing gender roles and values. It may be saying that you made a mistake, and then doing the right thing. It is the strength in your heart.[13]

---

2. Direct the relevant peer groups as follows:

Children. Split your peer group into boys and girls.

Caregivers. Split the group according to the sex of the caregiver's child (i.e. one group for caregivers of boys, and one for caregivers of girls). Caregivers who have children of both sexes may join either group.

All peer groups. Choose one of the situations in Box 3.e, or ask participants to suggest situations that require gender courage which are relevant to them or their children.

> **Box 3.e Examples of situations needing gender courage**
>
> *For boys aged 5–8 years*
> - Your friends are laughing at you because you want to play with a doll.
> - Your friends call you names because you like cooking with your sister.
> - An older girl invited you to have sex and you said 'No'. The other boys tease you.
>
> *For girls aged 5–8 years*
> - You want to wear trousers to school but people say you must dress like a girl.
> - You want to ask your brother to help carry water because you both have homework.
> - Boys say that girls' brains are not as good as boys' brains.
>
> *For boys aged 9–14 years*
> - Your friends say that you must prove that you are a man by drinking beer and paying a girl for sex.
> - Your friends tease you for being a 'girl' because you cried.
> - You want to help your grandmother with carrying wood for fuel but your friends are laughing at you.
>
> *For girls aged 9–14 years*
> - It's time for you to choose school subjects to specialize in and you want to do physics, but your teacher says that girls are no good at physics and that you had better do social studies.
> - Some boys are teasing your friend, whose period has stained her dress.
> - Your teacher asks a question about safer sex in class. You know the answer, but you feel shy to say it because the boys will call you a 'prostitute'.

3. Ask the participants to imagine that they or their child is in the chosen situation, and to discuss how they would show gender courage and mindsight. Ask them to prepare a role play to perform to the other half of their peer group.

4. Bring the group back together to watch the two role plays. After each one, ask:

'What gender role or belief did we see?'

'Who changed things in what way?'

'How did they do that? What courage did they show?'

'Who showed that they have mindsight?'

'How can we all support one another to develop courage and mindsight in these situations?'

SESSION 4 CHILDREN'S RIGHTS

Purpose: To increase understanding of the virtue of justice, rights for children, and sexual and reproductive rights; to identify how children's rights are being met and what supports them; to identify violations of children's rights and what we can do together to support these rights.

Contents	Materials required	Time required
Opening circle (see p.13)		15 mins
4.1 Joined pairs	Additional props can be used	20 mins
4.2 Justice		40 mins
4.3 Children's rights	Pictures on p69 and in Annex	45 mins
4.4 Promoting children's rights	Flipcharts from Exercise 4.3	60 mins
Closing circle (see p.14)		15 mins

About 3 hrs 15 mins

 EXERCISE 4.1 JOINED PAIRS

AIMS: To learn to respect each other's thoughts and feelings, and to express our own while working together.

DESCRIPTION: Participants work in joined pairs to complete various tasks.

Directions[14]

1. Ask the participants to pair up with someone of the same sex as them. Then ask them to hold one of their partner's hands, or place an arm around their partner's waist or shoulder, so that they each have one hand free to use.

2. Ask the pairs to complete various tasks together depending on their age, for example, taking off their socks, carrying a chair, or drawing a picture.

3. Add humour by asking participants to hold one another's ear or foot.

4. Discuss these questions with participants:

'How did it feel to be so closely connected to another person? Was it more or less difficult to do things?'

'What abilities can we use to help us to do a task with someone else?'

'How did you feel when you had accomplished the task with the other person?'

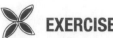 **EXERCISE 4.2 JUSTICE**

AIMS: To understand the virtue of justice and how to practise it.

DESCRIPTION: Participants make a mind map to show the meaning of justice and how we practise it.

Directions[15]

1. Explain that justice is a virtue, and that we are going to think about what it means and how we practise it. Make a mind map by drawing a circle in the middle of the chalkboard or on a flipchart, and write 'justice' inside the circle. Ask participants what they think justice means, and write or draw these ideas around the circle. Add ideas from Box 4.a if you wish.

Box 4.a What is justice?

We're practising justice when we:
- think for ourselves, and act fairly;
- avoid gossip and backbiting;
- see with our own eyes and don't judge something or someone by what other people tell us, or by their gender, race, religion, or health status;
- see people as individuals;
- own up to our mistakes and accept the consequences;
- share fairly with others;
- stand up for people's rights, including our own.

Without justice, people get away with hurting or taking advantage of others and keep on doing it. This is why justice is important for achieving rights. Without justice the world can be a cruel and dangerous place. When justice is practised, everyone has a fair chance to tell their side of the story and be listened to.

---

2. Ask participants, in pairs, to tell each other a story about a time when they practised justice.

3. After the pairs have heard each other's stories, invite everyone to add to the mind map what they did when they practised justice.

4. Discuss this quotation by Martin Luther King:

'True peace is not merely the absence of tension. It is the presence of justice.'

EXERCISE 4.3 CHILDREN'S RIGHTS

AIMS: To understand the meaning of the term 'rights', and the rights of children and caregivers.

DESCRIPTION: Participants learn about children's rights, then use role play to explore ways in which children's rights are not met locally, and how things could be different.

Directions[16]

1. Explain that we are now going to begin to look at some rights children have.

Ask participants to give their ideas on what a 'right' is, and to give some examples of children's rights (e.g. to go to school, to wear clothes, to have food and water).

2. Explain that human rights are about respect for everyone. They are about having our needs met, staying safe, and having a say in what happens in our lives. They also involve saying what we think and feel, and living life as we want to, as long as we act responsibly and respect the rights of others.

In 1989 almost all the governments in the world signed a special agreement called the Convention on the Rights of the Child. Governments should make sure that children enjoy all their rights, of which there are three types:

* rights to things children need, such as a home, food, health care, places to play and learn;
* rights to be kept safe from harm;
* rights to take part in deciding how they live their lives.

3. Show participants the pictures below, also in Annex, one by one, and ask:

'What do you see happening in the picture?'

'What right is being supported or abused?'

'Do children in our community have this right met?'

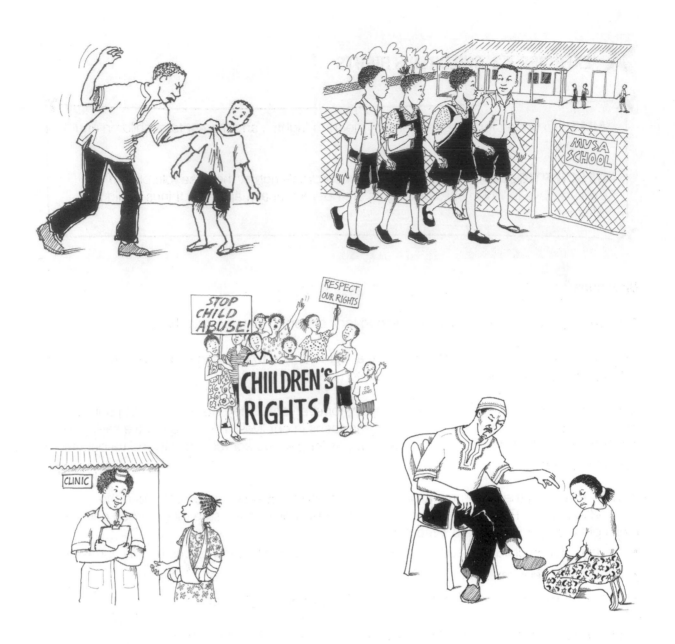

4. Now divide participants into three groups named A, B, and C, and invite each group to choose one right to consider from those listed within groups A, B, and C in Box 4.b.

Children. Ask them to give examples of ways this right is being met in their lives, and ways it is not being met. Make a note on flipchart paper of the examples given where the right is not being met.

Caregivers. Ask them to give examples of ways this right is being met in their children's lives, and ways it is not being met. Make a note on flipchart paper of the examples given where the right is not being met.

5. Repeat this exercise to consider one or two of the other rights listed within each group in Box 4.b.

Box 4.b Children's rights

Group A – Rights to things children need

- the right to life;
- the right to be healthy and to have access to health-care services;
- the right to information;
- the right to education.

Group B Rights to be kept safe from harm

- the right to feel well and happy in our body and our mind;
- the right to freedom from abuse, violence and exploitation (being used for another's benefit);
- the right to be protected from violence, and harmful practices;
- the right to refuse to have sexual intercourse or other sexual activity.

Group C Rights to take part in deciding how to live their lives

- the right to say what they think;
- the right to meet and talk with others;
- the right to confidentiality and privacy;
- the right to be part of important decisions that affect their lives.

6. Ask each group (A, B, and C) to create a role play to show a situation where one of these rights is *not* met. If any of the groups is made up of more than six participants, ask them to split into two groups.

7. Invite each group to show their role play to the whole peer group.

8. Invite participants to come up and change the role play, if they want, so that all agree that this right is met.

 EXERCISE 4.4 PROMOTING CHILDREN'S RIGHTS

AIM: To identify people, institutions, and collective strengths that can help work towards realizing children's rights.

DESCRIPTION: Participants engage in small group work to find ways of promoting child rights on the specific issues identified by peer groups. They practise talking about rights.

Directions

1. Explain that governments have a duty to give children support and protection in order to live safe, healthy, and happy lives. But many other people can also use justice to achieve children's

rights. They include caregivers, children, families, teachers, leaders, churches, communities, police, and health institutions.

2. Say: 'In this exercise we will look at some of the gaps in our rights, and how we can work together and get supporters to realize our rights more fully.'

3. Pin up the flipchart papers from Exercise 4.3. They show the gaps: the places where, in our community, children's rights are not met.

Divide the participants into small groups and ask them to select one gap each (so every group is working on a different gap).

4. Say: 'You have identified an issue. Now let's talk about what we can do. How can we support each other, and who can help us? How do we bring about change?'

5. After 15 minutes of discussion, ask the small groups to share the results of their discussions with the whole group. Each group should name one person or place that they could go to for support.

6. If necessary, explain that although issues can seem big, we can use our virtues of courage and justice to try and change things. For example, we can: discuss issues with our teachers and families and ask for their support; form groups and plan campaigns to speak about our feelings; and bring hidden challenges such as child abuse into the open.

7. Ask each small group to develop role plays to practise describing the gap in children's rights to their chosen supporter, and explaining the support or change that they want. Some group members act as the children and others act as the adult/s – for example, a teacher or health worker.

8. If there is time, invite the small groups to show these role plays to the whole group.

SESSION 5   THE TREE OF LIFE

Purpose: To picture and think about our lives using the idea of a tree; to feel supported by our history, where we are now, abilities, dreams, people who are important to us, and gifts we have given and received; to stand in a safer place, from where we can talk about our difficult experiences in ways that make us feel stronger.[17]

Special information: The peer groups come together for Exercises 5.2 and 5.3.

Watch out for children who feel upset or need extra help.

Contents	Materials required	Time required
Opening circle (see p.13)		15 mins
5.1 Making the tree of life	Prepared flipchart showing parts of tree and parts of life	90 mins
5.2 The forest of life		30 mins
5.3 The storms of life		30 mins
Closing circle (see p.14)		15 mins

About 3 hrs

 EXERCISE 5.1   MAKING THE TREE OF LIFE

AIMS: To picture and think about our lives using the idea of a tree. To feel supported by our history, where we are now, abilities, dreams, people who are important to us, and gifts we have given and received. To stand in a safer place, from where we can talk about our difficult experiences in ways that make us feel stronger.

DESCRIPTION: Participants draw and tell stories about their lives using the shape of a tree as a model. Encourage them to keep their trees for later exercises.

Directions

1. Explain that we will make a picture of a strong, beautiful tree to tell the story of our lives. We will think about our past history, our lives now, our future dreams, and the people who have supported us. We will each draw our own trees and then share them with our caregivers and children, and take them home if we wish.

2. Ask: 'What different kinds of trees do you know?'

'What are the different parts of a tree?

'Invite people to stand up and imagine that they are a tree. Say: 'Feel the weight of your feet and imagine they are growing roots. Shake your fingers like leaves. The sun is shining and you are making food with your leaves. The wind is getting stronger. Dance like a tree. It is raining; feel the water on your leaves and roots.

'Now imagine that the roots are where you come from, the branches are your hopes and dreams, and the leaves are important people in your life.'

3. Present the flipchart you have prepared showing the tree of life, including the parts of the tree and the parts of life. Demonstrate how you would draw your own tree on a flipchart, using some of the questions from Table 5.1.

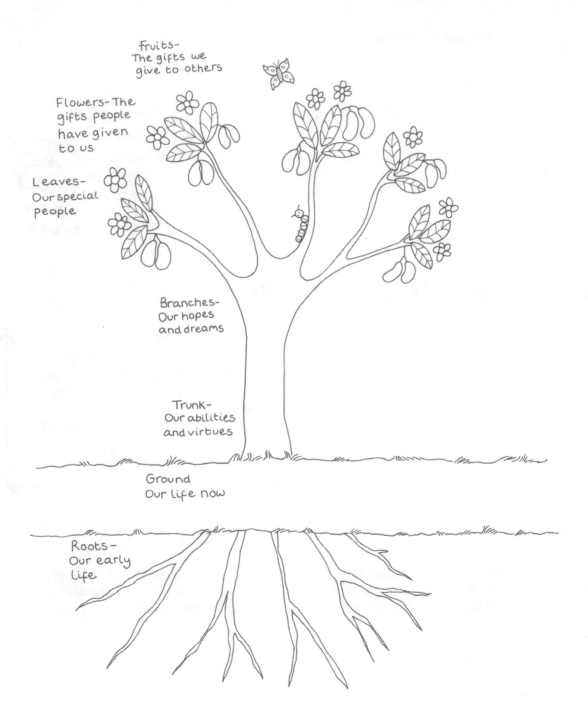

Fruits–
The gifts we
give to others

Flowers–The
gifts people
have given
to us

Leaves–
Our special
people

Branches–
Our hopes
and dreams

Trunk–
Our abilities
and virtues

Ground
Our life now

Roots –
Our early
life

Table 5.1 Parts of the tree of life

Part of tree	Part of life	Questions – draw or write answers on the tree	Extra questions – discuss in pairs, if there is time
Roots	Your history	Where do you come from? What is your family name? Where did your ancestors come from?	Who were your ancestors? Where are your extended family living?
Ground	Your life now	Who do you love the most? Who do you live with now? What do you do every day? What is your favourite place at home?	What is your favourite song? Why do you like that song so much?
Trunk	Your abilities (e.g. sport, maths, kindness, courage)	What are you good at and proud of? What do other people say you are good at?	Who taught you these abilities?
Branches	Your dreams and wishes	What are your hopes, dreams, and wishes?	What is the history of these hopes, dreams, and wishes? How are these hopes and dreams linked to important people in your life? How have you held on to them even through difficult times?
Leaves	People who are important to you (alive or dead)	Who is important to you in your life?	What is special about this person?
Fruits	Gifts that people have given you (material and non-material. e.g. love)	What gifts have you received in your life?	Why do you think the person gave you this? What did they appreciate about you? What do you think you contributed to their life?
Flowers	Gifts you have given to others (material and non-material)	What gifts have you given to people who are important in your life?	What do you appreciate about this person that led you to give them this gift? What do you think they have contributed to your life?

4. Invite participants to ask questions about the activity. Reassure them that the drawing is to help them tell their story. It will be special and beautiful because it is theirs.

5. Invite participants to draw their trees of life. Tell them that if they do not want to participate in the process, that is OK. Suggest that they think about the questions as the process goes on.

6. Say: 'Let's start by drawing our whole tree.'

7. For each part of the tree, read out questions in Table 5.1 column 3, one by one, and ask participants to draw or write their answers on their trees. Select and adapt questions according to the peer group. For example, for 5–8 year olds, use one or two questions from each part of the tree and make them very simple. You can use acting to help them answer questions such as, 'What are you good at and proud of?'

8. As going through all the parts of the tree will take time, you may want to break up the exercise by singing a song or doing a dance together to show solidarity.

9. When participants have finished answering all the questions, ask for a volunteer to share their tree of life with the group. Invite everyone to appreciate their abilities.

10. Invite people to get into pairs and tell each other what they wish about their tree of life. Ask them to listen actively to each other and appreciate each other's abilities. People who do not wish to share their trees and stories can listen to other people talking about theirs and join in the discussion.

  ## EXERCISE 5.2 THE FOREST OF LIFE

AIM: To understand why it is good for us to live together and support each other.

DESCRIPTION: Participants write words or pictures of encouragement on each others' trees.

Directions

1. Bring together the caregivers and children and sing a song to celebrate everyone's abilities.

Ask: 'What kind of trees live in a forest?'

Invite them to arrange their trees on the wall or floor or hold them up together to create a 'forest of life'.

2. Stand together and look at the forest created by all the trees.

Ask: 'Why is it good for trees to live together in a forest? Why is it good for us to live together?'

3. Encourage people to feel the strengths of their forest to support each other's hopes and dreams.

Say: 'Let's ask each other how our dreams are progressing, and what we and others can do to support our vision of the future.'

4. Suggest that people might invite other important people in their lives to join their forest of support when they get home.

Ask: 'Who might these people be? Those who are proud of us and want to see the best for us? People who have heard our stories and could accompany us on our road of life?'

Ask: 'Who else can we talk to and join with to support us in achieving our vision of the future?'

5. Invite people to choose a tree different from their own and, with permission, to write words or pictures of encouragement, support and appreciation on the tree. Give people time to walk around and read the trees and add their encouragement.

Ask: 'What caught your attention or captured your imagination? What made you think of your own life? How have you been moved by these stories?'

6. Ask people to go back to their own trees and read other people's responses to their stories.

7. Give people time to reflect on their experience and share a few thoughts.

  ## EXERCISE 5.3 THE STORMS OF LIFE

AIM: To invite people to talk about some of the challenges they may be facing in their life and how they are able to respond to them as members of the forest.

DESCRIPTION: Participants share how they have coped with a challenge in their life.

Directions

1. Ask: 'As beautiful and strong as the trees are in the forest, are they free from dangers and hazards? What are some of the dangers faced by trees?'

Participants might answer: 'the wind and storms may blow them down', 'they may get diseases', 'loggers may chop them down', etc.

2. Invite people to think about how strong we all are staying together in the forest if a storm comes. We have friends and support to help us through difficult times.

Say: 'Please get into pairs and tell each other about one challenge in your life. How does it affect you, and how have you been able to respond so far?'

3. Invite everyone to hug each other in a big group hug. Ask them to sway backwards and forwards together like trees in a storm, supporting each other.

4. Ask participants to keep their trees carefully because we will do more with them in Session 10.

SESSION 6 HOW TO BE ASSERTIVE

Purpose: To understand the virtue of assertiveness and how we can develop this virtue in our lives, rather than being passive (not able to say what we think or want) or aggressive (fighting).

Contents	Materials required	Time required
Opening circle (see p.13)		15 mins
6.1 Three ways to respond		50 mins
6.2 How assertive am I?		40 mins
6.3 Making 'I' statements		45 mins
6.4 Practising ways of staying assertive		45 mins
Closing circle (see p.14)		15 mins

About 3.5 hrs

EXERCISE 6.1 THREE WAYS TO RESPOND

AIM: To learn about assertive, passive, and aggressive ways of responding to situations, and to assess which is best.

DESCRIPTION: Participants create role plays to show passive, aggressive, and assertive behaviour, and practise responding in an assertive way.

Directions

1. Explain that today we are going to talk about and practise the virtue of assertiveness. Explain what this term means:

'*Assertiveness* means being positive and confident. It means being aware that we are worthy people with our own special gifts. When we are assertive we think for ourselves and ask for what we need. We have the self-confidence to tell the truth and the courage to seek justice.'[18]

Explain: 'We also use *passive* behaviour and *aggressive* behaviour. Let's look at each one in turn.'

2. We use passive behaviour to avoid trouble, to belong to a group, or to please people. Invite participants to give examples of passive behaviour. Add appropriate examples from the following list.

We behave in a passive way when we:
- are afraid to say that someone is hurting us;
- follow the crowd and give in to peer pressure;
- remain silent when we disagree or feel unhappy about something;
- put up with things we don't like;
- say sorry a lot, when we have done nothing to apologize for;
- find it difficult to say 'no';

- hide our feelings;
- do not start something new in case we fail;
- allow others to make all the decisions.

3. Explain that we may use aggressive, or fighting, behaviour to get what we want, take control, and show our anger. We might use unkind words to put people down, or push and hit people to make them afraid. Invite participants to give examples of aggressive behaviour, adding appropriate examples from the following list.

We behave aggressively when we:
- do what we want, with no thought for other people;
- try to control people;
- say we will do something bad to a person to get what we want;
- put ourselves first even though others lose out;
- make demands without listening to other people's ideas and needs;
- become angry quickly when others disagree with us;
- shout, push, or force people to do things they don't want to do;
- beat or act violently towards another person;
- make people feel that they need to defend themselves;
- make people look small so that we look big.

4. Ask people to give examples of assertive behaviour, adding from the following list as appropriate.

We use assertive behaviour when we:
- do not accept unfair or hurtful treatment;
- expect and give respect at all times;
- listen deeply to others;
- speak our own feelings and thoughts clearly and honestly;
- choose not to allow others to lead us into trouble;
- match our words to our body language;
- accept true suggestions for improving ourselves and learn from them;
- say 'no' without feeling bad;
- disagree without getting angry;
- say 'I feel angry' in a way that does not harm others;
- ask for help when we need it.

5. Ask the group to think of a challenging situation between two people that might happen to them. Ask for some volunteers to act out a role play about this situation. Explain that they will run through the role play three times, each time with the same beginning played out by the first actor, but with a different response from the second actor: passive, aggressive, and assertive.

For example: a boy beats his girlfriend. Her passive response is to accept it; her aggressive response is to pour boiling water on him; and her assertive response is to duck out of the way, shout 'NO!', and leave. Use an example suitable for your peer group.

6. After each role play, ask:

'Was the behaviour of the first person (e.g. the boy) passive, aggressive, or assertive?'

'How did that person feel?'

'Was the behaviour of the second person (e.g. the girl) passive, aggressive, or assertive?'

'How did that person feel?'

7. When you have talked about all the behaviours, ask:

'Which type of behaviour do you think is best, and for what reasons?'

'Are there any situations where aggressive or passive behaviour may be the safest response?'

8. In groups of three, ask people to share examples of a time when they behaved in an aggressive way, a passive way, or an assertive way. Ask: 'What happened next?'

9. Ask each small group to create a role play about a challenging situation in which one person was aggressive or passive. Then replay the story to show an assertive ending.

10. If you have time, ask one or two groups to present their assertive response as a role play.

 EXERCISE 6.2 HOW ASSERTIVE AM I?

AIM: To identify the kinds of assertive behaviour we practise and which we could do more often.

DESCRIPTION: Participants raise their arms to indicate how often they practise assertive behaviours.

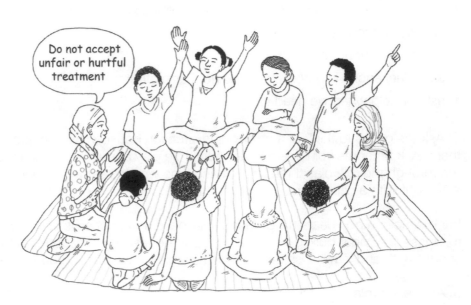

Directions

1. Ask participants to get into groups of three, and to chat for five minutes about the virtue of assertiveness. They can describe how they have seen it in others, how a public figure practises it, or how they practise it themselves.

2. Explain: 'We're going to find out how assertive we think we are. I'm going to read out some examples of assertive behaviour. I'll ask you to close your eyes and show me with your hands how often you practise each behaviour. Raise two hands if you do it most of the time, one hand if you do it some of the time, and keep your hands down if you only do it rarely. I want you to close your eyes so you can answer honestly, and without others seeing your answer.'

3. Say: 'Now please close your eyes', and read out the list in Box 6.a. Once you have asked these questions, you may add more behaviours from the list in Exercise 6.1, depending on which ones are most relevant to the group. Make a note in your Facilitator's Journal of how many hands are raised for each question. You may want to add comments.

Box 6.a Examples of assertive behaviour

How often do you:

- share your own ideas and feelings?
- tactfully tell others what you really think and feel?
- choose not to allow others to lead you into trouble?
- ask for what you want and need?
- not accept unfair or hurtful treatment?
- expect respect at all times?

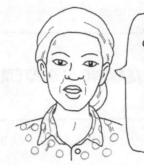

Aha, we find this difficult. In the next exercise we will practise ways of being assertive when we are treated unfairly

---

4. Share the results with the group: which behaviour got the highest score, and which behaviour had lower scores? The low scores show us where we can grow our virtue of assertiveness.

5. Invite people to get into groups of three, and give each group a challenging situation to role play with an assertive response. Make up situations which call for the type of assertive behaviour for which participants had a low score, or use the situations in Box 6.2. If you have time, invite each group to act out their best assertive response to the rest of the peer group.

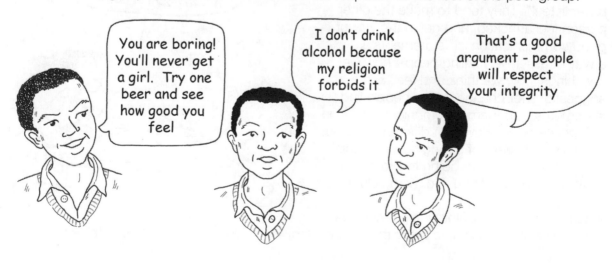

You are boring! You'll never get a girl. Try one beer and see how good you feel

I don't drink alcohol because my religion forbids it

That's a good argument - people will respect your integrity

Box 6.b Challenging situations

For children
How could you respond assertively if:

- you start to feel inferior around some popular children?

- an aggressive person starts to bully you?

- your teacher asks for your opinions about a story that you haven't read?

- a friend asks you to go somewhere you don't really want to go?

- a group tries to convince you to do something harmful?

- a stranger invites you to ride in his car?

For caregivers
How could you respond assertively if:

- your child has been rude and disrespectful to you?

- you fear that your child is drinking alcohol?

- a parent shouts at you, saying your child has hurt their child?

- you hear some children harassing a child, saying their parent died of AIDS?

- you have a partner who is aggressive towards your child?

 ## EXERCISE 6.3 MAKING 'I' STATEMENTS

AIM: To practise saying what we see, feel, want, prefer, or suggest through 'I' statements.

DESCRIPTION: The facilitator explains the four steps involved in using 'I' statements, and participants practise using them in different situations.

Directions

1. Explain: 'When we are upset we may use aggressive "you" statements, for example, "You always expect the worst of me!" or "You never listen!". They tend to make the other person feel attacked, and get in the way of good communication. "I" statements are a way of assertively telling people how we see things, how we think and feel, and our suggestions for change. Many people find "I" statements help them communicate in a kind and positive way. However, different cultures have different ways of saying how they think and feel. Today we are going to practise "I" statements to see if you find them helpful.'

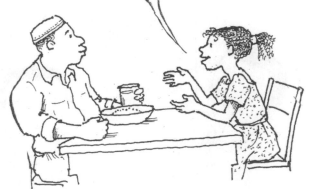

2. Explain the steps of the 'I' statement and read or act out an example using the story of Dabwiso in Box 6.c or ideas from Table 6.1.

Step 1: Explain the situation and your feelings about it. Be careful not to blame the other person. Just say how you feel and the reasons that make you feel that way.

Step 2: Say what you would like to happen.

Step 3: Ask what the other person feels about what you have said.

Step 4: If appropriate, agree on what to do. Not every conversation requires a resolution.

Box 6.c An example of assertive behaviour using an 'I' statement: Dabwiso's story[19]

Dabwiso has HIV and students at his school find out. They tease him and refuse to sit next to him.

Step 1: Explain how you feel about a situation and why you feel that way
'When you tease me and refuse to sit next to me, I feel very sad and angry because we are all human beings who might have HIV. I do not deserve to be treated this way.'

'Perhaps you are afraid of getting HIV, but I can't give it to you by sitting near you, or playing sport or eating together.'

Step 2: Say what you would like to happen
'I would like you to understand that HIV is just a health problem, like diabetes. And to see who I am, a human who would like to be friends.'

Step 3: Ask how the other people feel about what you have said
'What do you feel about this?'

Step 4: Reach an agreement on what to do next (if appropriate)
'I would feel happy if we could talk more about HIV and how to support all our classmates who have health problems.'

Table 6.1 Examples of 'You' and 'I' statements

'You' statement	'I' statement
Younger children *Boy to boy:* You are always taking my toy car over to the big boys. Give it back or I'll take your ball.	When you take my toy car over to the big boys, I feel worried that they might keep it or break it. I would like us to play with it together here. What do you say?
Older children *Child to caregiver:* You are always shouting at me so now I am shouting back!	When you shout at me I feel anxious because you are angry, and then sometimes I feel angry too. I would like us to speak more calmly and to listen to each other. How do you feel about that?
Child to caregiver: You are so ignorant, making me do the farming when I have homework to do!	When I don't have time to do my homework, I worry that I will fail my exams and not get a good job to help you. I would be happy if we could talk about how we can best support each other.

'You' statement	'I' statement
Caregivers *Caregiver to orphan:* All you do is fight or sit around moping! I'll throw you out to live with the street children if you don't behave better!	I feel sad when you fight and don't go to school. I think you are missing your mum. Come and sit with me and let's talk about the good times you had together. Would you like to do that?
Caregiver to child: You are so lazy, you sit around with your books while the farm grows weeds. If you don't work harder, I'll throw you out!	I'm worried that we won't grow enough food for the family this year. I would like us to talk about how we as a family can meet all our needs.

3. In groups of four, ask people to agree on a challenging situation that they want to solve, as a role play, using the four 'I' statement steps.

4. Read out each step, one by one, and ask the group to discuss what to say for their situation.

5. Bring the whole group together and ask each group to act out how they used this way of being strong. You might ask:

'What do you think about this way of behaving?'

'What do you like or not like about it?'

'Do you ever use it, and do you think you will?'

 EXERCISE 6.4 PRACTISING WAYS OF STAYING ASSERTIVE

AIM: To practise ways of staying assertive.

DESCRIPTION: Participants act out role plays to rehearse resisting pressure from others.

Directions

1. Explain that people often try to stop others from being assertive.

Ask: 'How might someone try to stop you from being strong and assertive?'

Add examples from Table 6.2 if needed.

2. Ask: 'Why do people want to stop us being assertive?'

3. Explain that, sometimes, having our assertiveness challenged can be useful, for example, if I were to insist my bicycle was safe to ride when it had no brakes! But often a challenge to our assertiveness is not for our good. Then we need to find ways to stay assertive, rather than giving in (being passive) or becoming aggressive.

Ask: 'How can we stay assertive?' Add examples from Table 6.2 if needed.

Table 6.2 Examples of ways of staying assertive

Ways that others try to undermine assertive behaviour	Ways of staying assertive
They deny that there is a problem – you are imagining it.	Repeat the 'I' statement, saying that you experience this as a problem. Ask them to imagine that something similar has happened to them – how would they feel?
They try to make you feel small for feeling that there is a problem.	Justify your feelings and ask them to imagine themselves in a similar situation.
They argue with your point of view.	Find something you can both agree on, a compromise. If this is not possible, finish the conversation by suggesting that you discuss it another time.
They don't respond to what you have said but attack you about something different.	Bring the conversation back to your concern, repeat the 'I' statement.
They give you false information to persuade you to change your mind.	Tell them the correct information.
They try to scare you by responding aggressively or with a threat.	If they become aggressive, leave.
They try to distract you by talking about something else.	Repeat how you feel and what you want to happen. Don't let yourself be distracted.

4. Ask the group to think of a situation relevant to them, in which one person tries to persuade another person to do something they don't want to do. Invite two people to role play the situation. Ask the rest of the group to watch and identify the methods each actor is using to get their way.

5. When the person persuading has run out of ideas, or the person refusing has given in, invite a new person to come from the group and try acting.

6. Continue changing the actors until everyone has run out of ideas.

7. Ask: 'Which methods did the persuaders use to make the other person agree?'

'Which methods did the person refusing use to resist?'

'Which methods worked well?'

8. Ask the participants to re-run the small-group role play they created at point 9 in Exercise 6.1. Using only the assertive response from that role play, they should practise what to do when the other actor tries to undermine their assertive response. If you have time, have one person persuading, one person refusing, and the third person assessing which strategies work best. Take it in turns to play each of the roles with a different situation.

9. Bring the peer group back together and ask: 'What did you learn from this activity? How might you use it?'

SESSION 7   ALL ABOUT VIRTUES

Purpose: To understand the meaning of virtues and cultivate them; to awaken the virtues that already exist in all of us; to learn to speak the language of virtues.[20]

Contents	Materials required	Time required
Opening circle (see p.13)		15 mins
7.1 Explanation of virtues	Virtues poster	30 mins
7.2 Virtues fruit salad		20 mins
7.3 Acknowledging virtues		40 mins
7.4 Using the language of virtues to guide us		40 mins
7.5 Using the language of virtues to correct ourselves	Flipcharts (Tables 7.4 and 7.5)	40 mins
7.6 Using language to lift us up		20 mins
Closing circle (see p.14)		15 mins
7.7 *Homework*: Inspirational walk		

About 4 hrs

  EXERCISE 7.1 EXPLANATION OF VIRTUES

AIMS: To introduce this session by explaining the meaning of virtues and looking at examples from the virtues poster.

DESCRIPTION: The facilitator explains the meaning of virtues and participants choose examples from the virtues poster.

Directions

1. Explain to participants that most of us want to use our strengths to make the world a better place, and to grow up as good people.

2. Stick the virtues poster (see Annex) on the wall and invite participants to look at it.

Ask: 'What is a virtue?' If needed, add information from Box 7.a.

Box 7.a Information for facilitators

Values are what we value and care about. They can be anything, and they can change. For example, we may value looking pretty, getting rich, having many children, becoming powerful, or being loved. Values vary between people, and across cultures and time.

Virtues are mainly shared by all cultures and religions, and are the same throughout our lives. Virtues are: the strengths in our hearts; the best aspects of our characters; the things that are kind and helpful, brave and fair about us; our power and energy for good.

---

3. Ask each participant in turn to read out one of the virtues on the poster and to give an example.

Explain: 'We're going to learn about virtues because they can help us develop our characters and how well we interact with others. Thinking about virtues is useful for everyone. We can learn and improve through our day-to-day activities. We find our best virtues in ourselves when we are "on our hub" (see Exercise 2.8).

'In fact, we are all going to work together with our virtues throughout the rest of this workshop. A few exercises ask us to discuss a specific virtue. In most sessions, though, we get to choose which virtue we wish to focus on during that session. At the end of the workshop you will each receive your own pack of virtues cards to take home with you.'

4. Say: 'Today we will learn more about our virtues and how we can support one another in practising them. But first we are going to play a game.'

 ## EXERCISE 7.2 VIRTUES FRUIT SALAD

AIMS: To teach the language of virtues, using whole body movement and connecting with people's life experiences.

DESCRIPTION: A high-energy game where participants position themselves in a circle, identify virtues that they have practised today, and change places. If they cannot find an empty place in the circle to move to, they become the leader in the middle.

GROUPS: Play either with caregivers and children together for high energy, or in peer groups.

Directions

1. Arrange chairs, mats, or other objects in a circle, with one for each person except the facilitator. You can also play the game standing up if you use something to mark each person's space.

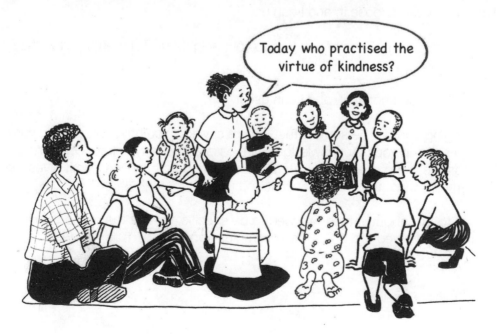

> Today who practised the virtue of kindness?

2. Explain the rules. Say: 'One person stands in the middle of the circle. They say a virtue they have practised today [or yesterday if this is a morning session], and how they practised it. Then they think of another virtue and ask who has practised it today/yesterday. If you have, you must leave your place and move to a different, empty place in the circle. If you have not, be honest and stay in your place. The person who cannot find another empty place becomes the next leader.'

3. Start as the leader, saying: 'Today I practised the virtue of (e.g. helpfulness), when I (e.g. helped my sister with her shopping).'

Then think of another virtue, and say: 'Who has practised the virtue of [...] today?' When others move, slip into an empty space. If participants get stuck trying to think of a virtue they have practised, remind them to look at the virtues poster for ideas.

4. The game continues until everyone has moved and laughed.

 ## EXERCISE 7.3 ACKNOWLEDGING VIRTUES

AIM: To learn how to encourage and reinforce virtues when we see them, and so build authentic self-esteem.

DESCRIPTION: Participants are given an explanation of the benefits of acknowledging virtues, and practise doing this.

Directions

1. Explain to participants: 'When you see a person showing or practising a virtue, it is good to acknowledge it out loud. This is like the ability-spotting that we have already been practising. It awakens the person's awareness that they have this virtue, that acting on it is a choice, and that they can choose to practise it in other situations. We can all say:

'I have this virtue. I can choose it, and I can use it.'

'Let's role play this quickly. Each of you turn to your neighbour. Tell them a virtue they have. Then they can reply:

'I have this virtue. I can choose it, and I can use it.'

'By acknowledging another person's virtue, we are saying, "You have this power, this capacity, and strength; I see it in you". Acknowledging virtues is particularly helpful when the person showing it finds the virtue challenging to practise. Hearing that they can do it gives them a boost, and reminds them they can choose it and use it.'

2. Explain that to talk about virtues we need to be specific, so that the person understands what they did that showed the virtue. Use examples from Table 7.1 as needed.

Table 7.1 Examples of general and specific comments on virtues

General comment	Specific comment
You're such a kind boy.	I saw you behaving in a kind way when you invited the new boy to sit next to you.
Good girl, you are reading for longer.	Annie, I see you are behaving purposefully. You have been reading for 10 minutes and really concentrating.
You're a nice auntie.	You made me feel so loved when I was crying, and you held me, and we talked about my mum.

3. Say: 'Get into pairs and take turns to acknowledge, in a specific way, how your partner has practised a virtue.

'Each partner can respond out loud: "I have [...] in me, I can choose it and use it."'

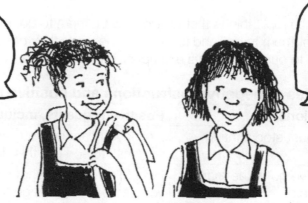

4. Then, speaking to the whole group again, say: 'Acknowledging a virtue supports us all. For instance, if we talk about peacefulness with our friends or our children, we can also benefit from our own sense of peacefulness.'

5. Explain that we are now going to practise acknowledging a particular virtue throughout the session. Ask one participant to choose a virtue from the poster to practise during the rest of this session.

6. Write the virtue up on flipchart paper and check that everyone understands what the virtue means.

7. Explain that every time anyone sees someone else using that virtue, they should tell them, and write the person's name next to the virtue on the flipchart.

Say: 'Everyone has virtues; we just need to look for them inside us, then shine a light on them, and use them. They can be especially useful when we are feeling stuck about something.'

EXERCISE 7.4 USING THE LANGUAGE OF VIRTUES TO GUIDE US

AIMS: To learn how to use the language of virtues to focus and guide behaviour.

DESCRIPTION: An explanation of using virtues as guidance, followed by examples and practice.

Directions

1. Explain that we can use the language of virtues to *guide* behaviour *before* any action takes place.

2. Say: 'We often tell people things that we *don't* want them to do, but it is more effective to say what we *do* want them to do, and to mention the virtue they need to do it. This also works when we are talking to ourselves.' Give examples from Table 7.2 as appropriate.

Table 7.2 Examples of negative instructions and positive requests

Negative instructions	Positive requests, including the virtue needed
You two children must stop fighting now!	I think you can use your virtues of *peacefulness* and *kindness* to sort out this disagreement between you.
Don't moan when we go to the market like you did last week.	I would love you to show me how *patient* and *strong* you can be when we go to the market.
Auntie, I don't want you to cook beans, I don't like them.	Auntie, I love your *thoughtfulness* when you cook eggs with bread for me.
I must make sure David doesn't find out that I broke his watch.	I will use *courage* and *honesty* to explain to David that I accidentally broke his watch.
I must stop losing my temper with the children.	I will try to be *peaceful* and *kind* when dealing the children. I will try to stay on my hub!

3. Explain that we can also use virtues to guide how we prepare to behave. For example, 'How can we *support* Mary after her mother's funeral today?'

Another strategy is to use virtues to thank others, and so guide how they behave with us in the future. For example, 'Auntie, I love it when you show *appreciation* through smiling at me and thanking me for helping you.'

4. In pairs, invite participants to create a role play, with one person saying what they don't want to the other, and then changing this to say what they do want, linked to a virtue. Take it in turns.

Ask: 'How did you feel? Which behaviour do you think would be more effective?'

5. Now ask participants to use the language of virtues in a role play to help prepare how to behave. For example, a caregiver might say to a child:

'At the clinic today, what will help you to be *patient* while waiting to be seen by the doctor?'

6. Explain that we can also ask others for their commitment to a virtue, for example, 'Who among us is ready to show *courage* and be *kind* to that boy who is getting bullied?'

Invite a few participants to ask for a suitable commitment from the group. For example, 'Please raise your hand to show you are ready to be *considerate*.'

 ## EXERCISE 7.5 USING THE LANGUAGE OF VIRTUES TO CORRECT OURSELVES

AIMS: To learn how to use virtues to stop misbehaviour, restore justice, and build conscience.

DESCRIPTION: Explanations of using virtues to correct behaviour, and the benefits of this with examples. Practice in using the language of virtues to correct someone rather than shaming them.

Directions

1. Explain to participants that we can also call on virtues when behaviour is out of line, or when improvement is needed. They can be used to *correct* behaviour *after* an action has happened that needs correcting. The aim is not to shame the person, but to call on the person's conscience and give them a moral reason to behave well. As before, you need to use specific language to have the best effect.

For example, 'How could the two of you have worked this out *peacefully*, instead of fighting?'

'When you correct behaviour by focussing on a virtue, you are acting *assertively*, not aggressively. You are modelling *justice*.

2. Act out the examples in Table 7.3, asking participants after each response: 'How would you describe that response? Does it educate the child?'

Table 7.3 Examples of aggressive and assertive ways of correcting behaviour

Aggressive, non-specific, shaming	Assertive, specific, using virtues
For children: 'I hate you, you're such a mean sister! No wonder you don't have any friends.'	'I felt hurt today when you said that mean thing about me. But you behaved *kindly* when you spoke up for Rabia. I wish you could show more *friendliness* to me.'
For caregivers: 'James, you're such a bully. I'm ashamed to be your relative!'	'James, you need to behave *peacefully*. How can you be a *friend* to other children even when you feel angry? How would a friend act? What kind of person do you really want to be with others?'

Note: Using the language of virtues to correct doesn't mean that the correction always happens! But it does give the person a clear and positive message.

3. Ask participants to imagine that a child is misbehaving; maybe she is refusing to share some food with a younger brother. Invite a few people to say what they would say to the child.

They might say: 'You're unkind and greedy. I'm going to tell your stepfather. You can't treat your brother that way.'

Ask: 'How would you describe this response? Does it educate the child?'

You might point out that this response is name-calling, labelling, shaming, and non-specific. It fails to educate.

A more specific response might be: 'Martha, you need to behave *generously*. How can you show compassion to your brother, even when you feel hungry too? How would a loving sister act? What kind of sister do you want to be?'

4. In the group, invite a few participants to role play a situation where behaviour needs correcting. The children's groups should think of what a child would typically say to other children, and the caregivers' groups what a caregiver would typically say.

Ask: 'How would you describe this response? Is it educative?'

5. Now invite a different group to role play the same situation, but using the language of virtues.

6. Explain: 'We are replacing shaming with naming virtues. When we fill our home, school or group with encouraging words, such as "compassionate", "courageous", "kind", and "self-disciplined", we are inviting and reinforcing those behaviours. We are building our characters and giving meaning to our behaviour.'

7. Ask participants to get into groups of three to do a role play.

For children. Say: 'Think of a situation in which there are two children, one who is behaving badly. Do a role play showing the bad behaviour, and how the other child would typically respond. The third one of you is the observer.'

Point to the flipchart and read out each character listed, and the questions linked to that character or observer. Explain that, after each role play, the characters in each group of three will answer the question related to their role while the others listen. (For younger children, it may work better to wait until groups have finished their role play, and then read out the questions for each character one by one, and share the answer with the whole group.)

Table 7.4 Flipchart showing characters and questions for children's role play

Character who answers the questions	Questions
1. The child whose behaviour needed correcting	How did you feel? What will you do?
2. The child who responded	How did you feel? What will you do?
3. The observer	How would you describe this interaction? Was it educative?

Now think about how the responding child could name virtues in their response. Run the role play again, using the language of virtues, and ask the same questions to each child.

Do the exercise twice more, using different situations, so that each child gets to play each role.

For caregivers. Say: 'Think of a situation in which your child is behaving badly. Do a role play with one person acting as the child, and the other as the caregiver, showing how you would typically respond. The third one of you is the observer.' Before the groups begin, explain the flipchart in table 7.5 and read out the questions. Explain that, after each role play, the characters in each group of three will answer the question related to their role while the others listen.

Table 7.5 Flipchart showing characters and questions for caregivers' role play

Character who answers the questions	Questions
1. The 'child'	How did you feel? What will you do?
2. The caregiver	How did you feel? What do you think your child will do?
3. The observer	How would you describe this interaction? Was it educative?

Now discuss how the caregiver could name virtues in their response. Run the role play again using the language of virtues and ask the same questions to each character.

Do the exercise twice more, using different situations, so that each caregiver gets to play each role.

8. Summarize by saying it is important that we specifically name the *action* that needs correcting, rather than naming the *whole person* as wrong.

Say: 'It does not help any of us to be shamed, blamed, or called names for making a mistake. We need to be held accountable, to be held responsible, and enabled to make amends and to focus on the virtue we were forgetting to practise. If the behaviour continues after the virtue has been named, we need to continue to support the person in practising the virtue, making amends, and restoring the situation to one of justice and peace. We will look more at discipline in Session 9.'

 EXERCISE 7.6 USING LANGUAGE TO LIFT US UP

AIMS: To create awareness of the power of our language to hurt or help us, to put each other down, or lift each other up. To practise using language to lift each other up.

DESCRIPTION: Participants are given an explanation of ways that we can use language to hurt or help people, and practise using language to lift each other up.

Directions

1. Explain about the power of words, and write the heading 'From Shaming to Naming' on a flipchart or chalkboard. Write and/or say: 'Sticks or stones may break my bones and words can break my spirit.'

2. Ask participants, in pairs, to think of a disrespectful name or a 'put down' that they have heard said to people like them (they or someone else might have said it).

3. Ask: 'Why might a person call someone that name, or say what they said?'

'How might the person who said it feel?'

'How might the other person feel?'

'What might the person have said instead to lift up the other person and make them feel included?'

4. If you have time, invite a few people in turn to call out their 'put downs', and then call out a corresponding virtue instead.

5. Ask for a commitment: 'How would our group, family, or school be different if we used virtues to lift each other up, rather than put downs, which hurt or embarrass us?'

6. Say: 'We all have seeds of every virtue inside us. How do we sow and water these seeds inside our friends? Remember the hub? Let us all support one another in nurturing and watering our virtues, so that they grow strong.'

Closing circle

Ask everyone to think of one small act of kindness that they would like to do for someone they like and feel close to, before the next session. It can be anything unexpected that the person would feel surprised and pleased by. They don't have to tell the group what it is unless they want to – this is their own secret. Just ask them to think of it as they go about their day, and to make sure they do it before the next session.

 EXERCISE 7.7 HOMEWORK: INSPIRATIONAL WALK

AIMS: To learn that we are all part of the living world, and that we can learn virtues from our planet's environment and all the living things in it.

DESCRIPTION: Participants go for a walk and find a living object to focus deeply on. They ask it questions and draw or write about it.

Directions

1. Ask participants, before the next session, to go for a walk alone or with a friend around their house or community. Say: 'Identify an object or living thing, such as a flower, insect, goat, leaf, or the sky, and focus your attention deeply on it. You might wish to write about it, draw it, or make up a poem.'

Ask participants to imagine asking the object/living thing the following questions to guide their thoughts: 'What are you saying to me? What lessons do you offer? What is your gift for me? What virtues do you show me?'

You might give participants this example: 'If you focus on ants, you might write a short poem about the virtues of *diligence* and *unity* and how they help you in your life at the moment.'

2. Invite participants to share their drawing, words, or thoughts informally before the next session, or at the start of the next session.

Ask: 'How did you feel doing this exercise? What did you learn?'

SESSION 8 THE POWER OF LOVE

Purpose: To learn about and practise the virtues of love, respect, and cooperation.

Contents	Materials required	Time required
Opening circle (see p.13)		15 mins
8.1 Cultivating a 'yes' state of mind		20 mins
8.2 What is love?		30 mins
8.3 The cooperating donkeys		30 mins
8.4 Treating each other with respect		30 mins
8.5 The singing fish		50 mins
8.6 The power of gifts	enough small gifts (e.g. flowers, fruits, sweets, crayons) for each participant to receive one	20 mins
Closing circle (see p.14)		15 mins

About 3.5 hrs

Box 8.a Information for facilitators

A strong loving relationship between caregivers and children is the most important factor in children developing as people with mental and social wellbeing. When caregivers and children have this relationship, they are better able to cope with challenges in life, to dream of the future, to stay on their hubs, and to use mindsight to understand themselves and others.

 ### EXERCISE 8.1 CULTIVATING A 'YES' STATE OF MIND

AIM: To support children and caregivers in creating an *open receptive* state of mind, rather than a *closed reactive* one, in order to be more receptive to relationships.

DESCRIPTION: Facilitator says 'no' and 'yes' several times, and people share how each word makes them feel. In pairs, participants take turns to say 'no' to each other in the same way seven times, and then to say 'yes' seven times. They share their experience of this.

Directions[21]

1. In separate peer groups, invite one or two people to share their small act of kindness towards someone they feel close to if they wish.

2. Explain that you're going to repeat a word several times, and that you want people just to notice what it feels like in their bodies.

3. Say 'no' firmly and harshly, seven times, with about two seconds between each 'no'. Pause. Then say 'yes' seven times, in a clear but gentler voice.

4. Invite participants to share how they felt in their bodies at hearing the 'no' and the 'yes'.

5. Ask participants to pair up and take it in turns to say 'no' to each other, as the facilitator did, and then to say 'yes' to each other.

6. Invite participants to share how they felt in their bodies at saying the 'no' and the 'yes'.

7. Explain that when we hear strongly negative words, we *react* by going into 'flight, fight, freeze, or appease' mode, using our lower brain. This makes it almost impossible to connect in an open, listening, and caring way with another person.

When we hear positive words, like 'yes', we become *receptive*. The upper part of the brain becomes active, and we have positive feelings, relax, and become more open to connecting with people.

 ## EXERCISE 8.2 WHAT IS LOVE?

AIMS: To nurture relationships based on love and a positive and stable emotional bond between children and caregivers.

GROUPS: Caregivers, children aged 9–14, and children aged 5–8, in separate groups first, and then together.

DESCRIPTION: Participants think of words for love between caregivers and children, and make a mind map. They identify ways in which caregivers and children show love to each other.

Box 8.b Information for facilitators

What is love?[22]

- Love is a special feeling that fills your heart.
- Love is putting yourself in someone else's shoes and caring about what they feel.
- Love is accepting and loving people just as they are, and caring about them enough to help them to do better.
- Loving helps others to feel important and happy, and become gentler and kinder.
- Sharing is a way of showing love. Share your belongings, your time, and yourself.
- You show love in a smile, a pleasant way of speaking, a thoughtful act, or a hug.
- Love is treating people as you would like them to treat you: with care and respect.
- Love is treating people with special care and kindness because they mean so much to you.

In this exercise, keep a positive focus on ways that caregivers and children show love or could show love to each other. Don't use the negative approach of asking about what caregivers do that shows a lack of love. We want to avoid blame and negative feelings among the participants.

Directions

1. Working with separate peer groups, ask the participants to think of as many words for love as they can between a caregiver and a child, and make them into a mind map.

2. *For caregivers*. Ask: 'What do you do to show your child that you love them? What does your child do to show that he or she loves you?'

For children. Ask: 'What do you do to show your caregiver that you love them? What does your caregiver do to show you that they love you?'

3. Add their answers to the mind map.

4. Bring all the peer groups together to share the mind maps. Ask: 'What is the same and what is different when comparing the caregivers' and children's mind maps?'

5. Ask: 'What other things would you like your caregiver or child to do to show that they love you, to strengthen your love?'

6. Keep the mind maps for Session 20: 'Relationships, love and sexuality'.

 ## EXERCISE 8.3 THE COOPERATING DONKEYS

AIMS: To help participants understand how useful the virtue of cooperation is in creating harmony and achieving goals.

DESCRIPTION: Participants engage in a role play, followed by a discussion.

Directions

1. Working with separate peer groups, invite two members of the group to act out the following scenario.

Say: 'Imagine that you are two donkeys' (or any other animal that fits the community, such as goats). Tie the two participants together around the waist with a short piece of rope.

Put out or draw some grass or leaves, one pile in each corner of the workshop space. Say: 'Try to go to the pile of grass nearest to you.' Explain that they should pull away from each other, but get no nearer to the grass.

Say: 'Imagine you are now frustrated, tired, and hungry. You sit down, and wonder what to do next.'

2. Ask: 'What advice would you give to the donkeys?' Invite participants to suggest answers to the donkeys, who act out their suggestions.

3. Agree on which suggestion works best and the reasons for this.

4. Ask participants: 'What virtues are being shown in this story? What have we learned from the story and how can we use it in our own lives?'

Say: 'Cooperation is working together for the benefit of everyone. Working together, we can make our community a peaceful and happy one. We can help each other, share the load, and do things that cannot be done alone.'

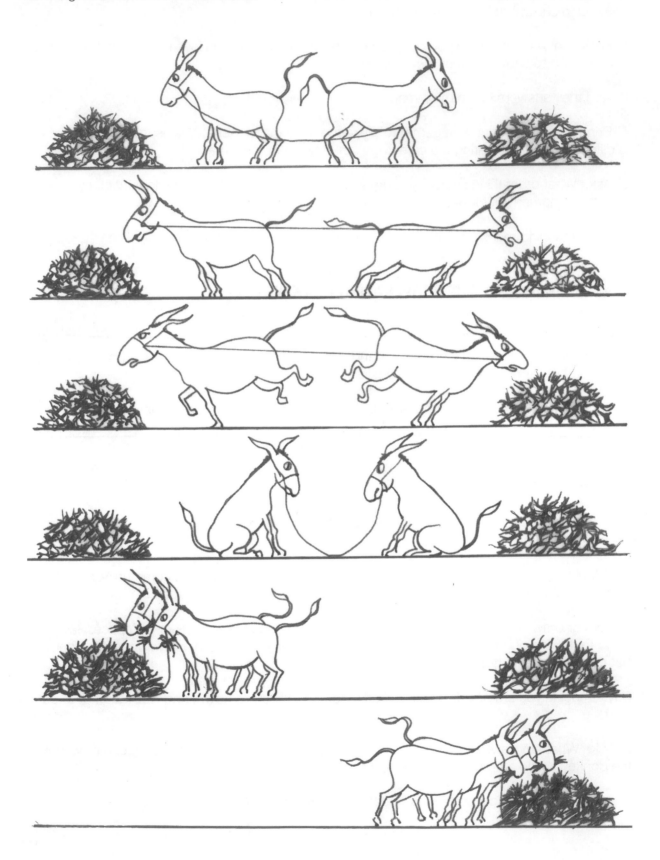

EXERCISE 8.4 TREATING EACH OTHER WITH RESPECT

AIM: To increase respect between caregivers and children.

DESCRIPTION: Participants prepare role plays, followed by a question and answer session and group discussion.

Directions

1. In separate peer groups, explain that we are going to talk about how we act on our virtues. Ask: 'What do we mean by the virtue of "respect"?'

Invite participants to give an explanation and a few examples of a child showing respect to an adult, and an adult showing respect to a child. If necessary, say: 'Respect is an attitude of caring about all people, whatever their age, gender, and health issues, and treating them with dignity. Respect is also valuing ourselves and others. We show respect by speaking and acting with courtesy. When we are respectful, we treat others as we would like to be treated ourselves.'

2. Ask participants to suggest a common interaction between a child and caregiver, for example, asking the child to do a task, or something related to school, friends, or appearance.

3. Divide the participants into two groups and ask them to prepare role plays:

Group 1. Prepare a role play of the chosen scenario which shows little respect and kindness between the caretaker and child. Ask the players to make it realistic.

Group 2. Prepare a role play of the chosen scenario which shows respect and kindness between the caregiver and child. Again, ask the players to make it realistic.

4. Invite Group 1 to perform their role play.

Ask: 'What was good about the interaction between the caregiver and the child? What didn't you like about their interaction?'

'What virtues did the caregiver show? What virtues did the child show? Which virtues would you like to have seen more of?'

'What was the outcome of the interaction?'

5. Ask Group 2 to perform their role play, and then ask the same questions.

6. After participants have answered the questions about both scenarios, ask: 'Which interaction did you prefer? What are your reasons? Why does one of them have a better outcome? How can we help each other respect one another?'

If there is time, invite Group 1 to do their role play again, this time showing a more respectful process.

EXERCISE 8.5 THE SINGING FISH

AIMS: To think about how caregivers may show less love to some of their children than others, and how children may show less love to some children in the household than others. To think about the causes and consequences of this, and how we can show love to all the children in the house equally.

DESCRIPTION: Participants listen to a story, then discuss it in groups. The story in Box 8c comes from Malawi. You could use a different story if you prefer.

Directions[23]

1. Invite the three peer groups to sit in a circle.

2. Read out the story in Box 8.c. Ask everyone to respond with a double-beat clap every time you pause and close your eyes.

Box 8.c The story of the singing fish

Once upon a time there was a 10-year-old girl named Tina, who was an orphan. Her uncle Zuze, who was her father's brother, took her into his home. But Zuze, who was a poor fisherman, did not allow anyone to eat in the home when he was away.
(Facilitator pauses and closes eyes. Participants double-clap here)

Now, Zuze's wife Namoyo was very different from her husband. She would go out and search for maize and sweet potatoes left over from harvesting. She would bring them home and prepare food for Tina and her own two children, making sure they had finished eating before Zuze came home. When Zuze returned, he would eat his fill before giving small amounts to Tina and her two cousins. But he always gave Tina less than he gave to his own two children. He expected Tina to work all day long in the house and garden while her cousins went to school.
(Participants double-clap here)

One day, as Zuze was fishing, he caught an extraordinary-looking fish. It was alive and kept looking at him with tears in its eyes. He was burning with curiosity, so he started talking to it: 'Why are you looking at me like that? You know I work hard to feed my family.'
(Participants double-clap here)

'I am Dimba, your brother.' Zuze was shocked. He thought he heard the fish sing! Someone must be playing tricks on him. But the fish kept singing: 'I have heard the cries of my daughter, Tina, whom you treat as a slave, Zuze. She deserves love and respect, as every child does. How could you treat our daughter like that?'

Zuze thought to himself: 'I must be strong. I'm not treating that girl so badly. Well, maybe I could give her a bit more food, but I must be careful in case my own two children think that I love Tina more than them.'
(Participants double-clap here)

But the fish continued: 'Why not love all three children equally, Zuze? Why not treat Tina as your own child? She has no one else but you in the world, and if you give love you receive love.'

Zuze was thinking. After all, Tina was part of his family now. His wife Namoyo seemed to like her, and so did his own children. So why not treat her the same? 'Dimba,' he called, 'you are right. I am really sorry for not being a loving father to Tina. Please forgive me.'

The extraordinary fish jumped back into the water, splashing Zuze as he did so, and reminding Zuze how he and his brother Dimba used to play with water when they were young. He started to smile and his chest seemed to swell with joy. He had not felt like this since before Dimba and his wife died. He decided that he didn't need to fish anymore today. He would go home to his wife and children and ask for their forgiveness, especially Tina's, for his selfish actions. He put his fishing equipment away and started walking home singing a cheerful song. 'Thank you Dimba,' he called out loud. 'I was losing my life, but you have brought me back my life and my family.'
(Participants double-clap here)

3. After reading out the story, give participants a short break to move about and think about it.

4. Divide into peer groups of older children, younger children, and caregivers.

5. With each group, ask participants to summarize what happened in the story, scene by scene.

6. Then start a discussion by asking these questions:

'Who in the story do you feel most empathy with? Why?'

'Can you explain why Zuze behaved in the way that he did towards his family?'

'Why did he give less food to Tina?'

'What did Tina feel when he behaved this way?'

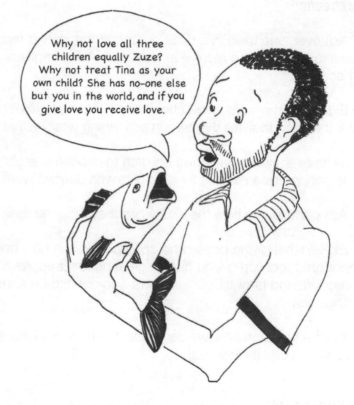

Why not love all three children equally Zuze? Why not treat Tina as your own child? She has no-one else but you in the world, and if you give love you receive love.

'How did Zuze's wife, Namoyo, show her love for her children and for Tina?'

'What did Zuze mean when he thanked the singing fish for giving him back his life and his family?'

For children. 'How do you feel if you think your caregiver shows more love to you or to other children? What would you like them to do?'

For caregivers. 'In our own families, do we sometimes show more love to some of our children than others? If so, what effect does this have on our children? What can we do to share our love more equally?'

7. Bring the caregivers and children together to share their thoughts about showing love equally between children. Ask each peer group to sing a song to show how they love their children or caregivers.

 EXERCISE 8.6 THE POWER OF GIFTS

AIMS: To experience how small gestures of kindness and appreciation can boost self-esteem. To develop ideas of specific actions that caregivers and children can take to strengthen each other's sense of self-esteem.

DESCRIPTION: Caregivers and children give each other gifts and tell each other one thing that they value or love about them.

GROUPS: Children and their caregivers together, sitting next to each other.

Directions[24]

1. Ask everyone to sit in a circle around a mat; on the mat, you have scattered enough small items for everyone to receive at least one. Ask caregivers and their children to sit next to each other.

2. Explain that everyone will choose one item and give it to their child or caregiver. As they hand over the item, they tell the person something positive that they value about them.

3. Invite all the caregivers and children to choose one gift to give each other. The pairs sit down together and give each other their gifts with positive words of appreciation.

4. Ask participants how they felt when they received their gift and encouraging words.

5. Explain that giving praise and appreciation can help boost our self-esteem. This is especially important for children who have a great need for approval and encouragement from their caregivers and family. But caregivers also need to be appreciated and feel good about themselves.

6. Ask for ideas on how we can boost each other's kindness towards ourselves through small, thoughtful acts of kindness.

Closing circle

Ask everyone to think of one small act of kindness that they would like to do for a family member before the next session. It can be anything unexpected that the person would feel surprised and pleased by. They don't have to tell the group what it is unless they want to – this is their own secret. Just ask them to think of it as they go about their day, and to make sure they do it before the next session.

BRINGING OUT THE BEST IN EACH OTHER

Purpose: To explore the virtue of compassion, including self-compassion; the characteristics and effectiveness of punishment and positive discipline; and to practise using positive discipline.

Contents	Materials required	Time required
Opening circle (see p.13)		15 mins
9.1 The virtue of compassion		30 mins
9.2 Punishment and discipline	Sets of punishment and positive discipline slips	40 mins
9.3 Problems with violent punishment		40 mins
9.4 Practising positive discipline		40 mins
9.5 Being a good role model	Sticky labels or safety pins	60 mins
Closing circle (see p.14)		15 mins
Additional exercise (children aged 9–14 years and caregivers only) 9.6 Our three voices		60 mins

About 4.5 hrs

Box 9.a Information for facilitators

We are going to talk about punishment in this session, as well as positive discipline. Physical and verbal punishment cause distress and sometimes severe trauma in children. See Introduction, 'HOW can we safeguard and protect children?', p.10. Discuss with your team how you will handle this, and make sure you are prepared before this session. Watch out for children who are disturbed and ensure that you have a trusted person available to support them. Give information about local services and counsellors who can support children and caregivers.

Preparation

Exercise 9.2. Photocopy Table 9.1 on p.107. Cut up as many rows as you need for your peer group, so that each slip shows one characteristic of either punishment or positive discipline. Mix them up. Make enough sets for each small group to have one.

Exercise 9.4. Use Box 9.h to learn about the Connect and Redirect tool, and to prepare a role play demonstrating a positive discipline scenario with your co-facilitator.

Additional exercise 9.6. If you do this exercise, you'll need to write up the sequence of voices and questions to guide participants through the activity. Also, think of an issue that you criticize yourself for, and use Table 9.3 to prepare to act out the three voices as a demonstration.

EXERCISE 9.1 THE VIRTUE OF COMPASSION

AIMS: To understand the meaning of compassion, and the importance of showing compassion to ourselves as well as others.

DESCRIPTION: Participants are given an explanation of compassion using a picture; and engage in a question and answer session and small group work with mind maps or role play.

 Directions

1. Invite one or two participants to tell the group about their one small act of kindness towards a family member if they wish.

Explain that our virtue for this session is compassion.

Ask: 'Who can tell us what *compassion* means?'

Explain that compassion is having kind feelings towards someone, including ourselves, who is troubled or hurt. It is caring deeply and wanting to help, even when we don't know the person. It is being kind and forgiving to someone who has hurt us. Using mindsight to be aware of what people are feeling and thinking supports us in practising compassion.[25]

Ask: 'What other words can we use to describe compassion?'

2. Direct the relevant peer groups as follows:

Children aged 9–14 years and caregivers. Ask them to form small groups and discuss: 'What are some signs that we are practising compassion successfully?'

Bring everyone together to draw or write the answers on a mind map, with 'compassion' drawn or written in the middle. Encourage participants to join up different parts of the mind map.

Children aged 5–8 years. Ask them to pair up and prepare quick role plays of an action that shows compassion to show to the whole peer group. If necessary, give examples from Box 9.b.

Box 9.b Examples of showing compassion to others
- We notice when someone is hurt or needs a friend.
- We imagine how someone must be feeling.
- We take time to show that we care.
- We ask how someone is and listen carefully.
- We forgive others when they make mistakes.
- We don't judge people when they fail.
- We do some service to help a person or animal in need.

---

3. *All peer groups*. Ask participants to pair up. Give each pair a way of showing compassion for others from Box 9.b and ask them to rephrase the example so it describes showing compassion towards ourselves (self-compassion) also.

For example: 'We notice when someone is hurt or needs a friend' becomes 'We notice when we are hurt and do something to comfort ourselves'.

4. Ask the pairs to discuss:
* What does compassion feel like inside?
* When have you felt compassion towards someone you didn't know?
* When have you felt compassion towards yourself?

5. Bring participants back into one big circle and invite them to share their ideas.

Use the information in Box 9.c to explain more about self-compassion.

Box 9.c Self-compassion[26]

Having compassion for ourselves (self-compassion) is the same as having compassion for others. Here's how to do it:

1. Instead of ignoring our pain, we stop to tell ourselves: 'This is really difficult right now. How can I comfort and care for myself at this time?'

2. We are kind and understanding about our personal failings. We may try to change, for example, to allow us to be in the river of wellbeing, but we do it because we care about ourselves, not because we are unacceptable as we are.

3. We accept that we will encounter frustrations, losses, and mistakes. We open our hearts to this reality instead of fighting against it. Many aspects of ourselves and our lives are not of our choosing, but come from outside factors such as our environment and the behaviour of others, which we have little control over. These are not our fault. However, how we respond to them in future is our responsibility.

4. We use our *mindsight* and *mindfulness* in self-compassion to take a balanced, open, non-judgemental approach to our negative emotions, so that we observe our thoughts and feelings as they are, neither denied nor made bigger. Just like the bug on the hub, we accept all these thoughts and feelings, without being thrown off balance by them. Remember the sky is always blue up high, even if the clouds are blocking our view of it. Goodness and peace remain within us all, even though there are difficult times.

---

6. Finish this exercise by saying: 'today we are going to look at the differences between punishment and discipline. During the session we may feel regret about how we have reacted to misbehaviour from the children in our care in the past. Remember self-compassion! We are all learning here together, and we need to be kind to ourselves and accept our past – and future – mistakes, while thinking about how we can also change things in future.

EXERCISE 9.2 PUNISHMENT AND DISCIPLINE

AIMS: To understand the difference between discipline and punishment.

DESCRIPTION: Participants use a sorting game to understand the characteristics of, and differences between, 'discipline' and 'punishment'. They vote on the best approach and identify benefits of positive discipline.

Directions

1. Explain that in this exercise we are going to look at the difference between punishment and positive discipline, and see the benefits of positive discipline.

Brainstorm the meanings of each term, and the differences between them. If necessary, add information from Box 9.d.

Box 9.d Information for facilitators: Punishment and positive discipline

Punishment aims to control behaviour through imposing *negative consequences for undesirable behaviour*. Punishments include physical pain, negative words, and denying things such as food, treats, or comfort.

Positive discipline aims to *teach ourselves and young people to behave in desirable ways*, both immediately and in the future. It teaches self-control and confidence by supporting us all in developing mindsight. It focusses on understanding reasons for the behaviour, what needs to be learned, what the person is capable of learning, and the best way of teaching it.

---

2. Divide participants into two or three groups, and give each group a set of statements from Table 9.1, including some from the 'punishment' column and some from the 'positive discipline' column:

Children aged 5–8 years. Give each group statements from four rows.

Children aged 9–14 years. Give each group statements from eight rows.

Caregivers. Give each group all the statements. Ask the groups to sort the pieces into two columns: one for statements relating to 'punishment', and one for those relating to 'positive discipline'. You can also give them some blank pieces of paper to add their own contributions.

Note. Do not tell the participants beforehand which column the statements come from. That is for them to decide themselves.

Table 9.1 Characteristics of punishment and positive discipline

Punishment	Positive discipline
Focus is on *what not to do*	Involves being guided on *what to do*
Physically and verbally violent	Physically and verbally loving and kind
Does not involve making amends	Involves making amends
Teaches people to follow rules only if there is a risk of getting caught breaking them	Teaches people to follow rules because the rules are useful and good
Gets people to follow rules because they have been threatened or bribed, or because we said so	Gets people to follow rules because they have discussed and agreed them
Involves denying or rejecting child's feelings	Connects with child by validating their feelings and empathizing
Involves rejecting child and sending them to a place by themselves	Stays with the child and shows we are on their side even when they are misbehaving
Reacts to undesirable behaviour	Encourages good behaviour and rewards efforts
Violates person's right to freedom from abuse and protection from harmful practices	Upholds person's right to safety from harmful practices, and to be part of decisions that affect their lives
Is directed at the person, rather than their behaviour, for example, *you* are very stupid, *you* were wrong	Is directed at the person's behaviour, for example, your *behaviour* was wrong
Controls, shames, ridicules	Provides consistent, firm guidance
Is negative and disrespectful	Is positive and respectful
Involves consequences often unrelated to the misbehaviour	Teaches skills by helping children think about their actions and set boundaries together
Involves immediate consequences	Waits until child is calm and ready to learn
May be inappropriate to the child's developmental stage of life, or individual circumstances and abilities; the child's needs are not taken into consideration	Understands individual abilities, needs, circumstances, and developmental stages
Involves a lot of telling off, which causes people to stop listening to us	Involves listening and understanding
Punishes mistakes without teaching	Teaches using mistakes as learning; offers opportunities to develop the brain and morality

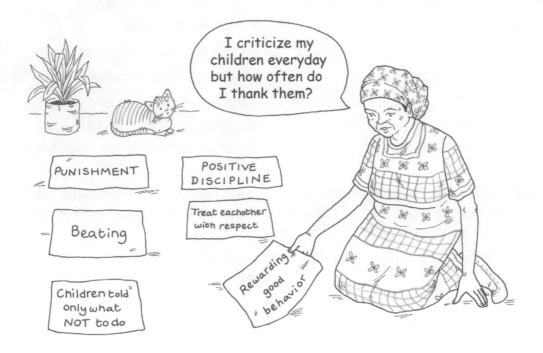

3. When the groups have finished, ask them to move around to look at other groups' columns. Bring everyone together to discuss the reasons for their decisions and any disagreements.

4. Ask participants to vote on which approach they prefer if the aim is to support people in behaving well – punishment or positive discipline? Explain that we will talk about punishment in the next exercise.

5. Ask: 'What are the benefits of positive discipline?' As needed, add information from Box 9.e.

Box 9.e The benefits of positive discipline
- It defuses difficult situations.
- It helps adults build relationships with children, as it communicates more clearly to the children how we love them and that they are safe even as we set boundaries.
- It builds the child's brain by strengthening the connections between the upper and lower brain. The way we interact with our children when they are upset significantly affects how their brains develop and, therefore, the kind of people they become, today and in years to come.
- It supports a goal of parenting that children become more insightful, empathetic, and able to make good decisions on their own.

---

6. Summarize the differences between the two approaches as ways of supporting people in behaving well.

EXERCISE 9.3 PROBLEMS WITH VIOLENT PUNISHMENT

AIMS: To understand the consequences of violent punishment for child and adult. To understand why violent punishment is not effective in helping people learn or change their behaviour. To assert the rights of all people, including children, to be protected from violent punishment.

DESCRIPTION: Participants engage in storytelling and discussion, agree the best approach to teaching virtues, and prepare a 'we statement'.

Directions

1. Explain that we are now going to look in more detail at *violent punishment*, which may be physical, or verbal and emotional.

2. Ask people to call out what *physical* punishments adults use on children. As needed, add information from Box 9.f.

Ask people to call out what *verbal* and *emotional* punishments adults use on children.

Box 9.f Examples of violent punishment

Physical punishments. These include hitting, kicking, shaking, throwing, cutting or burning a child; pinching or hair pulling; forcing a child to stay in an uncomfortable position; locking a child up; forcing a child to undergo excessive physical exercise or forced labour; withholding food, water or shelter; and forcing them to eat foul substances.

Verbal and emotional punishments. These include yelling and shouting; calling a child ugly, stupid, or bad names; saying 'no one loves you' or 'you should die'; making threats; blaming or belittling them; blaming their parents and saying hurtful things about people they love or loved.

All of these punishments violate children's rights as human beings to: respect, dignity, equal protection of the law, and protection from violence.

See Introduction: 'HOW can we safeguard and protect our children?' (p.10) for more information on violence towards children.

---

3. Direct relevant peer groups as follows:

Caregivers. Ask participants to sit in a circle facing outwards or to cover their eyes with a piece of cloth. Ask them to raise their hands and use their fingers to show how many times they have physically punished their child in the past week. If they have not done so, they keep their hands in their laps. Explain that if their answer is greater than 10, they should show all their fingers and thumbs and cross their hands over.

Record the number of fingers each participant shows in your Facilitator's journal, using 0 for someone who has their hands in their lap, and 10+ for someone with all fingers showing and hands crossed over each other.

Children. Ask participants to sit in a circle facing outwards or to cover their eyes with a piece of cloth. Ask them to raise their hands and use their fingers to show how many times they have been physically punished by their caregiver in the past week. If they have not been punished, they keep their hands in their laps. Explain that if their answer is greater than 10, they should show all their fingers and thumbs and cross their hands over.

Record the number of fingers each participant shows in your journal, using 0 for someone who has their hands in their lap, and 10+ for someone with all fingers showing and hands crossed over each other.

4. *Ask each peer group to form smaller groups of four or five, then direct as follows:*

Caregivers. Create a short story about a situation where a caregiver hurts a child when trying to improve their behaviour. The story should stop after the punishment has been given.

Children. Make up a story in which a child like them is hurt by a caregiver who is trying to improve their behaviour. The story should stop after the punishment has been given.

5. Invite one small group to tell their story to the whole peer group and then ask these questions:

'How do you think the caregiver felt? Why did they behave like that?'

'How do you think the child felt? How will they react to the hurt? What will happen to the relationship between them?'

6. Then ask these more general questions:

'Do you think it's OK for one person to hurt another person, to teach or control them? If there are times when it is OK, when is this and with whom?'

'What problems are there with trying to teach or control children by hurting them?'

As needed, add information from Box 9.g.

Box 9.g Consequences of violent punishment[27]

The results of violent punishment are unpredictable but always negative, and may include the following.

For the child's behaviour. The primary goals of discipline, which are changing behaviour and building the brain, are undermined. When children are hurt, they focus attention on the behaviour of the person hurting them, not their own.

The lower brain prepares itself for fight, flight, freeze, or appease. The link to the upper brain becomes disconnected so that the child is unable to connect with the upper brain. This means that all thinking and learning stops. The only learning that takes place is that the child feels the same strong emotions every time, and is unable to learn, or progress in practising virtues.

Punishment does little to help the child behave differently in the future; it results in social rejection and action to avoid pain, so it is not effective at encouraging positive behaviour, but rather encourages hiding and lying.

Punishments may become more severe, to the point when a child is injured, leaves, or fights back.

For the child's wellbeing. There may be physical and sometimes long-lasting impacts of injuries; emotional impacts (e.g. sadness, low self-esteem, anger, shame, guilt, desire for revenge, depression or anxiety), which may lead to aggressive behaviour, bullying, passive behaviour, nightmares and bedwetting, disrespect for authority, drug use, and stealing, for example.

For the relationship between the child and caregiver. There may be loss of trust and love, and creation of resentment and hostility; and undermining of the relationship owing to a focus on negatives rather than developing virtues. There is a conflict between the caregiver as protector from hurt and the caregiver as a source of hurt. The child's brain gets very confused about whether to run away, or go towards the caregiver for safety. This increases a hormone called cortisol, which is toxic to the brain.

For the caregiver. Practising violence conflicts with practising virtues, and often means that we've lost control of our emotions. This can undermine the caregiver's self-esteem and leave them feeling guilty. It spoils their relationship with their children. In some countries it also means they are breaking the law.

For the child when they grow up. Violence teaches the child that the only way to solve conflict is to inflict physical pain, particularly on someone who can't fight back. They are more likely to be violent to others, for example, their spouse and their own children; and are less likely to have developed into a rounded adult with virtues, skills, and emotional and mental wellbeing.

 EXERCISE 9.4 PRACTISING POSITIVE DISCIPLINE

AIMS: To understand the advantages for caregivers and children of using positive discipline. To practise using positive discipline approaches.

DESCRIPTION: Participants are given an explanation and demonstration of positive discipline using the Connect and Redirect tool, and practise positive discipline through role play.

Box 9.h Connect and Redirect as a tool for positive discipline[28]

Connect

We first connect with the child to:

- move the child from reacting in the lower brain, to being connected to the upper brain, and being open to their thoughts, feelings, and the outside world;
- build the child's brain;
- deepen our relationship with the child.

We connect by:

- *Communicating comfort.* We get down to the child's level, giving them a loving touch, a nod of the head, or an empathetic look; this often calms them down.
- *Validating.* Even when we don't like the child's behaviour, we acknowledge their feelings. For example, 'I understand that you are feeling angry.'
- *Stopping talking and starting listening.* When a child is out of control with big emotions, we don't explain, or try to talk them out of their feelings; we just listen, and look for the meaning and emotions our child is communicating.
- *Reflecting what we hear.* Once we've listened, we reflect back on what we've heard, letting our child know that we've heard them, which communicates comfort.
- *Letting go of background memories and feelings caused by past experiences and future fears for our children.* We are fully present, parenting only this child, based on the facts of this situation.

Redirect

When we are both ready to listen, talk, and learn, we can begin to talk about what happened.

Understanding why the child behaved as they did. We are curious about what's going on behind the actions: 'What is he or she communicating?', 'I wonder why my child did that?', 'What is she wanting here?', 'Is she asking for something?', 'Is she trying to discover something?'

We look for 'why?' rather than asking 'why?'. This is because it sounds judgemental, and younger children won't know the answer.

What lesson do I want to teach my child at this moment? This may be:

- insight: understanding their own feelings, responses to difficult situations, and how they are practising their virtues;
- empathy: practicing by reflecting on how their actions impact on others;
- repair: what they can do to make things right and grow their virtues.

How best to teach the lesson? We teach by:

- limiting words;
- accepting feelings;
- describing, not lecturing;
- engaging our child in the discipline;

- revising a 'no' as a 'yes' with conditions;
- focussing on the positive;
- being creative;
- teaching mindsight tools.

Directions

1. Explain that we are now going to use what we have learned in Exercises 9.2 and 9.3 to practise positive discipline.

Say: 'I'm going to demonstrate the use of positive discipline with a child, acted by my co-facilitator.' Ask participants to observe the role play carefully, thinking about these questions:
- In what ways is positive discipline being demonstrated?
- How did the caregiver connect with the child? What effect did that have?
- What lesson did the caregiver teach the child?
- How did the caregiver teach the lesson?
- What is the outcome of the discipline?

2. With your co-facilitator, get into character and perform the role play.

3. Stop the role play but stay in character. Invite participants to ask each actor to say how they felt at different points in the role play. For example, 'What did you feel when you were shouting at your caregiver?' 'I was feeling angry because […].'

4. Ask participants: 'What did I do to connect with the child?'

Add any additional points that the caregiver might have used from Box 9.h.

5. Ask: 'Do you think the child was ready to listen, talk, and learn?'

'Do you think the caregiver was ready?'

'What did the caregiver do to understand why their child acted this way and what they were feeling? What did they find out?'

'What lesson did the caregiver teach?'

'How did they teach that lesson?'

'What was the child's immediate response to the discipline? What other outcomes do you think there were?'

Directions for caregivers

6. Ask caregivers to form small groups and to think of a situation where a child is behaving badly, and where the caregiver is reacting to them emotionally, maybe angrily (see Table 9.2 for two examples). Ask each group to role play this situation in front of the others.

Afterwards, ask them to replay the situation using positive discipline.

7. Ask: 'What did the caregiver do that demonstrated positive discipline?'

Ask the person acting as the child: 'How do you feel now?'

Ask the person playing the caregiver: 'How do you feel now?'

Ask the whole peer group: 'What did the caregiver do to connect with the child?'

Add any additional points from Box 9.h.

Then ask these questions: 'Did you think the child was ready to listen, talk and learn?'

'Did you think the caregiver was ready?'

'What did the caregiver do to understand why the child acted this way and what they were feeling?'

'What lessons did the caregiver teach?'

'How did they teach those lessons?'

'What was the child's immediate response to the discipline? What other outcomes do you think there were?'

'Which approach worked best?'

Directions for children

8. Ask the children to form small groups and to think of a situation where a child – maybe a sibling or a friend – has done something that has made them feel angry or upset (see Table 9.2 for two examples).

Ask each group to role play, in front of the others, how they might typically respond to this situation.

Afterwards, ask them to role play it again using positive ways of guiding the child concerned to practise their virtues.

9. Ask these questions: 'What did the child do that demonstrated positive guidance?'

'How did the other child respond? How did they feel?'

'How did the child who guided the friend feel?'

'Which approach worked best?'

Table 9.2 Examples of responding with punishment and with positive discipline

Problem	Punishment	Positive discipline
For caregivers		
Child is in the habit of staying out late after choir instead of coming straight home as instructed. She is angry when her caregiver asks her where she has been.	Shout at child when she comes home. Forbid her from going to choir.	Connect with child. Find out why she is coming home late. Talk about the risks of staying out late and how she could be safe. Agree on a plan, for example, going to choir with a trustworthy person who will also accompany her home. If appropriate, agree a consequence if she doesn't follow the plan. Reward her with praise when she comes in on time.
Child has lied about breaking their brother's toy. He is upset when accused of lying.	Shout at child. Make them apologize. Send them to bed without food.	Connect with child. When he calms down, listen to his story, explore why he lied. Explain virtue of honesty and recall together times when he has used it. Discuss and agree how to make amends, for example, the child will make a gift for his brother, or replace the toy with one of his own.
For children		
Your brother or sister has worn your best clothes without asking, and stained them.	Shout and insult them. Take their clothes or other belongings. Fight.	Connect with your sibling and ask them why they did it. Explain that you want to have a trusting and honest relationship. Agree how to behave in the future, should either of you want to borrow the other's belongings. Agree how they can make amends to you, if necessary.
You have failed your maths test because you didn't study enough.	Tell yourself that you're stupid, and you'll never be any good at maths, and it doesn't matter anyway. Refuse to talk to your caregiver about it.	Use self-compassion to soothe yourself. Connect with your caregiver by talking about why you failed and the things that make it difficult for you to practise the virtue of self-discipline. Decide together that you will revise maths for 10 minutes a day to improve.

Directions for all peer groups

8. Give everyone a chance to practise using positive discipline through role play, to support a person who is out of control and misbehaving. Participants who are not acting one of the characters are observers.

9. Together, prepare a 'we statement': a request that this group can make to the other peer groups during the Closing circle. Practise performing one of the role plays to make the request.

 Record the 'we statements' in your Facilitator's Journal.

EXERCISE 9.5 BEING A GOOD ROLE MODEL

AIMS: To understand how caregivers' attitudes, values, and behaviour influence their children's attitudes, values, behaviour, health, and development. To identify the kinds of role models caregivers would like their children to be guided by, and the role models that the children themselves would like to be guided by. To enable caregivers to re-evaluate their own attitudes, behaviour, and spoken words, in terms of how these are likely to affect their children.

DESCRIPTION: Participants play a game, then work on a poem and draw a picture.

Box 9.j Information for facilitators

Remember to focus on the *behaviour* of the person, rather than *labelling* the person themselves. If participants label people (for example, as 'a lazy caregiver' or 'a naughty child'), you can remind them that our behaviour comes from our needs, fears, and past experiences, and we can change it.

Directions[29]

1. Explain that we are going to play a game called 'Guess my name'.

2. Ask the group to explain the meaning of the term 'role model'.

3. Ask the group to call out the names of famous people or fictional characters who have been admired for their virtues. Write each name on sticky labels or paper, and stick one (using safety pins if necessary) on each person's back without them seeing or hearing the name.

4. Ask people to mingle and try to find out the name on their back by asking questions of other group members. The only answers that can be given are 'Yes' or 'No'.

5. When most people have guessed the name of their person, ask them to tell the whole group their name and what they appreciate about that person's behaviour as a role model. Invite comments from other members of the group.

6. Invite participants to read the poem 'Mummy's footsteps' (see Box 9.k). Invite people to act out the poem as someone reads it.

Box 9.k Poem: Mummy's [or Daddy's] footsteps

Walk a little slower mummy
Said a little child so small
I'm following in your footsteps
and I don't want to fall

Sometimes your steps are very fast
Sometimes they're hard to see
So walk a little slower mummy
For you are teaching me

Some day when I'm grown up
You're what I want to be
Then I will have a little child
Who'll want to follow me

And I would want to lead just right
And know that I was true
So walk a little slower mummy
For I must follow you

---

7. Re-read the last line, 'For I must follow you', and ask what it means for us as caregivers, or as children. Bring out these factors: connecting with children through love; discipline; respect for individuality; and modelling of appropriate and virtuous behaviour.

Caregivers. Ask: 'What do you think your children are learning from you? What do you show in your own behaviour as messages to your children?

'Do you "practise what you preach?" Are there ways in which we could be better role models for our children?'

Ask the caregivers to split into small groups of males or females. Say: 'Please draw a picture of a man or woman as a caregiver. On one side, draw or write the way in which this imaginary caregiver positively influences children, and on the other the influences that you would like to change or improve. Discuss together why you would like to change them, and how you can make these changes.'

Children. Split into males and females. Say: 'Let's draw a typical caregiver (the boys should draw a man, the girls should draw a woman). On one side, let's put all the good influences this caregiver has on their children. On the other side, put all the things you think the imaginary caregiver should change or improve.'

Encourage the children to talk about this imaginary caregiver, rather than talking about personal experiences with their own caregiver.

Closing circle

Bring the caregivers and children together and share the 'we statements' from Exercise 9.4, and the drawings from Exercise 9.5.

Ask caregivers to pair up with their children. Say: 'Please tell each other one thing you will do to support each other in remembering and acting on the virtue of compassion.'

Note. Please remind everyone to bring their tree of life with them to the next session: Session 10 'Coping with loss and the tree of love'. Ask everyone to do one small act of kindness towards themselves before the next session. It can be anything pleasing that they don't usually do, for example, having a rest under a flowering tree after a hard morning weeding. They don't have to share this with the group unless they want to.

 ## ADDITIONAL EXERCISE 9.6 OUR THREE VOICES

We suggest that children aged 5–8 years do not do this exercise.

> **AIM:** To increase our self-compassion and learn to live with our critical voices.
>
> **DESCRIPTION:** Participants are given a demonstration of the three voices and practise using them.

Directions[30]

1. Explain: 'We often criticize ourselves for not doing well enough. This can be helpful if it leads us to do better and to make good choices. But it can make us and our children feel worthless and hopeless. As we have learned in this session, positive discipline is teaching done in a loving way, which addresses a particular behaviour at a specific moment, not a negative criticism of the whole person.

'In this exercise we are going to imagine that we have three voices in our heads: our self-critical voice; the voice of our criticized self; and the voice of our compassionate self. We will each speak for each of these voices in turn.' (See examples in Table 9.3.)

2. Ask: 'What sort of things do we criticize ourselves for?' Ask people to call out something that their *self-critical* voice might say.

Ask: 'What tone of voice are we using? What is our body language like?'

3. Invite people to call out something that their *criticized self* might say in reaction.

Ask: 'What tone of voice are we using? What is our body language like?'

4. Now invite people to call out what their *compassionate self* would say.

Ask: 'What tone of voice are we using? What is our body language like?'

5. Set out three seats and explain that each seat represents one of our three voices, as listed in Table 9.3.

Table 9.3 The three voices

Which voice?	Self-critical	Criticized self	Compassionate self
Which seat?	End seat (1st seat)	Other end seat (3rd seat)	Middle seat (2nd seat)
Tone of voice?	Cross, nagging	Sad, scared, discouraged	Friendly, gentle, strong, warm
Body language?	Stiff, tense	Slumped, frowning, miserable	Relaxed, assertive, balanced
Example for a caregiver	'You are always late – you are disorganized and forgetful, and people are fed up with you.'	'You are right, I'm useless and hopeless, and however hard I try I'm always late.'	'It's hard, but you have determination to organize your life. Let's list the things that make you late and change them, one at a time.'
Example for a child	'You can't read yet, you're really stupid.'	'Yes I know, I am stupid, even younger children read better than me.'	'I see that you are diligent and your reading is improving day by day. You had time off school when you were sick, but you are catching up.'

6. Explain that you are going to demonstrate.

Say: 'I'm thinking about an issue that troubles me, and that I often criticize myself for.'

For example: 'I'm so disorganized. I'm always late for work and meetings, and in getting the food ready.'

7. Sit in the first seat, the voice of the self-critic. Say out loud what the self-critical part of you is thinking and feeling about yourself. For example: 'You are always losing things and forgetting the time; everyone is fed up with you. You'll lose your friends and your job if you don't change.'

Ask participants: 'What tone of voice is my critical self using? How is it feeling? What is my body posture like?'

Tell participants what you are feeling right now, in the self-critical seat.

8. Ask: 'How do you think someone hearing that criticism might feel or respond?'

'Is the criticism helpful?'

'If the criticism is for protection or motivation, could you achieve these goals in another way?'

9. Move to the third chair, representing the criticized part of yourself. Tell people how you feel being criticized like this. Say whatever comes into your mind, directly addressing your inner critic.

For example: 'I feel useless and hopeless. I'm always going to be disorganized and late.'

Ask participants: 'What tone of voice is my criticized self using? What is my body posture like?'

10. Now imagine what a compassionate friend would say to your critical self in this situation. Sit in the middle seat, representing your compassionate self. Say that you are going to call upon your deepest wisdom, your creative brain, the wells of your caring concern, and talk to both the critic and the criticized.

Ask: 'What does my compassionate self say to the critic?'

For example: 'I see that you're frustrated, and you're trying to help me to be punctual. But you are making me feel useless, and even less able to organize my life.' Or: 'Shhhhsh, shhhsh, shshh', in a gentle way, as if soothing a baby. Explain that we can learn to read our self-criticism as a sign that we need to soothe ourselves.

11. Now ask: 'What does my compassionate self say to the criticized part of myself?'

Explain that this is where you try to relax, letting your heart soften and open. Say any words of compassion that naturally come to mind.

For example: 'I see that you're really hurting. But I see that you have it in you to be determined and organize your life. Let's list the things that make you late and change them, one at a time.'

Ask participants: 'What is the tone of my compassionate voice? What is my body posture like?'

12. Now put the palms of your hands on top of each other on your heart and say out loud, slowly and firmly, a compassionate statement of intent.

For example: 'I have it in me to be determined and organize my life. I'll make a start this evening by getting everything ready for tomorrow.'

Then say slowly and firmly: 'May I be happy, may I be safe and well.' Repeat this twice more.

13. After your demonstration, ask participants to pair up. One partner should speak in their three voices; the other should observe, ask questions, and comment. Then ask them to swap roles. Before they begin, check that participants are clear about what they are going to do. Remind them to: first, think of something that they often criticize themselves for; second, take it in turns to speak about their chosen subject using the three voices:

- statement by self-critical voice;
- reaction by criticized voice;
- intervention by compassionate voice;
- commitment to action;
- final assertion of 'May I be happy, may I be safe and well'.

14. Ask everyone to come together.

Ask: 'What have you learned about yourself in this exercise? Are you thinking about the situation in new ways that are more supportive?'

Then ask the relevant peer group:

Caregivers. 'What have you learned about disciplining your children?'

Children. 'What have you learned about giving feedback to your friends or family?'

15. Explain that punishment and criticism strengthen the critical voice; loving teaching or guidance strengthens the compassionate voice. Say that we should focus on changing a specific behaviour at a given moment, not the whole person.

Say: 'As you think about what you have learned, commit to relating to yourself and others in a kinder way in the future. Call a truce in your inner war with yourself and others; you can be at peace. Your old habits of self-criticism and criticizing others don't need to rule you forever. Listen to the voice that's already there, even if it's quiet – your wise, compassionate self. Whenever you criticize yourself or others, remember to put your hands on your heart and use your compassionate voice to talk kindly to yourself about your intentions (as in point 12 above). Then you can start to change things from a more positive position.'

Add that we can also commit to relating to our family, children, and friends in a kinder way that strengthens their compassionate voice and soothes their self-critical voice.

Finish by saying: 'Life is often hard, but we can be at peace with ourselves and not beat ourselves up!'

Purpose: To explore loss, death, and love in a way that builds support among participants.

Contents	Materials required	Time required
Opening circle (see p.13)		15 mins
10.1 Changes, losses, and gains in our lives		50 mins
10.2 Understanding death		20 mins
10.3 Using a picture to talk about death		30 mins
10.4 The tree of love – remembering people we love	Picture of boy and grandmother on p127 and in Annex. Participants' trees of life from Session 5	60 mins
10.5 Who is there for me?	Six different coloured lengths of wool or thread, or beads	30 mins
10.6 Loving kindness colour meditation		15 mins
Closing circle (see p.14)		15 mins

About 4 hrs

Box10.a Information for facilitators

This session can bring up a lot of emotions. Please have someone attending who can support any participants who become upset, while you continue to facilitate.

Please also adapt these exercises as needed to suit the participants' culture and religion. They have been used in different cultures around the world, but are just suggestions.

The exercises in this session invite participants to focus on positive and loving memories of someone who has died, but participants may also have negative feelings, such as anger, associated with their loss. As you facilitate the activities, be aware of the body language of participants and refer them to the support person if necessary. We will explore these mixed feelings in Exercise 11.2 on page 138.

 ## EXERCISE 10.1 CHANGES, LOSSES, AND GAINS IN OUR LIVES

AIM: To understand that adults and children are affected by different kinds of changes, including the death of people they love. To understand that many changes result in both losses and gains, and cause a range of feelings.

DESCRIPTION: Children listen to a story and answer questions about it. Caregivers think of changes in their own lives and interview each other about the resulting losses and gains.

Directions

1. Invite one or two participants to tell the group, if they wish, about their small act of kindness towards themselves.

2. Say: 'All of us have been touched by death or loss in our families. In this session and the next one, we will support each other in understanding death and our feelings, remembering our loved ones with sadness and joy, and finding ways of supporting ourselves and each other with loving kindness. Just like a bundle of sticks tied together, we can be strong in supporting each other. One stick can easily be snapped in half – but a bundle of sticks? Impossible!'

Explain that any participant can choose to drop out of the session at any stage if they feel too emotional to participate. They could spend time with the person who is available specifically to provide participants with support. Remind the group that participants are also able to support each other.

For children

1. Read the story in Box 10.b to the children, or ask a participant to read it. Adapt the story to suit your group and community.

Box 10.b The story of Amina[31]

Amina was born in a village. When she was little, she lived with her parents and grandparents. When Amina was five, she moved to the city with her parents. She missed her grandmother's food and her grandfather's stories. Then Amina went to school. She remembers crying on the first day, when she said goodbye to her parents at the gate. She was glad to see them each evening. Amina had a little brown cat whom she loved very much. One day, the cat was run over by a car and Amina cried all night. A few weeks later, her father found a stray kitten, which Amina took care of. When Amina was 10, her best friend left the school. Amina missed her.

Every year Amina went with her parents to the village where she was born to visit her grandparents. When Amina was 11, her grandfather died. Amina was very sad but she still remembered his funny stories, which made her smile. When Amina was 12, she left her primary school. The secondary school was a boarding school, so Amina only saw her parents once a month. She felt homesick at first, but things soon improved. She enjoyed school very much, but she also loved the holidays when she saw her parents again.

---

2. Say: 'Amina has had a good life so far, but she has sometimes lost, or spent time apart from, things and people she loves. Put your hands up if you have experienced the loss of an animal, or a relative, or a friend, like Amina.'

All the children will put up their hands. Please also put up your own hand.

Then you can say: 'Loss and sadness are things we all have in common, like Amina. Let's read the story again and listen carefully for those times when she experienced loss. Every time you spot a loss, put up your hand and call out what the loss is.'

As the children call out the losses, write them down as a list.

3. At the end of the story, say: 'Now we have a list of the different kinds of loss and separation that Amina has lived through. Let's look at each one in turn.'

For each loss, ask: 'How do you think Amina felt about this loss?' Invite a child to draw a happy or sad face next to the item on the list, to show how she felt.

'Were there any good things about this change or loss?' Invite a child to draw a face on the list to show any positive feelings.

You might also ask: 'How do you think Amina managed to cope? What happy memories did Amina have? If we were Amina's friends, what could we all do together to help her through this experience?'

5. Finish by asking: 'What have we learned?' Summarize by saying that it's normal to have change in our lives, including losses and gains, and that we can help each other cope.

For caregivers

1. Explain that we are going to look at changes, losses, and gains in our own lives.

2. Ask participants to divide into pairs. Give each person a sheet of paper, and crayons or coloured pencils to draw with.

3. Say: 'Think back over the last five years of your lives. Remember three or four events that changed your life in a good and/or challenging way.'

4. Next, say: 'Now turn your sheet of paper sideways, and draw or make a long horizontal line across it, representing the last five years. Mark your three or four events along this line. For each one, think about what losses resulted from this change. Use words or pictures below the line to show these. Then think about what good things resulted from the change, and use words or pictures to show these above the line.'

5. Invite the pairs to interview each other about their line, so that each participant explains each event, and then how they felt about it, to their partner.

6. Bring the group together and invite participants to talk about what they have learned from the activity and the interviews.

Then ask: 'What do you think this activity has shown us about change and loss in our lives?'

EXERCISE 10.2 UNDERSTANDING DEATH

AIMS: To help children understand the concept of death in a clear and simple way. To help caregivers know a range of ways of supporting children of different ages in understanding when someone they know dies.

DESCRIPTION: The children play the insect game to help them talk about the difference between a living and a dead creature, and to understand the concept of death. The caregivers review advice about how to support children in coping with the death of a loved one.

Directions

For children: the insect game[32]

1. Begin with a high-energy, fun song for togetherness and support.

2. Ask: 'Have you ever seen an insect? Show me what it looks like.' Let the children show you by drawing or acting.

Next, ask: 'Have you ever seen a dead insect? Now, show me what that looks like.' Again, let the children show you by drawing or acting.

3. Explain: 'Every living thing dies – insects, animals, and people. Tell me, when an insect is dead, does it breathe? Does it sleep? Can it eat? Can it play?'

Pinch yourself, and say: 'Can it feel a pinch?'

Summarize by saying: 'All these things are also true when a person dies. When someone dies, it is forever, and that person will not be coming back. But we can always remember the person we love in our minds. We can talk about them, think about them and remember the things they said or did.'

This game uses an insect, but you could use any creature.

For caregivers

1. Say: 'Children often understand death and react to it differently from adults, depending on their age, reasoning ability, and emotional development. Children of all ages need extra attention, physical and verbal love, and comfort after experiencing trauma or loss. In this brief activity we are going to review advice on how to support children of different ages in coping with the death of a loved one.'

2. Read out the pieces of advice listed in Box 10.c.

After each one, ask participants to raise two hands if they agree with the advice, one hand if they think it's OK, and keep their hands down if they don't like it. You don't need to count the hands, but use them as a rough indicator of agreement or disagreement. Note down which pieces of advice get low levels of agreement.

Box 10.c Advice about supporting children in understanding a death[33]

For children aged 5–8 years

- Give a simple, clear explanation of death: for example, 'Have you ever seen a dead insect? Tell me, can it breathe? Can it eat? It can't, because it's body has stopped working. That's what's happened to mummy. She can't eat, or walk, or play now, because she is dead. And she cannot come back.'

- Explain the cause of death, and that it was serious. Encourage them to ask questions.

- Help children to talk through their fears. Tell them that the death was *not their fault – nor anyone else's.*

- Reassure them about the future, and talk about the people who will be there to take care of them.

- Keep familiar routines going; they are comforting and necessary, for example, going to school, to church or to the mosque, and going out to play.

- Show encouragement, support, and loving praise at every opportunity, to build self-confidence.

- You may want to point up to the stars and say: 'Some people think that we all turn to stars when we die. The stars are always there, twinkling and watching over us and guarding us, even when it's daytime or when it's cloudy and we can't see them. We can't touch the stars, but we know they are always there, comforting us.'

- Tell a story that shows how things change in life, or die, but that new things come. For example, 'A flower gets old and the petals fall off. It leaves seeds behind, which fall to the ground and grow first into a seedling, and then into a whole plant. The plant has beautiful flowers and makes seeds of its own, and the cycle starts again. Even if there are no seeds, the petals become rich compost, which helps seeds from surrounding plants to grow well instead.'

For children aged 9–11 years

- Set time aside to talk and listen. Give simple and direct explanations about the death, as above, and tell the stars and flower stories as needed.

- The child may want to spend time alone, perhaps with the belongings of the deceased person.

- Be honest about how the death will affect their lives.

- They may wish to rely on friends for support as well as adults.

- Be sure that they still have time to play and be children; share responsibilities to give them some time off if necessary.

For children aged 12–14 years

- Set time aside to talk and listen to them. Use the stars and flower stories as needed.

- Encourage them to spend time with friends.

- They may express their feelings through risk-taking behaviours, for example, alcohol, other drugs, sex, self-cutting, or stopping taking their medication. Discuss the possible consequences of this and how they can feel supported in looking after themselves.

- Support teenagers who are caregivers in managing their responsibilities.

For children aged 5–14 years

- Involve children in planning the funeral, for example, by choosing a song liked by the person who died, putting that person's favourite flowers on the grave, or drawing a picture. Take them to the funeral if culturally acceptable, and if they would like to go.

- Help them think of a special place that reminds them of the person who has died, which they can go to in their mind any time, or a special song they can sing to themselves.

3. If there is time, revisit the piece of advice which had the least agreement. Discuss with participants what they suggest caregivers might do instead.

 ## EXERCISE 10.3 USING A PICTURE TO TALK ABOUT DEATH

AIM: To help caregivers and children talk about death and support children who have been bereaved.

DESCRIPTION: Each peer group uses a picture as a way of talking about death and feelings about death.

Directions[34]

1. Show the picture of a girl sitting with her grandmother, showing a thought bubble about her mother when she was alive, and one about her mother in a coffin.

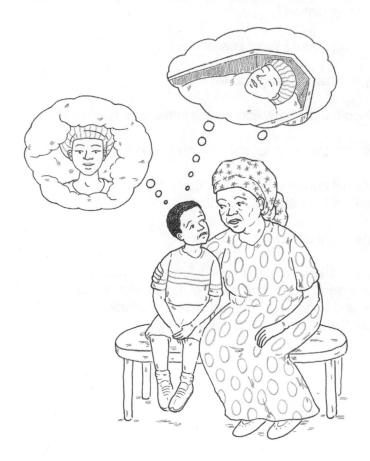

For children (divided into two or three groups)

Ask:

1. 'What do you see in this picture?'

2. 'What is the elderly woman saying to the girl?'

3. 'How does the girl feel?'

4. 'What is the girl thinking about?'

5. 'What questions does she have about the fact that the person she loves has died?'

6. 'What will happen to the girl?'

7. 'Will the person she loves come back again? Will she see this person again?'

8. 'Has someone you loved died? Do you know children who loved someone who has died?'

9. 'How can adults help children when someone they love dies?'

10. 'How can children like you help each other when someone dies?'

For caregivers (divided into groups of four)

Ask:

1. 'What do you see in this picture?'

2. 'What is the girl thinking about? What is she feeling?'

3. 'What is the elderly woman thinking and feeling?'

4. 'What questions does the girl have about her mother who has died?'

5. 'What are the important things to tell children when someone dies?'

6. 'What are the traditional beliefs in your community concerning death? Do any of these beliefs prevent adults from talking to children about death?'

7. 'What help does the girl need now?'

8. Explain that in some cultures people believe it is better to tell children that the dead person has gone away, rather than tell them that they have died. But not being told the truth can make children more anxious and angry. We now realize, through research, that it is better to tell children the truth about the death of someone they loved.

EXERCISE 10.4 THE TREE OF LOVE – REMEMBERING PEOPLE WE LOVE

AIMS: To remember and talk about the person we loved, and create a rich picture of our relationship with them to treasure and keep. To get strength from the forest of trees, as it creates close relationships and a community of support.

DESCRIPTION: Participants add to their own tree of life, which they drew in Session 5, focussing on a person they loved who has died.

Directions

1. Remind participants about Session 5, when they created their tree of life. Remind everyone what each part of the tree shows. Ask everyone to hold up their trees and stand together as a forest. Ask: 'How do we feel as a forest?'

2. Say: 'We have all sadly lost dear friends and relatives, who meant so much to us but who have died. As we stand together in our strong and beautiful forest, let us each think of one person who has died whom we want to think about. Today we are going to draw on our trees, and talk together about how much we loved the person who has died and what we remember about them. We will also talk about how we can support each other and still feel strong despite our loss and sadness.'

Say: 'Most people have happy and less happy memories about someone who has died. This is normal. In this exercise we are going to focus on our happy memories and the things we loved about the person who died. We will have a chance to look at our other feelings in another exercise.'

Say: 'It's good for us to express our feelings as we do this activity. It's fine to cry, or laugh, or remember without speaking. But let us only laugh at what others say if they also think it is funny.'

3. Say: 'Let's put our names on the tree, if we haven't already. Now draw a heart at the top of the paper to show love. Now, what is the name of the person you loved – did they have a favourite name that you liked to call them? Put this name on one side of your heart.

'Put your name on the other side; perhaps you can use a favourite name that made you happy when the person you loved used it for you. Join up the names across the heart to show how you will always love each other.'

Box 10.d Notes for facilitators

Please adjust the questions to suit the age of your peer group, and to fit with local culture. For example, if most children do not know the birthday of the ones they love, there is no need to ask that question. And if cultural or religious beliefs stop women and/or children going to funerals or graves, alter those questions.

When working with their trees of life, some participants may not have enough space on the paper to add as many words and drawings to it as they would like. In this case, they can stick more paper around the tree to make the sheet larger.

---

4. Say: 'Now we'll start talking again about the tree *roots*. The roots show how the person who died lives on in our lives, through us and our family, and in their spirit, maybe among their ancestors. We're going to draw on some of our memories of them.'

Ask: 'What did they look like? Draw a picture of them beside the roots. Do you see anything in yourself that looks like them? Perhaps the same nose or teeth, or hands or smile?'

After a few minutes, suggest that they add other pictures to help depict the person, using questions to prompt ideas. For example:
- 'What did they like to do? What things did you like doing together?'
- 'What were they good at? What qualities and abilities did they have? Do you have some of those qualities and abilities too?'
- 'Do you know when their birthday or name day was? If so, how did you celebrate their birthday or name day?'
- 'How old were they when they died?'
- 'What was their favourite song? What song did you both like?'
- 'What was the funniest thing the person ever did? What made them laugh? Can you remember a funny thing they did that made you laugh?'
- 'What made the person happy?'

6. Next, say: 'Now let's look again at the *ground*. This is the place where you live now, showing all the things that are found there and are going on there. Let's add some places that are special because they link us to the person we loved, or places that they would like if they were to visit us now.'
- 'Are there any special places where you were happy with them, or which have special meaning for you?'
- 'Did they have a favourite place, flower, or tree?'
- 'Do you go somewhere special to remember the person who died? If not, can you think of a place that you could go to, either for real or in your imagination, to remember them?'
- 'If you have moved, imagine what your loved one would think about the place where you now live. Where can you imagine being together? What would they like about it?'

7. Say: 'Now let's add to the *trunk*.'
- 'What are the things about you, your abilities, which your loved one would be proud to see?'
- 'What did they teach you? What skills, qualities, and knowledge did they give you?'
- 'How do you use that person as a role model now – in what ways do you try to be like them?'

8. Say: 'Now let's add to the *branches*.'
- 'What are your dreams for the future? What did the one you loved wish for you? What will make them happy as they follow your path in life?'
- 'At what points in your life would you like your loved one to see you, and be with you in spirit, as you grow up? What events would make them happy?'

9. Say: 'Now add to the *leaves*.

'Think to yourself: "Who are the new people in my life, who support me and care about me?"'

Ask participants to draw these people as leaves on the tree.

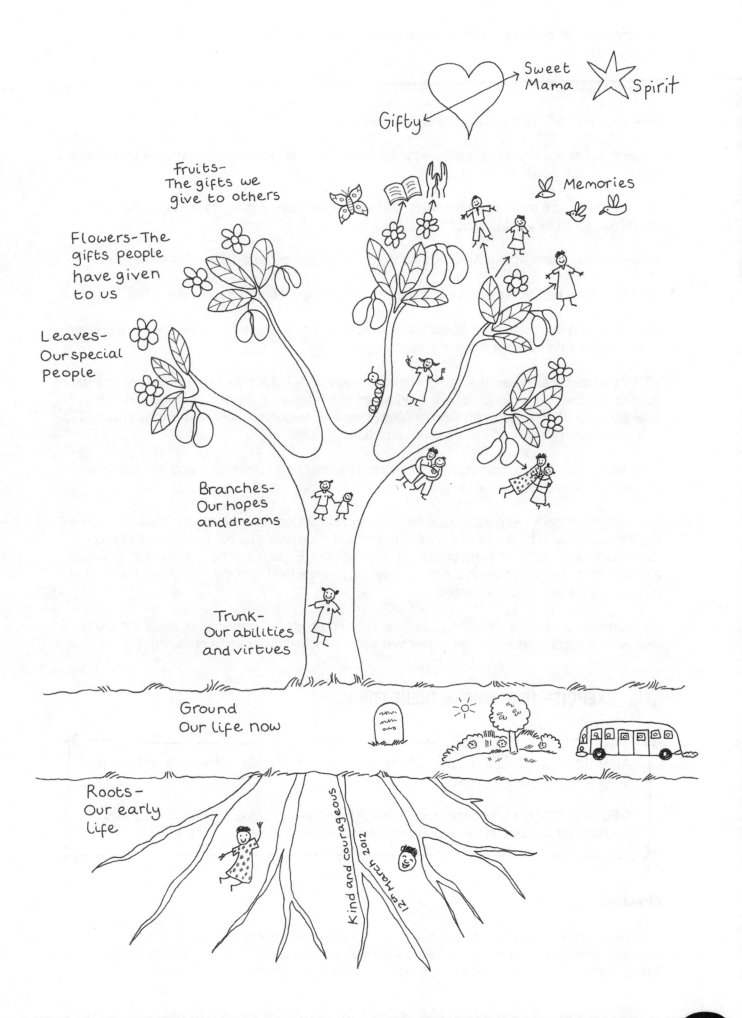

Ask them to ask themselves: 'How would the person I loved feel about my new family, siblings and friends?'

10. Say: 'Now let's think about the *flowers*.

'Ask yourselves: "What gifts did the one I loved give me?"

'Draw them as flowers on the tree, and write a word or symbol to remind you what you received and what these gifts meant to you.'

11. Say: 'Now let's think about the *fruits*, and ask yourselves: "What gifts did I give the one I loved? What did they enjoy about these gifts?"

'Draw the fruits, and write a word or symbol to remind you of the gifts you gave your loved one.'

12. Next, invite participants to draw some *birds*, *butterflies*, or *clouds* around the tree.

Say: 'As you draw them, think about some special memories you have of the person you loved, which float across your mind and make you cry or smile.'

13. Finally, say: 'Let's draw the spirit of the ones we loved. Think about where you imagine the spirit of the one you loved to be. Is it everywhere around you? In the stars? In the earth with your ancestors? In heaven with God or Allah? Use your favourite colour to draw the spirit of the one you loved, however you wish, on your picture.'

14. Invite participants to pair up with someone they feel comfortable with, and tell each other whatever they wish about their tree.

15. Then bring the three peer groups together and invite them to hold up their trees and come together again as a forest. Hold the trees higher and make them rustle. Sway together as if the wind is blowing. Be still and breathe quietly together. Explain that trees in the forest give us oxygen to breathe, and that, in the same way, we give each other hope and strength when we come together and love each other.

16. Invite caregivers and children to take their trees home and tell one another about the stories, if they wish. If anyone prefers to leave their tree with the facilitator or keep it private, that is also fine.

 ### EXERCISE 10.5 WHO IS THERE FOR ME?[35]

AIM: To make a bracelet using different colours, so that each colour reminds us of a person who cares about us.

DESCRIPTION: Participants each make a bracelet with coloured strands or beads, each colour symbolizing a person who cares for them.

Directions

1. Explain: 'When someone dies we can feel very lonely. Sometimes it feels as if there aren't any people who care, or that there are not enough people to talk to. But there are people in our family, friends, and other people at our school, clubs, or workplaces who do care.'

2. Say: 'Please think of all the different people who care about you, and count them up in your head or on your fingers. Now close your eyes, and hold up your fingers to show how many people you have thought of who care for you.'

Record all the males' and females' answers in your Facilitator's Journal.

3. Say: 'Now choose between two and five of those people who care about you. We are going to make a bracelet in different colours to remind you of them.'

Help any participants who held up very few fingers; perhaps suggest that they think of one or more people from among the group.

4. Ask participants to choose some pieces of thread, yarn, wool or plastic strip (all the same length), using a different colour for each person on their list. They could also have a thread for the person who has died, to show that this person is still with them in spirit. (Alternatively, if using beads, choose a different coloured bead for each person and thread these onto a bracelet.)

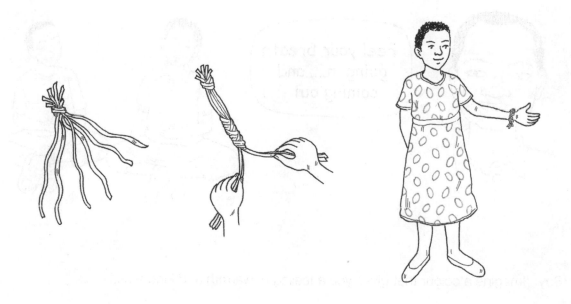

5. Ask participants to tie all the threads together at one end, and to tape the knotted end to a table or ask someone to hold it.

6. Next, invite them to twist or plait the threads together to make a pattern.

7. Suggest to participants that, when they have finished twisting/plaiting, they tie a knot at the end of the bracelet, and ask a friend to help them tie it around their wrist.

8. Encourage them to make bracelets at home using different colours and patterns.

9. Remind participants that it's OK to miss the person who died, but to remember that other people care about them too. You might say: 'We can wear this bracelet to remind us of the people who support us.'

EXERCISE 10.6 LOVING KINDNESS COLOUR MEDITATION

AIM: To learn a tool that we can use to soothe and calm us.

DESCRIPTION: Participants are led through a meditation on colour.

Directions

1. Say: 'We are going to do our breathing exercise, but this time we will imagine a colour. Please sit comfortably, close your eyes and relax. Feel your breath going in … and coming out.'

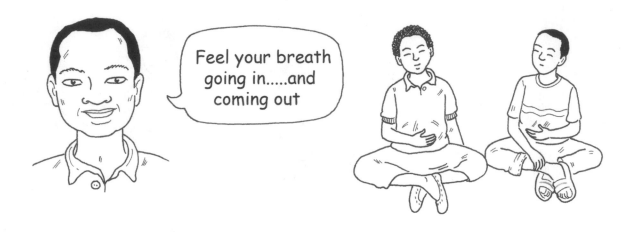

Feel your breath going in.....and coming out

2. Say: 'Imagine a colour that gives you a feeling of warmth and kindness.'

3. Say: 'Imagine the colour surrounding you.'

4. Say: 'Imagine breathing in the colour.'

5. Say: 'Imagine the colour entering your heart area, and spreading through your body. Imagine wrapping the colour around you so it keeps you warm and snug like a beautiful shawl.'

6. Say: 'Focus on the colour, warming and soothing you.'

7. Finally, say: 'When you are ready, open your eyes, and return your attention to your surroundings.'

Closing circle

Ask participants to do one small act of kindness, for someone they know a little bit, before the next session. Children should do this when there are people they know around; they should not go somewhere or arrange to meet with the person without telling their caregiver.

UNDERSTANDING DEATH AND COPING WITH OUR FEELINGS

Purpose: To learn more about recognizing and coping with our feelings after the death of someone we love, and how to respond to other people's feelings when they have lost someone.

Contents	Materials required	Time required
Opening circle (see p.13)		15 mins
11.1 Talking about feelings in a story		30 mins
11.2 Volcano	Card, newspaper, glue, sticky tape and paint, or local materials such as mud, leaves, and stones	75 mins
11.3 The wave game		20 mins
11.4 (*for caregivers only*) Supporting each other through the death of someone we love		75 mins
11.5 (*for children only*) Supporting each other through loss	Picture of two children visiting a sad child on p 145 and in Annex	45 mins
11.6 (*for children only*) Important dates		30 mins
Closing circle (see p.14)		15 mins

About 4 hrs

EXERCISE 11.1 TALKING ABOUT FEELINGS IN A STORY

AIM: To talk about how children show their feelings when someone dies, and how adults and children can help them express their feelings and heal.

DESCRIPTION: Participants listen to and discuss a story.

Note: We will cover talking about our feelings and HIV specifically in Session 13.

Directions

For caregivers[36]

1. Invite one or two people to tell the group about their small act of kindness to someone they know a little bit.

Read out the short story in Box 11.a.

Ask: 'Why is this girl misbehaving? How is she feeling?'

'What does she need?'

'How could her new caregiver help her?'

'How might she have behaved if she had been told the truth, in a kind way, about her mother?'

2. Share the information in Box 11.b as needed.

Box 11.b How to talk about feelings with a child

Make sure you are in a safe place. The child may become upset and want to run out.

Answer gently but honestly. For example: 'Your mother died from a serious illness', or 'You're going to stay with me now.' Uncertainty can cause a lot of anxiety. You can make the fact of death less harsh by saying, 'Mummy can't come back because her body doesn't work anymore, but she is still here in our thoughts and dreams.' You can also refer to the child's religious beliefs, such as talking about spirits and souls.

Help the child to express their feelings and thoughts. Sometimes it is enough to sit with the child and listen. You can also help by saying, for example: 'I know you miss your mother very much', or 'Your sadness tells me how much you loved your mum and how much she mattered to you.' Allow the child to cry. If you feel you also want to cry that is fine.

Allow children to express their sadness. It's OK for children to feel sad. Sometimes sadness may appear as anger or naughtiness. Explain this and try to comfort them. Use positive discipline to talk over issues, rather than punishment. Get down to their eye level and say that you also feel very sad.

3. If there is time, invite participants to share their reactions to this advice.

For children

1. Invite one or two children to tell the group about their small act of kindness to a person they know a little bit, if they wish.

Read out the short story in Box 11.c.

Box 11.c Short story for children

This is a story about a boy who is the same age as you. He loves to play running games. He is the fastest runner in the neighbourhood. Hardly anything scares him. He even taught his neighbour's dog to stop running after him and to stop growling.

But one day his mother died and he became very sad. No one told him where his mother had gone. He wished and prayed that his mother would come back. But she never did.

Then he decided that he would go to look for his mother. He started by looking under his bed. She wasn't there. Then he looked in all the cupboards. She wasn't there. He asked the adults where his mother had gone. Some people said she was in the ground. Some people said she was in heaven.

The boy didn't understand. He became very angry. He started to fight with all the other children. He even had fights with the big children. He would get into all sorts of trouble, and sometimes the adults would beat him.

He just wanted to see his mother again.

Ask: 'Do you know any children like this boy?'

'What happens to someone when they die?'

'How does the boy in the story feel?'

'What should we tell the boy about his mother?'

'How can you help this boy?'

'How might the boy have behaved if he had been told the truth about his mother in a kind way that he could understand?'

EXERCISE 11.2 VOLCANO

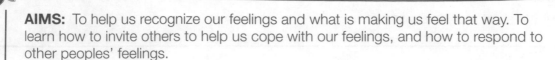

AIMS: To help us recognize our feelings and what is making us feel that way. To learn how to invite others to help us cope with our feelings, and how to respond to other peoples' feelings.

DESCRIPTION: Each participant makes a model of a volcano, writes their feelings and invitations on paper spirals, and sticks these on top of the volcano so they form an 'eruption'.

Box 11.d Information for facilitator

Most groups find this exercise very powerful.

If making a volcano is not practical or interesting to your group, create another way of doing the activity. For example:

- for each feeling, ask participants to draw a face showing the feeling, the reason for the feeling, the person they are inviting to help, and the good outcome;
- in pairs, act out the feelings one by one, including the reason, the invitation, and the person responding. Choose one of the feelings to perform to the whole group.

Whichever method you use, aim to follow up the feelings and invitations, if necessary, either in another exercise or through counselling and/or community action.

Directions[37]

1. Explain: 'When someone dies, we may have lots of different feelings inside us. For example, we may feel scared, sad, angry, or relieved. It's OK to have these different feelings. It can feel confusing – one minute we feel very sad, and the next we go and play, or chat with a friend, and feel happy again. It's like rain and sunshine, we see both in one day. This is all normal. Sometimes we may feel like a volcano, which is going to explode with feelings.

'Expressing our feelings is a way of communicating to ourselves and others what is happening to us and inviting them to support us. This helps us cope with our feelings. In this exercise we will name our feelings, and look at what makes us feel that way, and what changes and support we would like to help us cope with this feeling.

'Talking to people we trust about our feelings and asking them to help us cope with them is good, especially if someone in their family has died too.'

2. Explain that in this exercise, everyone is going to make their own volcano, with their feelings coming out of it.

Explain how to make the volcano:

i) Scrunch up paper into balls, or make balls of mud.

ii) Pile the balls up on your piece of card, sticking them onto the card with glue or tape.

iii) If there is time, paint or decorate the volcano with local materials.

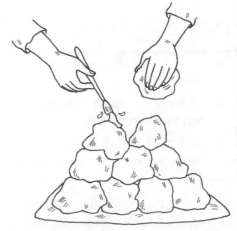

iv) Show participants how to cut out paper spirals. They will need three or four spirals each. They can colour them in if they like.

4. Invite participants to pair up (either with a peer, or pairing caregivers with children who are not their own).

Start to build up your volcano by sticking the paper balls onto the card

Explain: 'We are going to take it in turns to tell each other a feeling we have now, or have had recently.
It might be a nice feeling or a difficult feeling. Say the feeling, and what has made you feel that way. Then talk about what you would like to happen – either to help you cope with a difficult feeling, or to keep or increase a nice feeling – and who you would like to get support from.

'Begin with the feeling and what causes the feeling, and then state what you want and from whom. Let me give you some examples.'

Read out some appropriate examples from Box 11.e.

Box 11.e Examples of volcano statements

Caregivers
- I feel sad because I loved my daughter so much, and I miss her so. I wish I could talk about her more with my grandchildren, and cry with them if I want to.
- I feel angry that my husband died from cheating on me and left us with nothing. I wish I could talk to my imam about my anger and leave it behind.
- I feel guilty because I was judgemental towards my son and his wife before he died. I want to talk about it with her, and ask her forgiveness.
- I feel peaceful when I sit under my wife's tree by the river, and say a prayer and talk to her. I see her smile in the ripples and feel her spirit moving through the leaves. I want to bring my daughter here so she can feel the peace.

Children
- I feel scared about what will happen to me now. I would like my caregiver to explain who I will live with and what school I will go to.
- I feel safe when I'm with my sister. I want her to be my caregiver.
- I get confused when people tell me different things. I want my auntie to tell me if my father is coming back or if he is gone forever.
- I feel relieved that I can stay in school. I hope my cousin will let me work in his shop, so I can earn my keep and go to secondary school.

- I feel lonely when no friends come to play. I wish that Mary would invite me to play football with her.

- I feel worried because I think I might have HIV or TB too. I wish my grandma would take me to the clinic.

- I feel happy about my new home and school friends. I will feel even happier if my sister can live with us too.

- I feel glad that my dad will no longer beat me but I am worried that someone else will instead. I want my mum to protect me.

5. Explain to participants that when they have each talked about one feeling, they should each do two or three more. Then invite them to write each one on a spiral. They can be shortened to the feeling and the invitation, for example, 'Lonely: Mary please invite me to play football'.

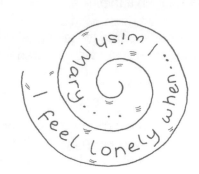

6. Explain to participants how to stick the spirals onto the top of their volcanoes, so that it looks as if they are erupting.

7. Invite participants to share their volcanoes with each other as they wish. They could take it in turns to talk about one spiral each.

8. Invite them to take their volcano home to keep if they wish.

9. Say: 'We can use the skills we have learned today to ask each other what we are feeling, the reason for the feeling, and what invitation we would like to make. We can also practise mindsight with each other in pairs by saying: "You seem to feel […]. Is it because […]? Shall we talk about what could make you feel better?" The other person can then say if their partner's mindsight is correct or not, and talk further.'

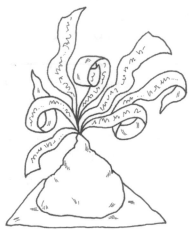

You might give participants this example: 'You seem to feel angry; is it because I can't afford to buy you those shoes? Shall we talk about what we can do to make you feel happier?'

 EXERCISE 11.3 THE WAVE GAME

AIM: To help people accept and live with the ups and downs of life, in calm and stormy weather.

DESCRIPTION: Participants are given a short explanation of the game, then act it out.

Directions

1. Remind participants: 'We have explored how change often leads to loss and gain. When someone dies we feel sad and painful feelings. These feelings are like waves on a sea or lake. There will be stormy times and then calm times again.' If participants find this hard to imagine, talk instead about a fierce dust storm or rainstorm, followed by calm and sunshine.

2. Explain that when someone dies we may go through different feelings. 'At first we may feel shock and think it can't be true. We may feel sad because we love the person and miss them. We may cry: our tears show how much we loved them. They taste of salt like the waves in the sea. Or we may not cry at all and just feel nothing. We may feel angry that they have left us, afraid of what will happen next, and helpless. Then we may start to feel better and grow into our new life. But we continue to remember the ones we love. We feel happy for the good times we spent with them and sad because we loved them. All these feelings are normal. There is no one way, or right way, for us to react to the news that someone we love has died. Our feelings can go up and down like the sun and the moon.'

3. Play a game about stormy and peaceful weather. Remind participants about their forest of trees, which can sway in the wind without breaking. Explain that we can support one another in swaying together, without any of us falling, during the storm. Then the wind will stop blowing and the trees will become calm again.

For example:

- Play a clapping and stamping game, where the sound of rain grows to a really loud storm, and then gets quieter until everything is peaceful again.

- Dance together to show a storm building and then calming down.

- Pretend you are in boats as a storm builds, holding on to each other for support as the boats rock, and then relaxing when it passes.

EXERCISE 11.4 SUPPORTING EACH OTHER THROUGH THE DEATH OF SOMEONE WE LOVE

For caregivers only. Children do Exercises 11.5 and 11.6.

AIM: To share the ways we help each other live through a death and flourish.

DESCRIPTION: Caregivers do ability spotting; mind mapping; and group work on helpful practices.

Directions[38]

1. Explain that this exercise enables us to think about helpful ways of supporting each other in coping with death in our lives.

2. Invite caregivers, in pairs, to interview each other and ask:

'Tell me about a time when you supported a friend or relative, adult or child, who had lost someone they loved. What did you do that you feel proud of to support them?'

Suggest that they interview each other using the helper questions (Who? When? Where? How? What? With what result?), and point out each other's abilities.

3. Back as a group, draw a big circle on flipchart paper. Write the following three themes on the circle (where the numbers 12, 4, and 8 appear on a clock), and explain them briefly:

- nurture and understand (this concerns helping each other express our feelings after a death);
- memory and ritual (talking about the person who has died, and using ritual to mark their passing);
- practical plans and building a future (dealing with the practical issues that arise when someone dies).

Discuss ways in which participants have supported people when someone they love has died. Draw or write each way on a small piece of paper. Then place each piece of paper under one of the three headings on the flipchart, between two of them, or in the middle if that form of support connects with all three themes.

4. Invite participants to add other ideas.

5. Explain that we will now look at the three themes in turn, to think in more detail about ways of helping each other.

Nurture, communicate, and support each other in expressing feelings after a death

1. Divide into three groups and give each group one idea from the circle activity (see step 3 above) for nurturing, communicating, and supporting each other in expressing feelings. Invite them to think of how they might put the ideas into practice.

2. Ask each group to describe or show their ideas to the wider peer group in whatever way they wish.

3. As needed, add additional information from Box 11.f.

Box 11.f Ideas on the theme of 'nurture and understand'

- Show them that we care about them and love them in many small ways.
- Let them know that sadness, tears, and even seeming indifferent, are normal. It's also normal to feel relieved or angry if there were problems with the person's behaviour, for example, if they were abusive.
- If we also have feelings of loss, show them.
- Say we are here to talk with them when they need someone to listen – and then be ready to listen.
- Be careful of the other person's feelings when talking about the person who has died. Instead of stating your own opinion, encourage them to talk and to say what they feel.

Supporting people in expressing feelings after loss

Explain that we show our sadness in many different ways and they are all OK. Children may feel sad one minute and cry, and then play and laugh soon after. They may feel angry and want to fight, be unable to concentrate, or be naughty. They may say they don't care that the person has died. This is normal too. Adults may also feel angry, feel nothing, or drink too much to forget their feelings. Say that these are all ways of expressing feelings after loss. We need to support each other in gradually accepting the death, and in using our virtues to move away from negative feelings and behaviours.

Memory and ritual

1. Explain that we are now going to focus on the theme of memory and ritual. Explain that we can help by:

- encouraging each other to remember the person who has died;
- supporting each other in using religious or spiritual rituals, for example prayers, to work through our feelings of loss.

2. Look at the pieces of paper under the 'memory and ritual' heading and talk in more detail about the ideas associated with this theme. Invite people to describe or show ways in which they remember people they loved, and use rituals. Invite people to add new ideas.

Ask: 'In what ways does it benefit us to remember the person who has died?'

3. As needed, add additional information from Box 11.g.

Box 11.g Ideas on the theme of 'memory and ritual'

Talking about the person who died again and again, and continuing to talk about them over many years is fine, and helps people keep their loving relationships alive. The people who surround the bereaved person need to think about what they say about the deceased when those who loved them are present. It can be very painful for the bereaved person to hear people saying cruel things about the person they loved. On the other hand, if the person who died was abusive, it can be supportive to encourage the bereaved person to talk about the suffering this behaviour caused with another person who also experienced it. Talking about how to get through negative feelings to achieve emotional wellbeing can also be helpful.

If children or adults have not had a chance to say goodbye – to see the person before they died, knowing that they are dying – then a ritual enabling them to do that can help. This could be a formal ceremony, such as a funeral or religious service; or it could be something informal, such as writing a letter or poem, singing a song, throwing a stone or shell or flower or goodbye drawing into a river, or going to a special place such as the grave.

Performing a ceremony or ritual gives us a chance to remember the person who has died and honour them. If done with others, it can give us a sense of comfort and support that we are not alone in our sorrow. It's important to let children take part, but make sure they are well prepared and are supported by an adult.

We can create simple rituals, such as lighting a candle to remember the person on certain days.

One way to focus memories is through a memory book, or a box or bag containing objects that bring back memories. These could be drawings, photos, bits of clothing or jewellery, letters, pressed flowers, or favourite things. We can use the items to help us talk about the person we loved, or spend private time remembering them.

Practical plans and building a future

1. Explain that we usually have to deal with practical issues after a death in the family, for example: arranging the funeral; sorting out any inheritance; and working out who will take care of the children, and where they will live and be educated.

In addition to these practical plans, there is the task of building the future: how best to cope with the loss; move on and live our lives; and support children in living theirs well.

2. Ask participants to look at the ideas placed on the circle nearest to 'practical plans and building a future'.

3. Ask: 'How can we all support one another in encouraging families and the community to support and protect children and adults who have lost someone they love?'

4. As needed, add additional information from Box 11.h.

Box 11.h Ideas on the theme of 'practical plans and building a future'

Explain to orphaned children any plans that have been made about their future care, and listen to what they feel, think, and want. Remember their right to be involved in decisions about their lives, and their rights to education, food, shelter, and love.

Give children honest information about how this death will affect them, for example, when discussing where they will live, or who will take care of them.

Support children in keeping family property and their possessions, particularly things given to them by the person who has died.

Support children in remaining with their siblings, and in being looked after by someone who knows them well and who knew the person who has died.

Build children's self-confidence and faith in the future. Encourage and praise their efforts rather than criticizing them. Talk to children about what they will do in the future, and encourage them to set goals.

---

5. Sum up the themes and ways in which we can support each other in living though the death of a person we loved, and flourishing.

 EXERCISE 11.5 SUPPORTING EACH OTHER THROUGH LOSS

For children only. Caregivers do Exercise 11.4.

AIM: To equip children with skills in supporting each other through loss, and in planning some actions.

DESCRIPTION: Participants discuss a picture and make a plan to help each other.

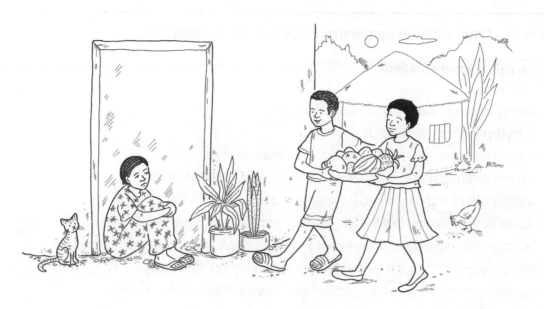

Directions[39]

1. Say to your peer group: 'Many of us have lost a person we loved, or have survived other big losses. Together as a group, in these sessions, we are supporting each other and building caring, trusting friendships. Let's think about how we can strengthen our support to each other and to others in the community who feel sad.'

2. Show the picture above and in the Annex of two children visiting a child who feels sad.

Ask: 'What do you think has made the child feel sad? What do you think would comfort and support the child?'

3. Ask the children to pair up and talk about the following questions:

'What help have you received from other children or from caregivers when you felt sad?'

'What help would you like to receive?'

'What help have you given other children or caregivers who feel sad?'

4. Ask each pair in turn to share one idea with the whole group. Write the ideas on flipchart paper, using symbols if necessary. Ask the children not to repeat any idea that has already been shared. Keep going round the pairs until all their ideas are on the list.

5. Say: 'Now we know lots of ways of supporting each other!' If there are gaps, you could suggest ideas from Box 11.i.

Box 11.i Ways children can support each other through loss

Being with a bereaved friend
- listening;
- sitting with my friend just to be with them;
- hugging and holding hands;
- encouraging my friend to talk and show their feelings;
- talking with my friend about the one they loved, who has died;
- being patient with my friend, giving them time to feel better;
- doing simple things, like bringing fruit or candles, to show I care;
- helping with household chores or farming, or playing with younger children;
- doing pleasant things together like playing, chatting, or singing;
- visiting other children and/or adults who have suffered bereavement.

Forming a group of friends to support a bereaved friend

When the time is right, we can encourage our friend to join our activities. Help them look forward and think about the future. The important thing is that those of our friends who miss someone do not feel alone or rejected by others. In time, they will be able to help other children who feel sad, because they know how it feels.

Helping a bereaved friend find an adult to talk to

We can find out which adults a bereaved child could go to for counselling, to share feelings of loss. This could be a kind teacher, a community or religious leader, or a person who is very caring. We can then take our friend to visit this person.

6. Say: 'Let's make a plan about what we will do.' The following questions can guide the plan:

'Who will we support?'

'How will we support them?'

'Where will we support them?'

'When will we support them?'

'Who will do what?'

'Who will support us?'

'What do we need to make our plan work?'

'How will we know how we are doing?'

7. Ask the children to sing a song and do things to show how *courageous* they are.

EXERCISE 11.6 IMPORTANT DATES

For children only. Caregivers do Exercise 11.4.

AIM: To give children a tool enabling them to keep remembering people they loved who have died.

DESCRIPTION: Children decide on one or more dates on which to remember the person who died, and on ways of remembering the person on those dates.

Directions[40]

1. Explain that after someone dies we can still remember them for as long as we want to. We can go on remembering them for years and years if we like.

2. Ask the children: 'Would you like to do this? If so, on which date or dates will you remember the person who has died? Let's write them down. Why is each date special? If you are not sure of a date, for example, the person's birthday, you could find out from other people in your family.'

If a child does not want to do this exercise, encourage them to do another activity, such as drawing a happy memory related to the person who has died.

3. Say: 'On these days we might like to do something special to remember the person who died. Here are some ideas:
- Go to the person's grave with some flowers or shells, or with a song to sing.
- Go to a place the person liked.
- Look at some photos.
- Light a candle (with an adult nearby to make sure you are safe).
- Have the person's favourite food for tea.'

4. Ask: 'What are your ideas?'

Encourage participants to draw their ideas next to the dates they have listed.

Closing circle

Before participants leave, invite them to write down all their questions about HIV and put them in the anonymous question box for use in the next session, 'All about HIV'. Invite participants who can't write to tell you their questions quietly, and then add these to the box for them. Use the questions to prepare the next session.

Ask everyone to do one small act of kindness for a stranger before the next session. It can be anything unexpected that the person would feel surprised and pleased by. They don't have to tell the group what it is unless they want to – this is their own secret. Just ask them to think of it as they go about their day, and to make sure they do it before the next session. Ask the children to do the act of kindness when other people are around; they should not go anywhere or arrange to meet the person without telling their caregiver.

SESSION 12 ALL ABOUT HIV

Purpose: To learn what HIV is; its effects on our bodies; how it gets shared between two people or it does not get shared; how we can look after ourselves if we have HIV; and how we can protect ourselves and other people from getting HIV.

Contents	Materials required	Time required
Opening circle (see p.13)		15 mins
12.1 What is HIV and how do children get it?	Questions from question box and small sweets for every child	30 mins
12.2 What does HIV do in the body?		45 mins
12.3 How can we stop (more) HIV getting into our bodies?	Props for HIV game. A piece of rope or chalk, selected statements from Table 12.1 written on paper	75 mins
12.4 How does HIV get around in the community?	Folded pieces of paper (some marked with '+'), plastic bags	60 mins
Closing circle (see p.14)		15 mins

About 4 hrs

Preparation

With the agreement of the peer groups, invite local caregivers or young people who are open about having HIV, and comfortable talking to others about it, to participate as members of the peer group. This can help the group feel comforted that they can live a 'normal', good life with HIV. (See guidance in Introduction 'Involving people who are living with HIV', p.10.)

At the end of Session 11 you will have collected participants' questions on HIV in the anonymous question box. Use these to prepare this session for the relevant peer group.

The following exercises require specific preparation:

Exercise 12.1. Have some small sweets or other small food items (the same number as there are participants in the group) ready to give to each child at the start of this exercise.

Exercise 12.3. Photocopy or draw the picture in Box 12.i to show group. Select suitable statements for your peer group from Table 12.1 (pp.157–8), and write them on pieces of paper. Also prepare pieces of paper which say: 'safe', 'mostly safe', 'unsafe', and 'don't know'.

Exercise 12.4. Prepare some small pieces of paper (the same number as the number of participants) as follows. Find out the prevalence of HIV in your area. If the prevalence is, for example, 20 per cent, draw a plus sign ('+') on 20 per cent of the pieces. Fold all the paper slips so no one can see what is written. Also gather a number of small plastic bags to match the number of participants.

Box 12.a Information for facilitators

Participants will be in different situations concerning HIV. Some caregivers and children may have been tested for HIV and others not. Some may have been told their HIV status and others not. Ensure that you facilitate in a way that includes everyone, whatever their HIV situation. It is important that you never ask anyone to talk about their HIV status in the group unless they have said that they are happy to be open about it with everyone.

If any participants are open about having HIV, whether caregivers or older children, it will be helpful if they are happy to share some experiences with their peer group.

Opening circle

Invite one or two people who feel comfortable doing so to tell the group about their small act of kindness to a stranger.

Say: 'Today we are going to learn about HIV. We are all affected by HIV, and quite a few of us may also have it in our bodies. By understanding HIV and supporting one another, we can all live happy, healthy, and fulfilling lives.

'Let's remember our ground rules and agreement about confidentiality. Also, let's be clear: none of us has to share personal information if we don't want to.'

 EXERCISE 12.1 WHAT IS HIV AND HOW DO CHILDREN GET IT?

AIMS: To learn what HIV is and how children get HIV.

DESCRIPTION: Participants engage in a question and answer session, using the questions below and others from the anonymous question box related to what HIV is and how children get it. Encourage members of the group to share their knowledge, and use information in Boxes 12.b, 12.c and 12.d after every question if you need to add to participants' answers.

Directions

1. Ask participants to act out being big, as if they are elephants. Next ask them to make themselves very small, like a mouse. Now ask everyone to stand in a line, with the participants at one end making themselves as small as possible, like a mouse, and gradually increasing in size until, at the other end of the line, they are as tall as an elephant.

2. Explain: 'The germs (bacteria and viruses) which make us sick are so tiny that we can't see them without a special instrument. They hide in different places in our bodies and we can't see them unless we search carefully.'

3. Give a small wrapped sweet to each child, and ask them to hide the sweet somewhere around their body; for example, in their hand, under their arm, or in a pocket. Ask: 'Can anyone see a sweet from where they are standing?'

4. Ask the children to pair up and take it in turns to find each other's sweet by pointing to the place they think it might be.

5. As soon as each pair has found their sweets, they should sit down. When all the pairs have found their sweets, get everyone to sit in a circle and ask: 'How does this game link to germs?' You might give this example: 'When we have a cold, germs hide in our noses and go from one person to another in the air when we sneeze. We can't see the germs because they are too small.'

Ask: 'Who can tell us about a germ that causes us to get sick, and how it can be shared between two people?' Participants might suggest, for example, diarrhoea or malaria.

6. Explain: 'All of us have tiny creatures hiding in our bodies all the time, which we can't see. Some of us have the HIV tiny creature hiding in us. Today we are going to talk more about HIV and the medicines that can keep us well, so that we learn from each other and can all understand more about it.'

7. Say: 'The most important thing to know about HIV is that we are all affected by it, whether we actually have it in our own bodies or not. By understanding HIV and AIDS and showing each other how much we care about one another, we can all live happier and healthier lives. We can have loving partners, if we want to, and healthy children, and grandchildren, whether we have HIV or not.'

8. Remind people that: 'None of us has to share personal information if we don't want to; instead we can talk about people like us, or discuss issues through stories. It's best only to talk about whether we have HIV or not if we have thought about it carefully. Ideally we will have agreed with our child or caregiver that it is OK to be open.'

9. Ask: 'Who can tell us what HIV is? What does HIV stand for?'

Box 12.b What is HIV?

HIV stands for Human Immunodeficiency Virus. It is a tiny creature called a virus. We can only see it through a microscope, a special machine which makes it look much bigger.

---

10. Ask: 'Where does HIV live? Where does it hide in our bodies?'

Box 12.c Where does HIV live in our bodies?

HIV lives in the largest amounts in these body fluids: blood, semen, vaginal fluid, and breast milk. There is almost no HIV in saliva, urine, or sweat.

Note: Please find appropriate ways of explaining these different fluids to the younger children, especially semen and vaginal fluid. They need to understand that HIV is in those fluids, but not in urine (see Exercise 12.3).

---

11. Ask: 'How do children get HIV?'

Box 12.d How do children get HIV?

Most children under 14 who have HIV got it from their mothers. HIV was shared with them as they grew during pregnancy, during birth, or through breastfeeding. Their parents did not intend to share HIV with them. They just did not have the knowledge, support, or medicines to stop the HIV being transmitted to their child.

Nowadays, women who have HIV can take medicines called anti-retrovirals (ARVs), which mean that, almost always, they can have babies free of HIV. Children who have HIV can also take ARVs when they need them, which means that they can stay well and, in due course, have their own babies who don't have HIV.

Most people understand that women want to keep their babies healthy. But some people blame women for sharing HIV with their babies. This is unjust and harmful. There are lots of reasons, to do with stigma and available services and harmful gender norms, why women may not get the medicines they need to protect their children from HIV. We will explore how to support each other in having children without HIV in Session 25.

Sadly, some children get HIV from older people who do sexual things to them. This is wrong of the older people. We will be learning about this and how we can protect each other from sexual abuse in Session 26.

EXERCISE 12.2 WHAT DOES HIV DO IN THE BODY?

AIMS: To learn how HIV damages the immune system and multiplies in the body, and how ARVs stop HIV from multiplying and keep us well.

DESCRIPTION: Participants ask questions about what HIV does in the body and how it can be treated. They then play a game to understand what happens when HIV gets into the body and how ARVs can stop it multiplying.

Directions

1. Ask questions about HIV and invite participants to answer them. Include questions from the anonymous question box which relate to what HIV is, and how it works in the body. Use information in Boxes 12.e, 12.f, 12.g, and 12.h after every question if you need to add to participants' answers.

For example, ask participants: 'Why is HIV called Human Immunodeficiency Virus?'

'What is the immune system?'

Box 12.e HIV and the immune system

The virus is called Human Immunodeficiency Virus because it damages and weakens the body's *immune system*. The immune system is the body's natural defence against disease. A person with HIV who is not taking ARVs gets sick and needs treatment more often than usual.

'What is the difference between HIV and AIDS?'

Box 12.f What is the difference between HIV and AIDS?

HIV is a virus. A person living with HIV can feel well and appear healthy for many years. But if they don't take medicine, HIV will gradually damage their body's immune system. Eventually, one or more serious illnesses develop and the person is diagnosed as having AIDS (Acquired Immune Deficiency Syndrome).

'How does HIV damage the immune system?'

Box 12.g How does HIV damage the immune system?

When HIV gets into the body, it damages a type of cell called *CD4* cells. They are a very important part of the immune system. HIV gets inside them and multiplies. The dying CD4 cell then releases more HIV into the body. The viruses move on to other CD4 cells. As more CD4 cells die, the body becomes less able to protect itself against germs. If a person with HIV gets other infections, the CD4 cells become more active to fight the infection. This activates the HIV in the CD4 cells to multiply, and the amount of HIV in the body fluids increases.

'Can HIV be treated? How does the treatment work?'

Box 12.h Treating HIV

HIV can be treated. Anti-Retrovirals are drugs that stop HIV cells from multiplying and spreading. They can massively reduce the amount of HIV in the body. This means that the immune system can recover, or stay strong. People with HIV who are able to take ARVs well can live longer and healthier lives.

By reducing the load of HIV in the body, ARVs enable mothers with HIV to give birth and breastfeed without sharing HIV with their babies.

We will explore how to live well with HIV in Session 14.

2. Explain that we are now going to play a game to show how HIV damages the immune system and how ARVs can stop HIV from multiplying.[41]

3. Ask participants to split into three equal-sized groups. Tell one group that they will pretend to be CD4 cells, another group that they will pretend to be HIV, and the last group that they will act as the ARVs. Ask the participants to find a way of showing which group they are in, for example, by all tying a piece of cloth on their heads, sticking a flower in their hair, pinning a label on themselves, or taking one sock off.

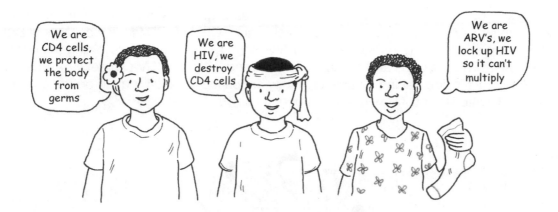

4. Make sure participants understand how HIV acts in the body. Ask them to tell you about it and explain again if needed.

5. Ask the CD4 cell group to form a circle, holding hands.

6. Say: 'When HIV enters the body, the CD4 cells try to protect the body from the virus. But in the end an HIV cell gets to the CD4 cell and climbs inside it.'

Now start directing the role play: 'First, let's see the HIV actors moving in. Two or three of you need to crawl under the hands of the CD4 circle and stand up inside their circle. Now, some of you CD4 actors should fall down. Each CD4 actor needs to be covered by an HIV actor, as HIV is stronger than the CD4 cell.'

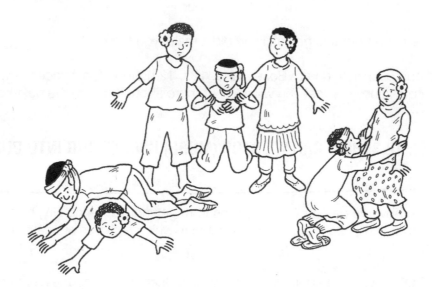

'Now HIV is taking over the body and multiplying. More HIV actors need to enter the circle! You can twist and turn and pull down the CD4 actors! Oh, now all the CD4 cells are down and the immune system has been overpowered.'

7. Thank everyone and ask them to stand up.

Say: 'Now let's do this role play again. CD4 actors, please get back into your circle. Now let's see two or three HIV actors crawling into the circle again. Oh, two CD4s have collapsed! But this time the person is going to take ARVs. So, let's have all the ARV actors joining the circle with the CD4s, filling the gaps and making it really strong. No more HIV can get in! And let's see the HIV actors inside getting smaller, until they are curled up and lying still on the ground. Together the CD4 cells and ARVs make a strong circle.'

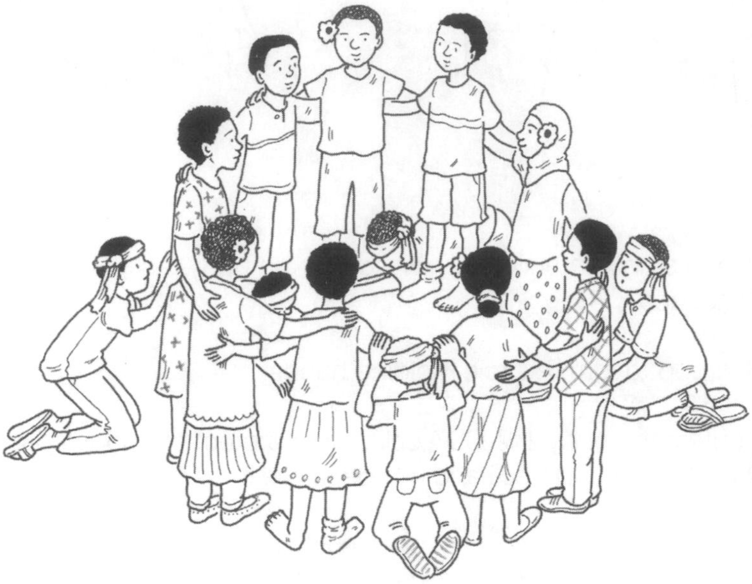

8. Thank everyone and say that we are now going to stop being HIV, CD4, and ARV actors. Ask the actors to say their names and their favourite colour.

Ask: 'What did we learn from this game? How did it make you feel?'

Summarize and add information from Boxes 12.e, 12.f, 12.g, and 12.h if necessary. If you cannot answer a question, say that you will find out more about it before the next session.

EXERCISE 12.3 HOW CAN WE STOP (MORE) HIV GETTING INTO OUR BODIES?

AIM: To learn how we can protect ourselves from getting or sharing HIV, or prevent more HIV from getting into our bodies, and identify which activities are safe, less safe, and unsafe.

DESCRIPTION: Learning about HIV transmission, then assessing the safety of various activities by placing them along a line according to whether they are safe, mostly safe, or unsafe in terms of HIV transmission.

Box 12.i Information for facilitators[42]

In this session, you will be focussing on everyday activities, and giving a summary of sexual transmission, and transmission from mother to child. You can tell participants that we will talk more about sexual transmission, safer sex, and condoms in Sessions 21 ('Our sexual feelings and sexual safety') and 24 ('All about condoms').

You need to be clear that for HIV transmission to take place, the *quality* of the virus must be strong, a large *quantity* must be present, and there must be a *route of transmission* for the virus to get shared between one person's body fluids and another person's body fluids.

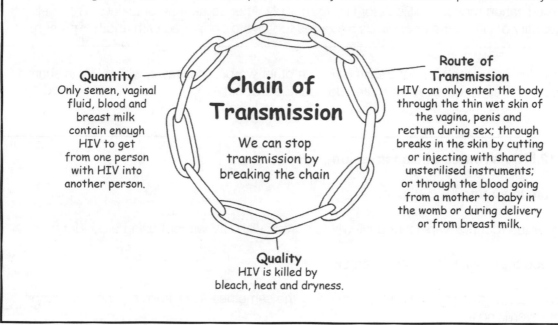

Quantity
Only semen, vaginal fluid, blood and breast milk contain enough HIV to get from one person with HIV into another person.

Chain of Transmission

We can stop transmission by breaking the chain

Route of Transmission
HIV can only enter the body through the thin wet skin of the vagina, penis and rectum during sex; through breaks in the skin by cutting or injecting with shared unsterilised instruments; or through the blood going from a mother to baby in the womb or during delivery or from breast milk.

Quality
HIV is killed by bleach, heat and dryness.

Directions

1. Explain: 'We are going to learn more about how HIV can be shared between one person and another. This is called transmission. There are three elements to HIV transmission. Without all three, HIV cannot be shared. Note that when HIV is shared between one person and another, it does not mean that the first person no longer has HIV, because there will always still be HIV in the first person's body fluids.'

The first element is *quality*: how strong HIV is. Do you think HIV is strong or not? What kills it?'

Use information in Boxes 12.j, 12.k, and 12.l after every question if you need to add to participants' answers.

Box 12.j Quality of HIV

HIV is not a very strong virus. It can survive for some time in blood outside the body, but there are no reports of people getting HIV from spillage of blood or semen on unbroken skin. HIV can live for one or two weeks in syringes in blood containing HIV.

We can kill HIV with fresh, full-strength bleach, and we can wash it away with three washes of water. HIV dies when it is exposed to heat above 60°C; for example, if someone with HIV bleeds into a cooking pot. HIV is killed by saliva and by the acid in our stomachs.

'The second element is *quantity*. Where is HIV found in the body in a large enough quantity to be shared with someone else's body?'

Box 12.k Quantity of HIV

HIV is found in large quantities in blood, semen, vaginal fluids, and breast milk. These are the fluids which contain enough HIV for it to be shared. HIV is not found in sweat, tears, or mosquitoes. It is found in tiny amounts in saliva, vomit, faeces, and urine, but not enough for there to be any risk of transmission, unless blood is present.

ARV medication makes it difficult for HIV to multiply. After some time of taking ARVs well, the quantity of HIV in the body fluids becomes too low to be shared with another person.

'The third element is the *route of transmission*, in other words, the way in which HIV is shared with another person's body. What routes do you know about?'

Box 12.l HIV's routes of transmission

There are four routes:

1) sexual intercourse (vaginal or anal) with a person with HIV without using a condom;

2) a blood transfusion using untested blood;

3) having an injection or cutting the skin using the same needle or knife as another person without sterilizing it;

4) from a woman with HIV to her baby during pregnancy, delivery, or breastfeeding.

HIV cannot be shared through unbroken skin, or even broken skin, very easily. The fluid that has HIV in it needs to meet with another person's fluid for sharing to be possible.

Summarize: 'So, now we know that for HIV to be shared, it needs quality (and it is only strong in bodies or in a vacuum); quantity (to be in blood, semen, vaginal fluids, or breast milk); and a route of transmission. If any one of these is missing, HIV cannot be shared. Let's play a game using this knowledge.'

2. Draw a line on the ground with chalk, or place a rope across the workshop area. Mark one end 'unsafe', the middle 'mostly safe', and the other end 'safe'. Mark an area away from the line as 'don't know'.

3. You should have pieces of paper ready marked up with selected statements from Table 12.1 (see 'Preparation', on p.148). Explain: 'We are going to discuss whether particular activities with a person who has enough HIV in his or her body fluids to share it with others are safe, unsafe, or mostly safe, both for the person with HIV and for the other person or people involved, who may or may not have HIV. Remember that a person taking ARVs correctly may have too few HIVs to share.

'There are different types of HIV, and someone who already has one type doesn't want to get other types as well, as that can make treatment less effective. They also want to avoid getting other germs, which can make the immune system and CD4 cells more active. This helps HIV multiply, but even the active immune system is not able to fight HIV.'

Table 12.1 Activity statements about HIV transmission

Statements (to be written on pieces of paper)	Points to consider
Holding or shaking hands with a person who has HIV	This carries no risk of sharing HIV, like any everyday social contact, e.g. hugs, kisses on the cheek, dancing together.
Cleaning up spilled blood	There are some other germs carried in blood which are more easily transmitted than HIV. If possible, wear protective gloves, or use a cloth or broom with water or antiseptic or mild bleach, rather than bare hands. If you don't have gloves, cover any cuts or sores on your hands.
A blood transfusion using blood which hasn't been tested for HIV	HIV and other conditions can easily be transmitted like this.
Using unsterilized needles or razor/knife blades, or getting needle-stick injuries	We should always use sterilized or new needles, razors, or knife blades for any procedure which breaks the skin. If people need to re-use needles or razors they should wash them with fresh bleach and clean water. In group cutting situations (for example, circumcision), each person should bring their own clean razor or knife.
A boy being circumcised	This is safe for the boy if all the instruments used are new or sterilized, and if the cutters do not cut themselves and bleed into the wound. The boy should still use a condom for proper protection if he has sex. See Session 19 ('When we are growing up') and Session 24 ('All about condoms').
Pregnancy and birth	If a woman has HIV and is not given the right care, support, and treatment, there is a 33% chance of the baby being born with HIV. With the right treatment and support, this risk can be reduced to 1%.
Breastfeeding	If a woman has HIV and breastfeeds her baby without taking ARV treatment, she may share HIV with her baby. With ARV treatment and support, this risk is greatly reduced. (Check the latest guidelines from your Ministry of Health.)
Sex using male or female condoms	Male and female condoms form a barrier which stops HIV being shared between one person and another during sex. If used correctly, and for every instance of sexual intercourse over one year, both male and female condoms offer an 80–90% rate of protection against HIV. This is because condoms sometimes break or slip during use. It's important to use condoms which are in date and which have been stored in a cool place. We will learn more about condoms in Session 24.
Kissing and licking	Kissing on the body is safe if the skin has no cuts or sores. Kissing on the mouth is safe if neither person has any cuts, ulcers, or bleeding gums. Kissing on the vagina or penis is less safe, because the quantity of HIV is higher in semen and vaginal fluids.
Cleaning or bathing a person with HIV	This is a safe activity and provides much support for the person with HIV, if done with love and care.

Statements (to be written on pieces of paper)	Points to consider
Sharing cups, plates, cutlery, food, sheets, towels, and clothing	It is safe to share any of these items. Just follow normal hygiene rules.
Using toilets	It is safe to share toilets. Faeces and urine do not carry enough HIV to be risky, as long as there is no blood in them. However, faeces do carry other germs.
Sleeping in the bed or room of a person with HIV	This is completely safe if there is no sexual intercourse.
Bites from mosquitoes or fleas	Insects cannot transmit HIV. They can transmit other germs, such as malaria and dengue fever.
Meeting and chatting with visitors to the house	Social contact that does not involve sex is completely safe, and can help people with HIV feel loved, cared for, and supported.
Playing with other children	This is a completely safe activity. Children love running and playing together!
Inclusion in family events, discussions, and decisions	This is completely safe and highly important, so that people with HIV continue to be valued as full family members. This helps protect them from depression, anxiety, and stress, all of which can affect the immune system.
Cooking for family and friends or a business	Cooking is a completely safe activity and many people with HIV are cooks. HIV would not be transmitted even if blood got into the food, because it would be killed if the food is heated, by saliva, and in the stomach.
Cutting meat	This is safe. Even if the cook got cut and bled on the meat, washing the meat and cooking it would kill HIV. In any case, HIV cannot get into the body through the stomach.
Road traffic or other accidents	This is safe if there is no blood from the accident. If there is blood, the person caring for others should wear gloves or cover any cuts or sores on their hands. This is to protect them from various diseases which are carried in blood, including HIV.
Sexual intercourse without a condom	This is not safe, unless ARV treatment means the HIV is not found in the blood of a person with HIV. *For children.* Children should not have sex until their brains and bodies are developed enough to cope with the psychological and physical consequences of doing so. *For adults.* It is always a good idea to use a condom and another contraceptive, such as the pill, to avoid other sexually transmitted infections and unplanned pregnancy.

4. Ask participants to pair up. Divide the statements out among the pairs. Ask them to discuss where they would put each activity along the line from 'safe' to 'unsafe', or 'don't know'.

5. Invite participants to take it in turns to place their activity along the line and explain why they have put it there.

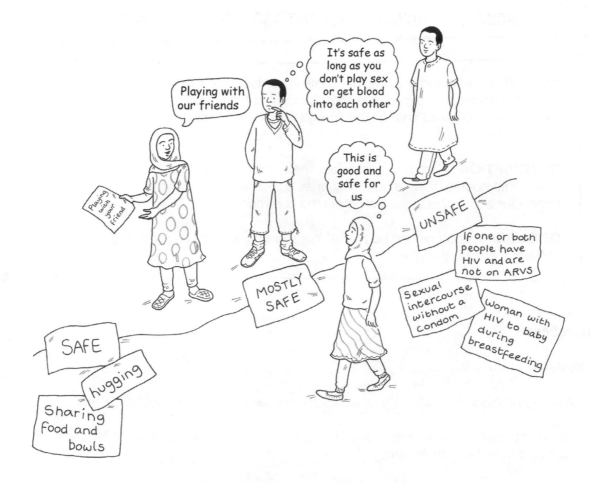

6. Invite the other participants to comment, ask questions, or suggest moving the paper to another place along the line. When you reach agreement, put the paper in the agreed place.

7. When all the pieces of paper have been positioned, ask if there are any situations that the participants would like to add to the game. If there is a situation you are unsure about, you can say that you will research it and share what you find out in the next session.

8. Ask: 'What have you learned about HIV with this game?'

Ask the following questions (using the SIFT tool introduced in Session 2 'Using our brains' as a reminder):
- S 'What Sensations do you have in your body?'
- I 'What Images do you have in your mind?'
- F 'What are your Feelings?'
- T 'What are your Thoughts?'

Emphasize that there are many things that people with HIV can do which are absolutely safe.

9. Ask: 'What is your favourite safe activity?'

10. Summarize that for HIV transmission to take place, the *quality* of the virus must be strong, a large *quantity* must be present, and that the virus needs one of four *routes of transmission* to get from one person's body fluids into another person's body. There are only four ways that HIV might get shared between one person and another (see Box 12.1).

EXERCISE 12.4 HOW DOES HIV GET AROUND IN THE COMMUNITY?

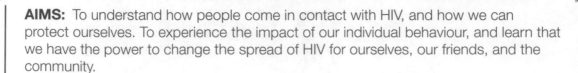

AIMS: To understand how people come in contact with HIV, and how we can protect ourselves. To experience the impact of our individual behaviour, and learn that we have the power to change the spread of HIV for ourselves, our friends, and the community.

DESCRIPTION: Participants simulate the spread of HIV, shaking hands to represent sexual intercourse, then change how they shake hands to simulate how changing behaviour affects the spread of HIV in the community.

GROUPS: This game can be played in separate peer groups, or with the two children's groups together.

Directions[43]

Round 1

1. Ask all participants to take one of the folded pieces of paper, but not to open it.

2. Ask participants to walk around the room and, when you clap, to shake hands with one other person and remember their name.

3. Repeat, so that again participants walk around, you clap, and they shake hands with another person and remember their name.

4. Repeat once more, so that everyone has shaken hands three times.

5. Say: 'Some of us have a "+" symbol on our paper. For this game, we are *pretending* that these are people who have HIV. This is only for the game; it is just chance who has a "+" symbol and who does not. The "+" symbol does not have any meaning outside of this game.

'Now, before we open the paper slips, can we say how many of us have HIV, and how many of us have come into contact with a "+"? We can't. Let's find out.'

6. Ask everyone to open their slip of paper, and invite the people with the '+' symbol to come forward and sit in the middle of the workshop space.

7. Ask everyone who shook hands with a '+' person after the first clap to sit in the middle.

8. Ask everyone who shook hands with a '+' person after the second clap, or with any of the people already sitting in the middle, to join them.

9. Ask everyone who shook hands with a '+' person after the third clap, or with any of the people already sitting in the middle, to join them.

10. Ask: 'What activity is the handshake pretending to be?' Stress that you can share HIV through sexual intercourse, and that for this game we are pretending that shaking hands is having sex. But in reality, we cannot share HIV through shaking hands.

11. Ask: 'How many people have been "in contact with HIV" through shaking hands in the game?'

Count these people. Explain they have been in contact with HIV, but that we do not know whether the HIV got out of, or into, their bodies. HIV does not always get shared with another person, even when it has the opportunity. For example, there are many couples where one person has HIV and the other does not, even though they have sex without a condom. We might get HIV in our bodies the first time we have sex, or the 50th time, or not at all.

12. Ask: 'What did those of us who are standing up, do to stay free of HIV in this game?'

Explain that those people didn't do anything, because they were told to shake hands and nobody knew who had a '+' and who did not. It was chance whether or not we had HIV, and whether or not we shook hands with someone with HIV. In real life, people can have HIV for several years without any signs or symptoms. So HIV can spread in our communities without us knowing.

Round 2

1. Collect the folded paper slips. Explain that we are going to play the game again. This time, participants can choose not to share their HIV, and not to get HIV. Ask how they will do this. Make sure they include all the options in Table 12.2, and explain how to act these out in the game. Point out where the plastic bags are.

Table 12.2 Ways of avoiding sexual transmission of HIV

In real life, we can avoid getting or sharing HIV by:	In the game, we can avoid getting or sharing HIV by:
Not having sex	Refusing to shake hands
Always using condoms when having sex	putting a plastic bag over the hand before shaking hands
Only having sex with each other if neither of us has HIV. (If both of us have HIV, we might share a different strain of HIV with each other, which could make treatment less effective)	Shaking hands with the same person each time – with or without a plastic bag
Enjoying sexual activities without intercourse, which do not allow semen or vaginal fluids to pass from one person into the other	Shaking hands using fingertips only

2. Ask everyone to decide on their strategy and prepare.

3. Hand out the paper slips again, asking people not to look at them. Remind them to follow their own strategy, regardless of your instruction to shake hands.

4. Repeat the process of instructing participants to walk around until you clap, and then shake hands; do this three times, as before.

5. Ask everyone to open their slip of paper, and invite the people with the '+' to come forward and sit in the middle of the workshop space.

6. Ask everyone who, after the first clap, shook hands with a person with a '+' to join the people in the middle, *unless* they were wearing a plastic bag or touching fingertips.

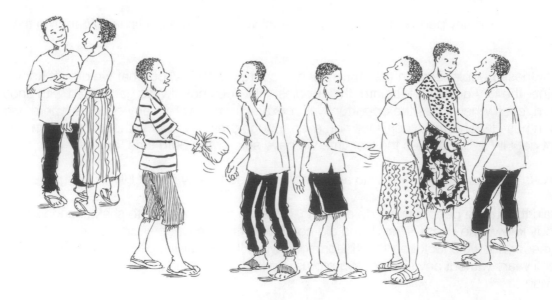

7. Ask everyone who, after the second clap, shook hands with a person with a '+', or with any of the people already sitting in the middle, to join them, *unless* they were wearing a plastic bag or touching fingertips.

8. Ask everyone who, after the third clap, shook hands with a person with a '+', or with any of the people already sitting in the middle, to join them, *unless* they were wearing a plastic bag or shook fingertips.

9. Ask: 'How many of us have been in contact with HIV this time?' Count the people sitting down. Say: 'Let's find out why so many more of us are still standing this time.'

10. Remind everyone: 'Some of us used bags to shake hands, which is like using a condom for sex in real life.' Then ask: 'How many of us used bags?'

'How did you feel when you shook hands with the bag on?'

'How did other people feel shaking hands with the plastic bags? Did anyone say anything, or laugh, or go to another person?'

'Did the people using a bag for every handshake come into contact with HIV?'

If needed, explain that they didn't. Those with a '+' did not get any more HIV, or share HIV with anyone, though they still have HIV. They did not get any other STIs either.

11. Ask: 'Did any two people only shake hands with each other, with one or both of them wearing a bag?' Explore what happened.
- If they were both '+', then they still have HIV, but have not got more HIV from each other.
- If one was '+', then they have protected themself from getting more HIV and the other person will still be HIV-free.
- If neither had '+', then they are both HIV-free.

12. Ask: 'What were the people who refused to shake hands doing?' (If needed, remind participants that they were not having sex.)

'Do they have HIV?' (Yes if they had a '+'; no if they didn't.)

'How did you feel when you refused to shake hands?'

'How did others feel when they refused to shake hands?'

'How do you feel now?'

13. 'What were the people who touched fingertips doing?' Remind participants that they were enjoying sexual activities without intercourse, such as caressing.

Ask: 'Did they share HIV?' If needed, explain that they didn't, because they were using safe sexual activities where no semen, vaginal fluids, or blood got on to the sexual organs.

14. Summarize: 'Almost all the people who used the new strategies were able to avoid contact with HIV or sharing HIV. The only exception was if someone shook hands, without a condom, with the same person each time, but that person had HIV".'

15. Make sure that the participants are all clear about the statements in Box 12.m.

Box 12.m Things to know about HIV and sexual transmission

We can't know who has HIV and who does not. Opening the paper slip is like having an HIV test: that is the only way to know. Many people do not know if they have HIV, or if their partners have HIV.

We can protect ourselves from getting HIV, and avoid sharing it, by: not having sexual intercourse; enjoying sexual activities without intercourse; or by always using condoms.

If we are only having sex with one person, and they are only having sex with us, we can use condoms until we have both had an HIV test. We can keep using condoms after the test if one person has HIV, or if we want to prevent other STIs and pregnancy. We might decide not to use them if we both have HIV, if we are both taking ARVs, and if we both have a very low viral load count; but using them will prevent us from sharing and getting different types of HIV from each other. We might also decide not to use condoms if neither of us has HIV, and if we are willing to trust each other to be faithful.

---

16. Remind everyone how many people came into contact with HIV in round 1 compared with round 2. Provided the number has reduced, congratulate them: 'Give yourselves a big clap!

'This game shows us how each one of us can reduce the spread of HIV through our community.'

17. Ask: 'What did we learn and how will we use this knowledge?'

Ask: 'What virtues will help us use healthy behaviours, such as using condoms?'

Explain: 'We can use our virtues of love, caring, mutual respect, and personal responsibility towards each other, irrespective of whether we have HIV or not. When we recognize that HIV affects us all, and is the responsibility of us all, we can keep each other safe, including our babies when we are ready to have them.'

Closing circle

1. Invite participants to get comfortable, close their eyes, and focus on their breathing for about a minute.

2. Now say: 'Imagine how we will act responsibly to protect ourselves and others from getting HIV into our bodies.'
'Think about the different ways we will do this.'
'Imagine telling our friends and family how they can protect themselves and others around them from HIV.'

SESSION 13 TESTING FOR HIV AND TALKING ABOUT IT

Purpose: To understand the HIV test and how to talk about it with children; and to gain courage and skills in talking to children about having HIV.

Contents	Materials required	Time required	
Opening circle (see p.13)		15 mins	
13.1 'Prrr' and 'pukutu' game		10 mins	
13.2 Talking about HIV, trust, and confidentiality		30 mins	
13.3 How can we know whether we have HIV?	Map of HIV testing services	45 mins	
13.4 HIV testing for children		45 mins	**About 3.5 hrs**
13.5 The story of Martha and Mark		60 mins	
Closing circle (see p.14)		15 mins	
Exercises for caregivers only			
13.6 Fears and benefits of telling a child that they have HIV	Two prepared flipcharts	30 mins	**About 2.5 hrs**
13.7 How to tell a child that you or they have HIV		60 mins	
13.8 Providing emotional support after a child learns that you or they have HIV		45 mins	

Preparation

Exercise 13.3. Research where HIV testing services are locally available and at what cost, and make a map to show them.

Exercise 13.6. Write out the questions at points 3 and 4 onto two flipcharts.

Exercises 13.6 to 13.8 are for caregivers only. Please make appropriate arrangements with caregivers for the care of the children.

Box 13.a Information for facilitators

Be mindful that some caregivers and children in the group may have been tested for HIV and others not. Some may have been given the results and others not. Some may be anxious about testing themselves or their child, or feel worried about possible consequences, such as violence, loneliness, and rejection. Some may need help in telling their child that they or their child has HIV.

If any facilitators or participants are happy to be open about having an HIV test or talking about having HIV, it would be very helpful for others to talk with them, ask questions, and get support. Try to identify younger and older people who are comfortable talking about their experiences before you run this session. You could also involve people who aren't participants, such as members of an HIV support group. Explain to visitors that you would like them to contribute to the conversation while participants do the activities, rather than give a separate speech.

If participants feel any topic is not relevant to them, suggest they still engage with it to get better at helping others, or because they might be in this situation in the future.

EXERCISE 13.1 'PRRR' AND 'PUKUTU' GAME

AIM: To make everyone laugh and relax.

DESCRIPTION: Everyone stands in a circle and reacts to what is called out.

Directions

1. Say: 'Let's all stand in a circle. We are going to pretend to be two kinds of bird. If I call 'prrr', then you will stand on your tiptoes and wiggle your wings and your tail. If I call 'pukutu', then you will stand still!'

2. Make the two bird calls. After a few practice calls, explain that people who move when they shouldn't, or who stay still when they should move, have to drop out of the game. Everyone should have fun and clap the few people who are left in the circle at the end.

 ## EXERCISE 13.2 TALKING ABOUT HIV, TRUST, AND CONFIDENTIALITY

AIMS: To discuss how we feel about talking about HIV in our own lives, and agree on how we want to share information in our group.

DESCRIPTION: Each group discusses and decides how they want to organize themselves for the later exercises.

Directions

1. Explain: 'In the next exercises we are going to talk about the possible consequences of taking an HIV test, and of knowing whether we have HIV or not. We will also talk about how we can support each other in talking about the test results. These are issues that we need to think carefully about.'

2. Say: 'Remember that one of our virtues is *kindness*. How can we all use our kindness together today to talk about something which affects so many of us in the world?

'Let us remember that we are in different situations, with different feelings, but we are all here to support each other. None of us has to talk, inside or outside the group, about whether we or our child/caregiver have had an HIV test, nor about the result of the test, unless we want to. We will talk together about these issues, but make our own decisions about what to share and what not to share in relation to ourselves.'

3. Say: 'Let's get a sense of how we feel about this. Please close your eyes, and raise two hands if you feel comfortable talking about these issues; one hand if you are quite comfortable; and keep your hands down if you feel uncomfortable.'

Count the hands and then, with everyone's eyes open, tell the group how many people felt each way.

Ask: 'Does anyone want to talk about how they feel?'

'Does anyone have ideas about how we can help each other feel comfortable? For example, instead of talking about ourselves, we can talk about people like us.'

4. Say: 'Let's discuss how to handle confidentiality in these discussions. What are our suggestions for confidentiality within our own peer group? What about between our peer group and our child's/caregiver's peer group?'

Offer caregivers and their children a few minutes to agree privately on what to share about HIV testing and talking about results during the session.

5. Summarize what the participants have decided.

 ## EXERCISE 13.3 HOW CAN WE KNOW WHETHER WE HAVE HIV?

AIMS: To understand that an HIV test is the only way to know whether a person has HIV. To understand how the HIV test is done, and our rights regarding testing.

DESCRIPTION: Participants engage in a question and answer session.

Box 13.b Information for facilitators

Participants may have doubts about having an HIV test or testing their children. *Never* try to persuade people to have a test. Support them in understanding how the test works, and the benefits and challenges of having a test. We should all take as much time as we need to make our own decision, and be supported in whatever decision we make.

Please adapt questions and answers as needed for children's peer groups. Keep them simple and reassuring.

Directions

1. Say: 'Some illnesses have the same signs and symptoms as other diseases, and doctors can't tell them apart without testing the person's blood. HIV, malaria, and diabetes are like this. Also, some illnesses don't show any signs or symptoms at first, but can still harm our bodies and be passed on to other people. HIV is like this.

'Today we are going to talk about the test which shows whether we have HIV or not. For those of us who have already taken an HIV test and know our results, this exercise can help us to support our friends better if they are thinking of having a test.'

2. Ask participants to get into groups of four. Ask them to discuss: 'What questions do (did) we want to ask before we make (made) a decision about having an HIV test ourselves, or for our child?' Ask them to write their questions on slips of paper.

3. Using participants' questions, facilitate a question and answer session about the HIV test, so that people can learn from each other; you can add further information if necessary. You may

want to invite a resource person, such as an HIV support group member, an HIV counsellor, or a doctor, to help with this exercise. Make sure the topics in Box 13.c are covered.

Box 13.c Information about HIV testing

What are our rights regarding HIV testing?

We have the right to high-quality services for HIV testing. These are as follows:

- We decide whether to have an HIV test or not: it is *voluntary*. No one has the right to force us, or our children, to be tested. In most countries, caregivers need to give their *consent* for their child to have an HIV test, and the child gives their *assent* (agreement). Sometimes, older children can give their consent without their caregiver. Check the rules in your country.

- We have *counselling* before the test (to help us decide whether to have the test) and after the test (to help us cope with the results, whatever they may be, and get support). The counsellor should adapt how they work to suit us, especially when counselling children.

- We are offered support after testing, including *care and treatment* if we need it.

- The test and results are *kept secret* unless we say we are willing to tell others. No health worker should tell our partner, children, family, or colleagues about any of our health issues without our consent.

Quality services will help protect us from violence, blame, and stigma.

Where is testing available locally?

Facilitators should prepare a map of the area, showing HIV testing services. If possible, maps should also show other services such as counselling, home visiting, and treatment. Explain to participants where, when, and at what cost services are available. Point out which ones cater for children.

Who should have a test?

Anyone who wants to know whether they have HIV. We may particularly want to have a child tested for HIV if:

- either of the child's parents has HIV, is sick with AIDS-related illnesses, or has died of AIDS;

- a child is frequently sick, or has signs and symptoms of AIDS-related illness;

- a child is sexually active, or has been sexually abused;

- a child has been injecting drugs using unsterile needles, or has been cut using unsterile blades.

How is the test done?

- We should be counselled before the test about the possible result of the test; the meaning of a positive and negative result and how the result might affect us; what we will do if the test is positive or negative; whom we trust to share the result with; and what support we can get.

- We may have several sessions of counselling before we decide whether to have the test or not. We may have the test and decide not to go for the result. This is fine. We should only have the test and go for the result after we have had time to make an informed decision.

- If we have the test, a nurse takes a small amount of blood from a finger or vein in our arm. The blood is mixed with a liquid that changes colour if we have HIV antibodies in our blood.

What does an HIV test establish?

The HIV test is testing for antibodies to HIV. The body makes cells called antibodies to control any germs that enter the body. They are part of our immune system.

What does it mean if the test is positive?

If the test is positive it shows that we have antibodies to HIV. This means that HIV has got into our blood. We may be well, because HIV has not yet harmed our immune system. We may stay well for a long time without treatment, or start to get sick more often. Or we may already have signs of low immunity, such as frequent sickness and the illnesses associated with AIDS. Once it is known we have HIV, doctors monitor our health and our number of CD4 cells, and advise us when to start taking ARVs. These reduce the amount of HIV in our blood so we start to feel well again.

What does it mean if the test is negative?

A negative result usually means that we do not have HIV. However, it can mean that we have only recently acquired HIV and that our body has not yet produced the antibodies against HIV. This is called the window period. It is the time between when HIV enters the body, and when the test is able to detect the antibodies. It lasts for about three months. During the window period, we can have HIV in our blood and share it with others, even though the test shows negative. If someone has a negative result, but may have been in contact with HIV recently, they will be asked to retake the test in three months and avoid risky activities.

What does it mean if the test is inconclusive?

This means that the test result is not clear and we will be asked to repeat it.

How long does it take to get the results?

Some tests give the results on the spot. For others, clients have to wait and come back for the result. Provide information about the tests available in your locality.

What happens when we get the results?

The counsellor asks us if we are ready to receive the result and, if so, reminds us about the meaning of a positive and a negative result. The counsellor tells us the result, and gives us a chance to express our feelings and reactions to the news.
- If the result is negative, the counsellor supports us in making a plan to protect ourselves from HIV or, if necessary, to come back in three months for another test.
- If the result is positive, we may feel afraid, angry, or distressed, or we may feel relieved that we know what is the matter with us. All these feelings are OK and normal. The counsellor should support us in expressing these feelings, getting support and living positively. We can talk about what to do immediately, whom we might want to tell about the test result, and where to get practical and emotional support.

EXERCISE 13.4 HIV TESTING FOR CHILDREN

AIMS: To think and talk about the benefits and challenges of children having an HIV test. *For caregivers*. To think about and practise talking to a child about having an HIV test.

DESCRIPTION:
Caregivers. Participants make mind maps on fears and benefits linked to having an HIV test, and create role plays involving talking to a child about having an HIV test.

Children aged 5–8 and 9–14 years. Participants role play discussing the benefits and challenges of having an HIV test, and make a mind map.

Directions

Caregivers

1. Say: 'We are going to talk about our fears about, and the benefits of, HIV testing for our children. How shall we do this? Do you want to form small groups, or discuss in one big group?'

Ask: 'What do we fear about our children having an HIV test? What might happen?'

'What can we do to reduce these fears?'

'What are the benefits of our children having an HIV test? What can we do to make these benefits happen?'

2. Make mind maps showing positive things about having a test, and turn fears into positive things.

3. Invite anyone who is happy to share their own experience of having an HIV test, or of supporting their child in having an HIV test, to talk about it and answer questions. Share tips from Box 13.d as needed.

Box 13.d Tips for caregivers about talking to children about having an HIV test

- Explain to children how having an HIV test can help them and the family, and ask for their views and questions. If they feel that the test will help them, they will manage much better.

- Give information suitable for their age and level of understanding. Be attentive to how they respond and support them if they get upset.

- Be aware that secrecy around HIV can make children feel worried and fearful, and fear that they have been bad and that HIV is their fault. For children over 12 years old, especially, we encourage you to discuss HIV openly, so you can support them in understanding. The more normal you make HIV, the more your children will be able to feel normal about HIV.

- Many children fear having an HIV test because they believe that if they test positive, they will become very sick and die young; they are afraid they will be stigmatized and will not be able to study, work, marry, or have children.

---

4. Ask caregivers to form groups of six, if possible grouping those who have children of roughly the same age. Ask them to role play talking to a child of that age about having an HIV test.

Ask: 'What questions do you think a child may want to ask you before having an HIV test? What would you want to reply?'

Tell each group that one member needs to act as the child. They should try out different ways of talking to the child, and different responses, and work together until they feel pleased with their role play.

5. Come together, so that each group can show their role play to the other caregivers.

Separate peer groups of 5–8 and 9–14 year olds

1. Ask the children to form groups of five or six and to act out a role play where they are talking about the positive and negative points of having an HIV test. Some characters do not want a test; some think it's a good idea; and some are not sure.

2. Bring the groups together and ask them to use their ideas from the role plays to draw a mind map of all the positive and negative points about having an HIV test. Explore how the negative points could be made into positive points.

3. If a child in the group is open about having had an HIV test, invite them to share their experience.

 ## EXERCISE 13.5 THE STORY OF MARTHA AND MARK

AIMS: To understand the benefits of talking with children about caregivers or children having HIV, and good and supportive ways of doing this.

DESCRIPTION: Participants read a story and discuss questions.

Box 13.e Information for facilitators

Share as appropriate with participants.

Fears: reasons we may not wish to tell our child that we or they have HIV

We may:

- not feel ready; for example, if we have not accepted that we or our child has HIV;
- feel guilty or ashamed of having HIV (ask participants: 'Is this feeling reasonable?'), or worry that if we tell our child, they will feel unhappy, afraid, or angry;
- think that our child is not ready to cope with the news;
- think that our child will not understand;
- be afraid that our child will blame us;
- be afraid that our child will talk about having HIV at school or with neighbours, and that family and neighbours will be unkind or violent towards them and our family.

Benefits: reasons it is good to tell our child that we or they have HIV

- We can give our child correct information and make sure that they have understood it.
- We can share the news in a caring and loving way. If we don't tell them, they might find out in an unkind way, or when there is no one to help, support and comfort. They may not tell us and suffer in silence without help. Children can also feel resentful towards us for not telling them. They may self-harm and stop taking their ARVs.
- We will not have to keep secrets from the child. Keeping secrets is stressful. Children often guess or fear the reason why they or we have to take medicines every day. If we don't talk about it, they may feel that it is a terrible secret, or blame themselves.
- We want our child to trust us, and being open about something so important will strengthen that trust.
- Knowing they have been trusted with the truth can help children cope and encourage them to keep taking their ARVs as they grow into their teenage years. They can get full information and be involved in decisions about their health care.
- When they know, children can be important partners in managing treatment for themselves or family members with HIV. They may take their medication themselves, or remind us when it is time to take their medicine. They have strategies for keeping it a secret.
- We can help children understand and cope with possible discrimination against them.
- As children grow up with HIV, we can teach them how to keep healthy and manage their emerging sexuality safely.
- Children can meet and make friends with other children who have the same experiences. They can then support each other and know they are not alone.
- Children have the right to know important information about their own bodies and lives when they are old enough.
- A relationship of openness, caring, and sharing between a child and their caregiver can make both your lives easier and happier in many ways.

Directions[44]

1. Explain that we are going to read a story in five parts. It's about Martha, a caregiver who has HIV, and her son Mark. Please adapt the story as needed for the peer group you are working with.

2. If appropriate, invite members of the group to read the story aloud. After each part, read out the questions and discuss what happened.

Box 13.f Martha and Mark: Part 1

Martha finds life a struggle. Her husband died two years ago from an illness related to AIDS. She is bringing up her four children by herself. She often feels tired and sick. Last month she had an HIV test and found out that she has HIV. She worries about how she will find enough money to feed the children and send them to school. She does not feel ready to tell them that she has HIV, but wishes that her eldest son Mark, who is 12 years old, was more understanding. He is always asking for money for school stuff and sometimes gets angry when there is no food ready after school. Martha sometimes thinks it would be

---

good if she told him that she has HIV. He would help her more and let her rest. The health worker says that she needs to rest and eat more to take her ARVs safely.

Mark is also anxious. He is afraid that his mother might have HIV. She seems so tired and is often sick. He sees her hiding pills and taking them when she thinks he's not looking. He thinks his father died of an AIDS-related illness. How would he and his siblings cope if his mother was not there? How would he look after them all? Might he or his siblings also have HIV? He wishes he could talk to his mother about his feelings. Sometimes he feels bad because he gets angry and doesn't help his mother on the farm. He wishes that he and his mother could talk openly about what is really happening in their lives.

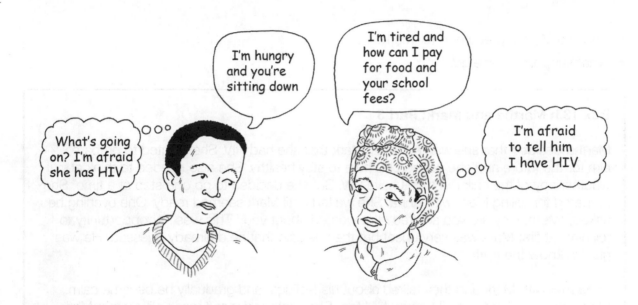

- What is Martha worried about?
- What is Mark worried about?
- Why would Martha not want to tell Mark that she has HIV?
- Why might Mark want to know whether his mother has HIV?
- What would be the advantages for Martha and Mark of talking openly?
- Are there any disadvantages to talking openly?
- What kind of support does Martha need?
- What kind of support does Mark need?
- How could Mark find out if he or any of his siblings have HIV?

Box 13.g Martha and Mark: Part 2

Martha heard that there were some women in her community who had formed a support group for women with HIV. Because the women in the group talked openly about having HIV, they were able to support and advise each other and seek medical help openly. Martha went to visit Anna, the group leader. Anna invited Martha to come to some meetings to help her decide whether she wanted to tell Mark and her family about her HIV or not. There were many consequences to think about, but she could choose who she wanted to tell, if anybody.

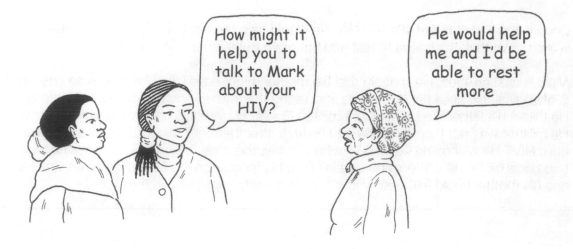

- How did Martha prepare to tell Mark?
- What support did she get?

Box 13.h Martha and Mark: Part 3

Martha decided that she wanted to tell Mark that she had HIV. She wanted to prepare him for the future and she needed his help to stay healthy. She also needed to think about whether any of the children might have HIV. But she decided to go one step at a time. She prepared for telling Mark with Anna. She waited until Mark seemed ready. One evening he asked, 'Mum, why are you so tired? I'm worried about you.' This was her opportunity to tell him. At first Mark was very upset but then he said that he'd already guessed. He was glad to know the truth.

Anna met with Mark and they talked about his feelings, and gradually he became calm. Mark then decided to ask if he had HIV too. She explained that it was unlikely that Mark had HIV, as he was 12 years old and rarely ill. Anna also had a son of her own, John, aged 14. She asked Mark if he would like to meet up with John. Mark agreed and met and talked with John also. Mark was surprised that he recognized John from school. They played football together, which felt great.

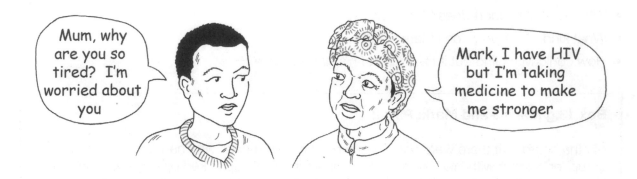

- What did Mark do well when he asked Martha?
- How did Mark react when Martha told him that she has HIV?
- What support did Mark need to help him become calm?

Box 13.i Martha and Mark: Part 4

It is now a few months later. Martha's health is much improved. She is more relaxed because she is no longer trying to keep her HIV a secret. She goes to meetings with other women, which encourages her. The women support each other in getting treatment at the health centre. Mark is also now calm and feels happy that his mother decided to trust in him. He helps his mother on the farm so that they can eat healthy food. Mark also gets the younger children to help more about the house, so his mother can rest. He talks with his mother a lot. He also sees John regularly outside school. Mark is glad to see his mum looking so much healthier and happier.

Martha is writing a memory book so that she and Mark can record past memories and plan for the future. She has written a will so that Mark will know about his inheritance. But for now, Martha feels very positive. She is getting stronger day by day, and Mark is feeling happier too because they can share their concerns and their minds are at ease. He also knows that John understands too and is his friend. There is song and laughter again in the house.

- How does Mark help Martha now?
- Do you think Martha was right to tell Mark? Why? Why not?
- What are the advantages and disadvantages of talking openly about HIV in the family?

Box 13.j Martha and Mark: Part 5

Mark is worried that he or his siblings might have HIV. He talks to his mother about his worries.

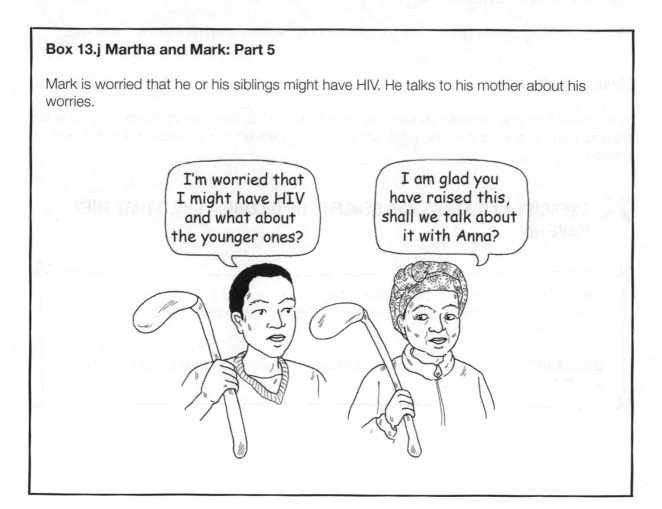

3. Invite participants to continue the story: 'What happens next?'

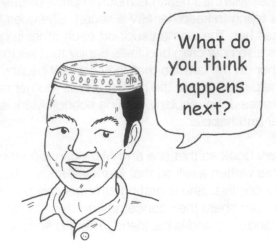

What do you think happens next?

4. Explain to participants: 'This same story is being shared with all three peer groups at present. Maybe you would all like to reflect on this story over the coming days, and see if you think it might help anyone you know?'

This will give participants time and space to reflect on the story and link it to their own lives.

Closing circle

If caregivers continue immediately with exercises 13.6 to 13.8, they can do the closing circle at the end. Remind everyone to bring their ability-spotting necklaces from Session 1 to the next session.

 EXERCISE 13.6 FEARS AND BENEFITS OF TELLING A CHILD THAT THEY HAVE HIV

AIMS: To explore fears and benefits relating to telling a child that they have HIV. To share positive experiences of talking about having HIV and ways of overcoming challenges.

DESCRIPTION: Caregivers discuss questions on fears about, and benefits of, telling a child that they have HIV.

Box 13.k Information for facilitators

Your role as a facilitator is to create a safe place for participants to talk about the subject, where everyone feels safe and their confidentiality is respected.

Please note the following:

- Telling children that they have HIV is a very important and personal decision.
- There is no 'right' way for everyone. It is each person's choice.
- Telling children that they have HIV is something you can't undo.
- We can't control whom children tell that they have HIV, once they are informed.
- We can't be sure that children won't find out from someone else.
- Sometimes it makes sense not to tell children because the circumstances are not right.

Remember that a child who tests negative for HIV, but who has other family members with HIV, also needs love and support. They may feel guilty for not having HIV and may somehow feel that they are to blame.

Directions

1. Explain: 'Some caregivers see the benefit of having their child take an HIV test, but think that it is best not to tell the child the results. We are going to talk about our feelings about telling a child that they have HIV. This is a sensitive issue and we will support each other, remembering what we have agreed about confidentiality.'

2. Appreciate or introduce anyone in, or visiting, the group, who is open about having HIV or caring for a child with HIV. Warmly invite them to support others by sharing their experiences.

3. Ask participants to move into groups of five. Ask each group to discuss these questions (which you have previously written on a flipchart, see 'Preparation'), using their own experience if they wish:

- What do we fear might happen if we tell our child that they have HIV?
- How can we lessen the chance that the things we fear will happen?
- How will we support our child in coping with the big feelings that are common when they learn that they have HIV?
- When might *not* telling the child that they have HIV be the best option?

4. Ask the groups to discuss who would benefit from telling a child about their HIV status. Put up a flipchart showing the following questions, and ask them to make a mind map:

- How could it be helpful and positive for *the child* to be told that they have HIV?
- How could it be helpful and positive *for us* to choose to tell our child about their HIV status?
- How could it be helpful and positive for the child's *family and friends*?
- How could it be helpful and positive for the *community*?
- In what ways do different parts of this mind map join up?

EXERCISE 13.7 HOW TO TELL A CHILD THAT YOU OR THEY HAVE HIV

AIMS: To recognize and develop abilities in caregivers to tell children that they have HIV, or that the child has HIV. To enable caregivers to make informed, responsible decisions about whether to tell their child that they or their child have HIV, and if so when, where, and how.

DESCRIPTION: Caregivers do ability spotting.

Directions[45]

1. Explain: 'We are going to get into groups of three to look for abilities and skills that will help us tell a child that we have HIV, or they have HIV. For 10 minutes, one of you will be the storyteller, one the interviewer, and one the observer. We will swap roles, so you each play each role. None of us has to share stories about HIV; we can talk about doing other things that took courage.'

2. Say: 'I invite each of you, when you are the *storyteller*, to tell about your experiences of one of the following situations:
- telling a child or children that you have HIV;
- telling a child that they have HIV;
- deciding actively that you would not tell your child that you or they have HIV;
- telling another person that you have HIV;
- listening to someone who told you that they have HIV;
- telling someone some difficult news;
- telling someone something that took a lot of courage and strength.'

3. Add this option if you think it would be useful: 'Would anyone like to form a group of three with others to focus on a certain situation? Otherwise, we can just form the groups of three, and see what stories emerge.'

4. Once the groups are formed, ask the *interviewers* to use the helper questions (who, what, where, when, how ...) to understand the situation and expand the story.

Ask them to question what the person was thinking about before telling someone something challenging, such as having HIV. They could ask:
- 'What did you see as the advantages and disadvantages?'
- 'Who did you talk about it with?'
- 'How, when, and where did you tell the child?'
- 'How did the conversation go when you told your child?'

5. Say to the groups: 'Some of your stories will be positive, and some may be difficult and painful. With difficult stories, please focus on how the person coped with the difficulties and the strengths they showed, rather than the pain. Let's focus on what worked well and what we can all learn from the stories.'

6. If a person has actively decided not to tell their child, the interviewer should support them in talking about what stopped them and appreciate their abilities. For example, they might

recognize that the caregiver was insightful, and responsible for the feelings of their child and their safety in a family or community that treats people with HIV badly.

7. Ask the *observer* to spot the skills, abilities, and strengths, and to write them down for the necklace; for example, courage, sensitivity, confidence, competence, sense of humour, kindness, generosity. The *interviewer* may also mention these; for example, 'That showed quick thinking!'

8. Ask the groups to do their first round; then to switch roles and repeat; then to switch for the final time. Explain that you will clap your hands after 10 minutes and that is when people should switch roles.

9. After everyone has played each role, ask participants to stay in their small groups. Invite one or two people, who feel comfortable about sharing their story, to share their abilities and strategies with the whole group.

10. Summarize by asking for the main ideas that have emerged about telling children that you have HIV or they have HIV: how to do it, where to do it, and when to do it.

11. As needed, add information from Box 13.I.

Box 13.I Tips for telling your child that they have HIV[46]

Adapt as needed for telling your child that you have HIV.

1. Prepare your child by giving them information in small chunks. Start off with simple information about viruses and how the immune system protects us against diseases.

2. Choose a time and place where you will not be rushed or disturbed. Make sure that the child cannot run into the street, or get lost if they are upset.

3. Tell someone whom the child likes and trusts what you plan to do, and ask them to be available.

4. Be prepared with the basic facts: how HIV is transmitted; the difference between HIV and AIDS; and how support, care, and treatment can keep people well for many years.

5. Reassure them that they are/can be well, and can do all the things that other people do.

6. Try not to make it a big thing. Say something along the lines of: 'You have HIV, it's a virus that makes your immune system weak, so it is harder to fight off infections. When you need to, you can take medicines that make your immune system strong again, so you can do the same things as other people.'

7. Ask them to tell you any questions they may have, at any time. Find out the answers to questions you are not sure about.

8. Explain why it is important to think about who to tell about having HIV. It is not a secret; just personal information that is best kept with trusted family members, friends, and health workers, because some people may not understand.

9. Tell them about other family members or friends who know that they have HIV and who would be happy to talk with them about it.

10. Link them in with support from a local HIV support group and counsellor.

EXERCISE 13.8 PROVIDING EMOTIONAL SUPPORT AFTER A CHILD LEARNS THAT YOU OR THEY HAVE HIV

AIM: To be prepared to support a child who learns that you or they have HIV.

DESCRIPTION: Caregivers discuss and practise supporting a child who learns that their caregiver or they have HIV.

Directions

1. Say: 'Whether we talk to our child about having HIV, or they find this out from someone else, we need to be prepared to support them emotionally.'

Ask participants: 'What feelings might a child have after learning that they or their caregiver has HIV? How might they behave?'

If needed, add information from Box 13.m.

Box 13.m Children's reactions to learning that they or their caregiver has HIV

A child might:
- say nothing and be quiet and withdrawn;
- be upset, with tears and wailing;
- show anger towards caregivers or other family members;
- refuse to speak to caregivers;
- act as if nothing has happened;
- be anxious, concerned, and not leave their caregiver's side;
- show a need for comfort;
- be relieved that they know what is happening and that the caregiver has trusted them enough to tell them the truth;
- ask lots of questions.

---

2. Ask: 'What questions might a child ask after being told that they have HIV?'

Participants might say:
- Do I have HIV or AIDS?
- Can I be cured?
- Will I be healthy?
- Will I grow up?
- Can I study?
- Can I work?
- 'Can I have a boy or girl friend?
- Can I get married?
- Can I have HIV-free children?

At a *Stepping Stones with Children* workshop, a boy asked his caregiver: 'Do I have HIV or AIDS?' His caregiver replied: 'You have HIV, because you are taking your ARVs so well, and that keeps you happy and healthy.' The boy responded, 'OK, that's fine then.'

3. Ask: 'How can we support our children emotionally to accept that they have HIV and live well with it?' If needed, add information from Box 13.n.

Box 13.n: Tips for supporting children emotionally

- Try to stay calm and on your hub.
- Be available to talk about the issue frequently, and to repeat the same information.
- Give a lot of love and praise to reassure children that they have support, and to raise their self-compassion.
- Read their body language and listen to what they say, so you can use your mindsight skills to understand how they are feeling. First use your virtues of compassion and empathy to help them cope with the feelings that may be overwhelming them.
- Then help them to think about what is happening in a calmer way.
- Talk about the situation positively to help children to lay down positive memories of what happened which will help them cope with the situation. Point out how strong and brave children have been; how many people are living well with HIV; and how medicine, when our bodies need it, can keep us healthy, even with HIV.
- Talk about how your child will probably live for a long time. With medicines, your child can get married and have their own children free of HIV.

If the child found out from someone else

- Check what they think they know or have found out. Give them correct information as needed. Tell the truth.
- Explain why you did not tell them earlier. For example, 'I didn't want to put a burden on you, but now I know you are becoming so mature and wise, we will use our courage and strength to cope with this together.' If appropriate, apologize: 'I'm sorry you are hurt. I did what I thought was best.'

4. Ask participants to divide into threes. Explain that each group member will have a turn at role playing a caregiver, a child, and an observer (who gives feedback to the caregiver). Ask the groups to think of situations in which a child responds in different ways to learning that they have HIV. Ask each person to imagine individually that they are this child, and to think about how they might feel and behave when they learn that they have HIV.

Invite one person to play the child they have imagined, one person to play the caregiver, and the other the observer. The caregiver connects with the child and helps them tell a positive story and think about a positive future. The child and the observer give feedback to the caregiver about what they did that was helpful and their suggestions. The group members take it in turns to play these roles with their imagined children.

5. When the groups have finished the role plays, invite them to share what they have learned from the activity with the wider group.

6. Remind participants of Exercise 2.9 'Getting back on our hub'.

Purpose: To support caregivers and children in keeping healthy and living well with HIV, including keeping clean, eating well, managing stress, and taking medicines correctly.

Contents	Materials required	Time required
Opening circle (see p.13)		15 mins
14.1 Game, dance, or song		15 mins
14.2 Keeping healthy	Ability necklaces	30 mins
14.3 Safety in the house	'Chain of HIV transmission' picture from Session 12, chalk, at least four puppets or toy figures	60 mins
14.4 Keeping clean		30 mins
14.5 Eating well		60 mins
14.6 How to manage stress		60 mins
14.7 Taking medicines correctly		45 mins
Closing circle (see p.14)		15 mins

About 5.5 hrs

Preparation

Exercise 14.2. Find out which local treatments and prophylaxis are offered to children and adults in your area.

Exercise 14.3. Make sure you know how HIV is, and is not, shared between people (see Exercise 12.3).

Exercise 14.7. Choose which story to use with 5–8 year olds. Find out when people with HIV are started on ARVs in your country.

Box 14.a Information for facilitators

Session 14 contains very important information and support for participants who are living with HIV and/or caring for a child or caregiver with HIV. It is essential to do Sessions 12 and 13 before doing this session, because those sessions provide essential information about HIV. They also enable participants to become comfortable with the idea that some, or all, caregivers and children may have HIV, and that it is equally fine to be open about this or to keep this knowledge confidential.

Note that we will learn more about using the health service in Session 15.

 EXERCISE 14.1 GAME, DANCE, OR SONG

Invite participants to choose a local game, song, or dance, which you can all do together, to give the session a lively and fun start.

EXERCISE 14.2 KEEPING HEALTHY

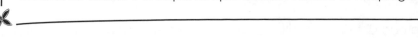

AIM: To understand how to strengthen the immune system and what actions to take to keep healthy.

DESCRIPTION: Participants spot abilities related to keeping healthy.

Directions

1. Explain: 'In this session we will talk about what actions to take to keep healthy, for example, to protect ourselves and other people from illnesses caused by germs. This is important for us all, but particularly for those of us with HIV, because our immunity may be weak and illnesses allow HIV to multiply in our bodies. For all of us, illness makes the immune system work harder and it takes time for it to recover. This can set off a downward cycle – we may feel better, but if our immune system is still weakened, our body is more vulnerable to germs. If we get sick again before our immune system has fully recovered, the illness is usually more serious and recovery takes longer.'

2. Ask: 'What ways do we know of strengthening our immune systems and keeping healthy?' As needed, add information from Box 14.b.

Box 14.b Ways in which caregivers and children can work together to strengthen their immune systems

- We can try to keep ourselves and our home extra clean.
- We can try to eat healthy food, frequently during the day.
- We can try to get enough sleep (at least 7–8 hours) and rest every day.
- We can try to do moderate amounts of physical work and exercise every day, as this strengthens the immune system. However, too much can weaken it. We can dance, play sport, and walk together, but we shouldn't feel exhausted from it.
- We can go to the best clinic or doctor that we can get to, for regular check-ups.
- We can go straight to the clinic or doctor for treatment if we are ill.
- If the medicine does not help within a few days, we can go back to the clinic – there may be other medicine that will help.

In addition, if we have HIV:

- We can get the usual immunizations except for live vaccines, for example, polio and yellow fever.
- We might be given vitamin A injections twice a year and multivitamin drops to take daily, though these are not necessary if we have a good diet.
- We might be given Co-trimoxazole (Bactrim) if our CD4 count is low. This helps prevent chest infections and malaria. This drug is dangerous during pregnancy.
- We can ask for painkillers if we are uncomfortable or in pain.

Note to facilitators: adapt the above information to the local treatments and prophylaxis available for children and adults in your area.

---

3. Invite participants to pair up and interview each other about what they do to keep healthy, or to support their child in keeping healthy. Ask them to spot abilities and put them on their ability-spotting necklace.

For children. Ask: 'What actions are you taking to strengthen your immune system and to keep healthy?'

For caregivers. Ask: 'What actions are you taking to support your child in having a strong immune system and keeping healthy?'

4. Facilitate the whole peer group drawing or writing their actions on a mind map. Ask: 'What more would you like to do from now on?' Draw or write the new actions in a different colour.#

Explore how different parts of the mind map link up. Put the mind map on the wall to share with other peer groups later.

5. Summarize and explain that in the next exercises, we will look in more detail at emotional health, protecting the household from HIV and other germs, keeping clean, eating well, managing stress, and taking medicine correctly.

✿ EXERCISE 14.3 SAFETY IN THE HOUSE

AIMS: To support caregivers, children, and members of the household in understanding how HIV might be transmitted in the household. To reduce their fears about transmission. To learn what we can all do to protect one another.

DESCRIPTION: Participants talk about fears of HIV transmission, map houses and fears, assess safety, and find ways of making activities safer.

Directions

1. Explain: 'Despite our knowledge of how HIV is and isn't shared, it's not unusual for us to worry about transmitting HIV through everyday activities (not sex) in the house. We may stop doing things which are safe, because we fear that we will give HIV to another person or that they will give it to us. As one mother said:

> "Sometimes my son comes and puts his mouth on mine. I told him not to do that. I can't kiss him or share spoons, as I did with my other children when I didn't know I had HIV. With him, I often look at my hands to see that I have no wounds before I touch him."[47]

'In this exercise, we will talk about our fears, like this mother's, and use our knowledge from Session 12 to see whether they are grounded in reality. If they are not, we can let go of those fears.'

 Explain that you would like to learn how much this exercise helps participants feel safe, by finding out how safe they feel now about living with someone who has HIV. We will use our 'fingers up' method, and ask the same question again at the end of the workshop. Ask participants to sit in a circle facing outwards, or to cover their eyes. Say: 'On a scale of 1 to 5, how safe would you feel if you were living with someone who has HIV?' Explain that 1 is not safe at all, 2 is a little safe, 3 is quite safe, 4 is safe, and 5 is very safe. Ask participants to show their answer with their fingers and thumb. Record each number in your Facilitator's Journal.

2. Use chalk to draw a map of a typical house on the floor, and label all the rooms and outside space. Make it big enough for the participants to walk around the different rooms and spaces.

3. Invite participants to think quietly about their own fears of HIV transmission in their home. These fears may be both about sharing HIV and getting it.

4. *For children.* Show some toy figures or puppets, and ask the children to give them characters in an imaginary family. Include a child with HIV, a caregiver with HIV, a child who does not have HIV, and an adult who has not been tested for HIV. Hand out the figures or puppets to the children (they will all get a turn to hold one and role play its character).

Invite all the children to walk with you into a room in the house. Ask them to talk about and act out how, in this room, the puppets might pass HIV on to another person (except through sex), and how they might get germs from others to make them sick. Write each idea down on a separate piece of paper and lay it on the floor. Do this for every room and space, with the children taking it in turns to hold the puppets.

For caregivers. Invite participants to walk around the house, stopping in each room or space to think of any fears they have about the transmission of HIV in that space. Ask them to say their fears out loud, while someone draws or writes each fear on a separate piece of paper and puts them on the floor. For example, if someone fears sharing or getting HIV through blood in the toilet, write 'blood in toilet' and put it in the space which represents the toilet or latrine.

5. Ask everyone to stand outside the house plan, and to look at how many slips of paper there are. Now remind them how HIV needs quality, quantity, and a route for it to be shared. Put up the picture showing the chain of HIV transmission and invite people to explain what it means. Say: 'We are now going to use our knowledge to think about how HIV may and may not be transmitted in our household, and what we can do to make sure that we are all safe.'

6. Repeat the walk around the house, and get the participants to assess each concern in turn. Support them in thinking about the quality and quantity of HIV, and if it has a route of transmission, to decide: 'Is this action safe, mostly safe or unsafe?'
- If the activity is safe, ask someone to rip up the paper and throw it into the air. It is something we don't need to worry about!
- If the activity is unsafe or mostly safe, ask: 'How can we make it safer?' Write the safer way on paper in another colour, and place it over the first piece of paper. The children can use the puppets to act out the safer way of behaving.

7. Repeat this in all the rooms and spaces. There is no need to repeat activities that might happen in more than one room or space.

8. Ask everyone to stand outside the house to see how many pieces of paper remain.

Ask: 'How are your feelings and thoughts about HIV in your house now? What has changed, if anything?'

If some participants are still feeling anxious, explain the following as needed.
- The next exercise is about cleanliness, and this may help them feel less anxious.
- Our main concern for caregivers and children with HIV is not that they will share HIV with others (as that's hard to do), but that they need protecting from germs. There are lots of germs around; they are much easier to share and get than HIV is, and they can make people living with HIV sick.

- In Exercise 14.7 we will learn about taking medicine correctly. If people are able to take their ARVs correctly and the ARVs work well, the quantity of HIV in their body fluids falls so low that they cannot share it with another person.

9. Invite everyone to close their eyes and listen to their breathing. Ask them to imagine a peaceful place where they have no worries.

10. Ask them to imagine their bodies with plenty of CD4 cells on the alert to deal with any germs which come near or into their bodies.

11. Invite people to say together: 'If I can teach one person something about HIV, I will have done well.'

 EXERCISE 14.4 KEEPING CLEAN

AIMS: To understand the importance of cleanliness for everyone, including people with HIV. To be motivated to keep ourselves, our homes, and our environment clean, and to know how to do this.

DESCRIPTION: This exercise builds on the previous exercise on safety in the home: participants add ideas to the house maps drawn in that exercise, and tell stories: 'We can be clean'.

Directions[48]

1. Explain that in this exercise we will talk about cleanliness of ourselves, our home, and our environment.

2. Ask: 'Why is it important for people with HIV and those around us to be extra clean?'

Share ideas and as needed, add information from Box 14.c.

Box 14.c The importance of cleanliness for those with HIV

There are many different germs in our bodies and all around us. Usually we are not aware of them because our CD4 cells control them and stop them harming us. When a member of our family with HIV has a low CD4 count, and is not on ARVs, they may have low immunity. This means that germs can more easily attack them and make them sick. They get sick more frequently, and more severely, than people with strong immune systems. It takes them longer to get better. So everyone needs to be extra careful about cleanliness to reduce the harmful germs as much as possible.

---

3. Draw a picture of the body and talk about the places that we need to keep very clean.

For children. You can make this more fun and reinforce the actions by acting each one out, for example, 'Let's all pretend we are scrubbing our hands! Let's get them nice and soapy. Goodbye germs!'

As needed, add information from Box 14.d.

Box 14.d How to keep our bodies clean

Protect the skin and it will protect you. Keep skin clean and free from cuts and rashes, so it keeps out germs. You can use skin cream to make your skin feel lovely and soft again if it is dry.

Cleaning our hands. Wash hands with soap often, especially before cooking, before eating, after using the toilet, and after handling dirty items. If you don't have any soap, scrub the hands well with clean water and rinse well by pouring water over them. If you have no soap, it is best to use running water if you can, as using still water in a basin, or cloths, can spread germs.

Cleaning our fingernails. Keep fingernails clean and short. Take care not to damage the skin under the nails. Wash clippers in hot soapy water.

Checking our mouths and throats. Check every day, when you brush your teeth. White patches in the mouth or throat are thrush, and need to be treated at once with medicine.

Cleaning our mouths. Drink clean water after any milk or sugary drink because germs can grow if these drinks stay in the mouth.

Protecting our teeth. Brush teeth twice a day after meals. Use fluoride toothpaste or tablets. Every member of the family should have their own tooth stick or toothbrush, and should *only* use their own one. Limit sugary foods, like sweets, because they can make teeth decay.

4. Go back to the plan of the house and outside spaces, and discuss which places need to be kept very clean. As needed, add information from Box 14.e.

Box 14.e How to keep our homes clean

We all make dirt, create rubbish, and have germs in our bodies – this is normal. We just need regular routines to keep germs under our control. We can control germs with high and low temperatures; with water, bleach and soap; and by drying out the moist places in which they multiply.

In the latrine. Faeces contain many germs, which can cause diarrhoea and vomiting. Put them in a latrine, flush them down the toilet, or bury them deep so nothing can dig them up.

In the bathroom. Germs love damp and dirty cloths. Give each person their own cloth or towel to use. Wash these every week and, if possible, hang them in the sun each day to dry.

In the kitchen.
- Wash hands before preparing food.
- Rinse vegetables and fruit with clean water before eating.
- Cover any cooked food that you are storing for later – store in a cool, dry place.
- Reheat food until it is bubbling hot (just warming food may not kill germs).
- Add a tablespoon of bleach to the water when washing dishes and wiping your kitchen surfaces.

- Let dishes drip dry rather than drying them with a cloth.
- Boil dishcloths, or wash them very well, and hang them in the sun to dry.

Drinking water. If the water does not come from a borehole or safe tap, either boil it for one minute, or add bleach as instructed on the bottle, or put it in a clear bottle in the sun all day to kill germs. Cover water to stop dirt getting into it.

Cleaning up blood spills. All blood can carry germs and viruses, most of which are much easier to get than HIV. Blood may also be found in diarrhoea or urine. It is good practice to:
- wash away blood spilled on the floor with bleach or hot soapy water, or cover it with sand.
- protect your hands with rubber gloves or plastic bags if touching blood or any body fluids. Cover any broken skin, such as sores, with plasters. Wash hands thoroughly with soap afterwards.
- rinse any cloth that has blood on it (for example, sanitary cloths) in very hot soapy water or water with bleach in it, and soak overnight. If you are throwing them away, put them in the pit latrine, bury them deep, or burn them.

5. Ask participants to imagine a very clean house, where the household members have worked together to keep dangerous germs safely inside a bin with a tight lid. Then say: 'Let's imagine ourselves feeling freshly clean and washed, with clean hands and clean bodies.'

Invite participants to say together: 'May we all be safe in our clean homes, with our clean families, because we can overcome the germs together.'

 EXERCISE 14.5 EATING WELL

AIMS: To understand how to eat to keep the body healthy and our immune systems strong. To understand how to feed a sick child.

DESCRIPTION: Drawing foods, and sorting foods according to their nutrients, seasonality, cost, and pleasure. Participants create dishes and snacks for caregivers and children with HIV and those on ARVs. They share ideas on helping sick children or children on ARVs to eat.

Directions

1. Explain that in this exercise we will look at how what we eat affects our immune systems and health. Give each person three or four pieces of paper and something to draw with. Ask them to draw one item of food (something they eat in their community) on each piece of paper.

2. Lay a piece of flipchart paper on the floor and divide it into quarters. Using information from Box 14.f, put one of the food-type headings in each quarter. Explain what each of them does, and give examples.

Box 14.f Foods for a healthy diet

Carbohydrates

These are the main food for *energy*. These staple foods are quite easy to digest. The healthiest kinds are 'unrefined', such as brown rice and brown bread. This means that the outer husk of the grain is included, which is good for us. This group includes rice, maize, millet, wheat, sorghum, bread, yam, cassava, and potatoes.

Proteins

These help us *grow* and develop strong bodies, keep our immune systems strong, and repair our bodies after illness. This group includes certain plant foods such as cereals (wheat, rice, millet, maize, and sorghum) and legumes and nuts (beans, seeds, peas, lentils, soybeans, and groundnuts); and animal foods such as eggs, milk, cheese, yoghurt, fish, chicken, insects, meat, liver, and snails.

Vitamins and minerals

These are things in foods that support our bodies in *keeping healthy* and overcoming diseases. We can get different vitamins and minerals by eating lots of different *fruits* and *vegetables*. Foods that are particularly helpful for people with HIV and HIV-related illnesses include: spinach and other dark green leafy vegetables, squash, carrots, green beans, okra, tomatoes, oranges, papaya, mango, bananas, shea-nut fruit, guavas, and baobab fruit.

Fats

These give us *extra energy* and also help the body absorb nutrients from other food. People living with HIV may have to eat fats a little at a time because they can cause diarrhoea, but they are still important for energy. Seeds and nuts contain healthy fat. Avocado is the only fruit which contains fat as well as protein and vitamins. Oil, butter, margarine, whole milk, and fatty meat are also rich in fats.

3. Invite participants to put one of their pictures in one of the segments, and explain why they put it there.

4. Ask them to use the food pictures to show meals or snacks that people like them might have eaten this week.

For each meal or snack, ask: 'What nutrients does this dish or snack contain?'

'What foods could you add to it which would make it more complete?'

5. If there are no foods available to complete the dish, discuss how participants could grow or obtain them. For example, if there are no vegetables in the dry season, how could they grow them? Are there any fruits available at that time?

6. Invite participants to lay out the dishes and snacks they might eat in one day.

Ask: 'Are there any foods from the food groups which are missing from these meals and snacks for the day? What are they? How could they be added?'

7. Ask participants to think about how they feel when they are hungry.

Then ask: 'When you are sick, do you feel like eating? What might encourage you to eat more when you are sick?'

8. Ask: 'How can we support sick children in eating enough food to get better?' Bring together everyone's ideas in a mind map. Explore how different parts of the mind map link up. As needed, add ideas from Box 14.g.

Box 14.g Encouraging a sick child to eat

Children need to eat, even if they don't feel like it, to keep up the level of sugar in their blood. If they get too hungry, the level drops and they can get upset or angry. They are not being naughty; they just need a snack to raise their blood sugar levels and calm them down. Dates, raisins, or other fruits are good sources of natural fruit sugar.

Children who are not well often do not feel hungry, but need to be persuaded to eat. Losing weight and getting thin is one of the biggest problems for a child living with HIV. Here are some ideas to try.

- Give food that the child likes, and try to make it look and taste good.
- Let them eat small meals, often, and rest after eating.
- Encourage and praise them when they eat.
- Give them fluid between meals, not with meals.
- Make mealtimes a pleasant and friendly time for the child by eating with them. Having other children to eat with may help a sick child enjoy the meal and want to eat.
- If the child is eating alone, tell stories, sing songs, and play games.
- When children are not hungry and refuse to eat, make sure they drink more during the day, especially a nutrient-rich drink such as sour milk, milk, yoghurt, custard made with milk, or soup.

If sores in the mouth make it painful for a child to eat:

- give paracetamol half an hour before eating to reduce the pain;
- give soothing drinks such as milk, yoghurt, and thin porridge;
- avoid sour foods like orange juice, tomatoes, and spinach;
- give soft and mashed food, as it is easier to eat;
- give food that is warm but not too hot;
- give cold foods such as ice cream, lollies, or ice made from clean water to suck;
- give plain food without salt, spices or chilli, which will make the pain worse;
- help children to feed themselves – cut food up small, thicken porridge, or give them a smaller spoon – and help the child more than you would normally.

If the child feels as if they may vomit, or is vomiting:

- cold foods might be better than warm foods;
- dry toast, crackers, or rusks can help to relieve nausea;
- try giving bread, thick porridge, or plain rice, without gravy;
- give extra fluids to replace losses from diarrhoea and vomiting;
- give sugar/salt solution ('oral rehydration salts') to stop children getting dried out (dissolve 1 teaspoon of salt and 1 tablespoon of sugar in 1 litre of warm water, wait for it to cool and encourage the child to take sips of it little and often);
- do not give food that is too sweet or too fatty, nor tea, coffee, milk, milk products, or spicy foods, until the child has stopped vomiting or feeling nauseous.

EXERCISE 14.6 HOW TO MANAGE STRESS

AIMS: To understand what stress is, and its effects. To identify the causes of stress in our own lives. To try out different ways of becoming more relaxed and peaceful.

DESCRIPTION: Children explore stress through a child's story; caregivers play the SIFT game and draw a flow chart. All peer groups practise different ways of reducing stress.

Directions

For children

1. Read Ama's story.

Box 14.h The story of Ama

Ama is 13 years old. Her mother has HIV, but she is on ARVs and she is strong. Ama's father has gone away. Ama is helping to care for her three brothers and sister while her mother is away on the farm. Everyone helps with the planting and weeding. The food in the store is almost finished and the price of food is increasing. The rains have brought malaria, and her little sister has a fever. Ama hopes to go to secondary school. It is time for exams and paying fees. If her mother doesn't pay her fees she will be thrown out of school.

Ama wakes in the night and thinks about all their problems. Her heart beats fast and she shakes. Sometimes she has bad dreams that her mother is dead, they have no food or money, and the children are hungry. She finds herself shouting at the little ones and slapping them. They are shocked; she is usually so kind. Why is their sister behaving like this?

---

2. After reading the story, ask: 'What is Ama suffering from?'

As needed, add information from Box 14.i.

Box 14.i What is stress and how does it affect us?

If we feel so anxious that it gets in the way of our everyday life, we are said to be suffering from stress.

Stress affects us in different ways. It can make us feel tired, miserable, bad-tempered, angry, and tearful. It can lead to panic attacks, not being able to sleep, depression, and physical problems such as migraine, asthma and eczema.

Over a long time, stress weakens our immune system. We may also be more vulnerable to negative influences, for example, using alcohol to cheer ourselves up, or allowing others to bully us or behave violently towards us because we feel overwhelmed by the thought of challenging them.

Caregivers

Stress also negatively affects the way that we relate to our children, so it's important to understand why it happens, and how our actions make our children feel. Only then can we take steps to manage the stress in our lives and reduce the harm that our children may suffer.

Remember that children can also suffer from stress, with all its effects. They also learn from us: if they see us getting upset and angry when things don't go right, they will probably react in a similar way to difficulties in their own lives.

3. Ask: 'What are the signs that Ama has too much stress?'

'What are the causes of Ama's stress?'

'Does this happen in our community?'

'How could you support Ama in coping with her stress?'

4. Invite the children to get into small groups, and think of all the things that make them feel stressed.

5. Next, ask: 'What ways have you found to cope with stress?'

Ask each group to make a mind map of these.

6. Ask the small groups to share their mind maps with the rest of the peer group.

For caregivers

1. Ask participants: 'What is the meaning of stress? What effects does it have on us and our relationships with our children?' As needed, add information from Box 14.j.

2. Say: 'Remember a time when you were stressed, or think of a situation which makes you feel stressed.'

Ask participants to pair up and act out short mimes, statue-shapes, or role plays to show what happens to their mind and body when they are stressed.

3. Then, with that situation in mind, ask participants to play the SIFT (Sensations, Images, Feelings, and Thoughts) game from Session 2 'Using our brains'. Read out the questions below, and ask them to show the actions that help remind them of the brain's different parts.

'What Sensations do you have in your body?'

'What Images do you have in your mind?'

'What are you Feeling?'

'What are your Thoughts?'

Ask participants what they have learned about stress from the SIFT game.

4. Ask participants to divide into groups of six. Ask them to write 'stress' in a circle in the middle of a piece of flipchart paper. Then say: 'Add in all the things that are making you feel stressed at the moment. Link up the different causes of stress across the flow chart.'

5. Stick the flow charts on the wall or place them on the floor. Invite the whole group to compare their similarities and differences.

For all peer groups

Reassure participants that a certain amount of stress is normal and motivates us to make an effort to do well and improve our lives. Explain that we are now going to explore ways of reducing harmful levels of stress. You will ask them to work in pairs and change partners after each activity.

Box 14.j Note for facilitators

If you are short of time you could select one or two of these ideas and suggest that participants try the rest at home, or you could use them in opening or closing circles for other sessions.

---

1. *Congratulate each other for coping.*

Ask participants to pair up and take it in turns to tell a story about when they coped really well with a difficult situation and managed to reduce their stress. Ask them to interview each other to get the full story, and spot abilities for their necklaces.

2. *Talk and listen.*

Explain that communication is the key to all good relationships. We need to say 'I am feeling stressed right now', ask for what we need, and say what we think. Being open to each other's needs and our children's needs is important.

Invite participants to get into new pairs, and practise saying 'I'm feeling stressed right now about […], and I need […]'; the other person should respond with empathy and support.

3. *Get organized.*

Explain that planning ahead can help us identify and find ways of dealing with situations that we expect will make us feel stressed.

Say: 'In new pairs, talk about what may make you feel stressed tomorrow, and find ways to reduce the stress.'

4. *Take time off.*

Explain that it can help to take a break from everyday tasks. For example, going for a walk, spending time with a friend, listening to music, or meditating. All these can help us relax and give us something to look forward to.

Ask people, in new pairs, to imagine how they will take a break over the next week. Ask: 'What will you do and when? What do you enjoy about that place or activity?'

5. *Get moving.*

Remind participants about the effect of physical movement on how we are feeling, as discussed in Session 2 'Using our brains'. For instance, we can dance a lively dance to some happy music, skip with a rope, juggle some balls, or go for a walk.

Ask participants, in new pairs: 'What physical movements could help you when you feel stressed? Act out these movements.'

6. *Change things around you.*

Explain that sometimes we feel overwhelmed by our problems, partly because many of them are outside our control. But there are always some things that we can control or change, even if it's only 2 per cent of the total. If we take control of that 2 per cent, it can grow, and give us confidence in controlling more things.

Ask participants, in new pairs, to tell each other about a difficulty they have, which they feel they have no control over. Ask them to interview each other to identify what small steps they could take to gain control over 2 per cent of the situation.

7. *Get help.*

Explain that getting help is a positive and useful step to take and not a sign of weakness.

Invite participants, in new pairs, to think of one thing they feel stressed about at this time.

Ask: 'Who could you ask for their support with this problem? What would you like that person to do?'

8. Finish the exercise by reminding participants about using wheels of awareness to gain perspective and to get back on their hubs (Exercises 2.8 and 2.9), and using meditation (Exercises 2.9 and 10.6).

 EXERCISE 14.7 TAKING MEDICINES CORRECTLY

AIMS: To understand how medicines work and why it is important to take them correctly when our bodies need them. To find practical ways of supporting each other in taking medicines correctly.

DESCRIPTION: The young children have a choice of two stories, while older children and caregivers in separate groups learn about taking medicines and drug resistance; all peer groups then identify strategies to support each other in taking medicines correctly.

Directions

1. Explain that 'we would like to measure how much this exercise helps participants use medicines correctly. At this point we will ask you how well you use, or have used, any medicines, for example: ARVs, antibiotics, or anti-malarials. We will use our 'fingers up' method, so please get into an outward-facing circle or cover your eyes.

2. When everyone is in position, say: 'First, if you have medicine to take every day, please use your fingers to show how many days out of the last seven (one week) you took your medicine in the correct amount and at the times you are instructed to take it. For example, if you took the medicine correctly every day show seven fingers; if you took it correctly on three days show three fingers. If you do not have medicine to take every day, please leave your hands in your lap.'

Record the fingers shown by each male and female in your Facilitator's Journal, putting a 0 for those with their hands in their laps.

Reassure participants by saying: 'Please do not blame yourself if you have not been able to take your medication correctly, because many of the challenges are not under your control.'

3. Next, say: 'Second, thinking more generally about how you usually manage when you need to take medicine – taking it on time, and finishing a course of medicine – how well do you think you do it on a scale of 1 to 5? Show 1 finger for not very well at all, 2 for not very well, 3 for OK, 4 for well, and 5 for very well.' Record the scores for each male and female in your Facilitator's Journal.

For 5–8 year olds

1. Tell the story you have chosen (from either Box 14.m or 14.n), with the children taking part by drawing or acting.

Box 14.I Story 1: Keeping the lid on the drinking water

Say: 'Once there was a family like any other, who stored their water in a big container without a lid.' Draw or act out using the big pot.

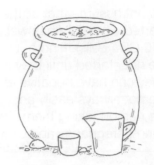

Ask: 'What could happen to make the water dirty?' (If needed, explain that mosquitoes and cockroaches can get into the water pot, and that dust and dirt can get in, including from the latrine.)

Draw or act out that the water is now dirty.

Ask: 'What might happen if someone drinks the dirty water?'

(If needed, explain that they might get sick from diarrhoea.)

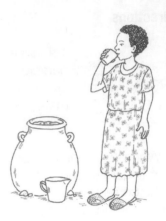

Ask: 'What if the mosquitoes lay their eggs in the water?' (If needed, explain that their eggs grow into larvae. The new mosquitoes come out of the larvae and bite us and give us malaria. They can also fly to another water pot and lay their eggs there too.)

Ask: 'How can the family keep the water clean, so that no one gets sick?' (If needed, explain that they need to cover it tightly.) Draw or act out fitting a lid on the pot.

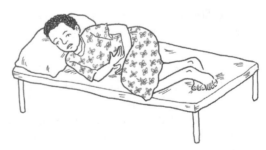

Ask: 'What do we learn from this story?' Then explain: 'This story teaches us how to store water well. But it can also remind us about HIV and ARVs.

'HIV damages our good CD4 immune cells, which keep us well, but ARVs can cover them up and protect them, like a lid. When the ARV lid is there, HIV can't enter the cell, multiply, and destroy it. If we stop taking our ARVs, we are removing the lid. The cells are uncovered and HIV can enter them. Then HIV can multiply, come out of the cell, and go into new cells.'

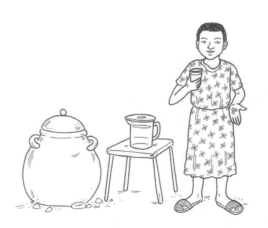

Box 14.m Story 2: Is HIV like a termite in our house?

Termites are insects that live in the thatch and wood of our house. They like to hide and slowly eat these parts of our house. At first we don't know that anything is wrong.

But the roof and walls get weaker and weaker. Sometimes, by the time we see what is happening, the roof and walls are already falling down, destroying our house.

If we look carefully, we can see the termites before they do too much damage. If we spray them with medicine regularly, we can keep them under control and stop them weakening our house. It's the same thing with HIV: it is like a termite. Taking our medicine regularly is like spraying regularly; it stops HIV from multiplying and weakening our immune system.

2. If you have time, ask the children, in threes, to talk about 'what is HIV like?' and to draw a picture to show the wider group. Invite them to make up a story about their HIV picture, to explain why we have to keep taking our ARVs.

For 9–14 year olds and caregivers in separate peer groups

1. Explain that if we need to take ARVs, it is very important to take those medicines correctly, exactly as they are prescribed. This is true of all medicines. We need to take them for a certain period of time, until the germs are dead or not able to harm us. Examples are:

Malaria. We take the pills for three days and all the malaria parasites are killed.

Tuberculosis (TB). We take the pills for six months and the TB germs are killed.

Ask: 'Is this the same for HIV? Can we take the pills for a time and kill HIV?' As needed, add information from Box 14.n.

Box 14.n Can pills kill HIV?

If our immunity is weakened too much by HIV (our CD4 count is less than 350), then we have to start taking ARVs. We must keep taking them for the rest of our lives, because ARVs can't kill HIV. Instead, ARVs lock HIV up in our CD4 cells and stop them from multiplying.

A pregnant woman with HIV and a high CD4 count only needs to take ARVs during pregnancy, to prevent HIV passing from mother to baby in the womb or during delivery.

Ask: 'What happens if we stop taking ARVs?' As needed, add information from Box 14.p.

Box 14.o What happens if we stop taking ARVs?

When we stop taking ARVs, HIV is able to multiply, to escape from the CD4 cells, and damage new CD4 cells. We may become ill as HIV weakens our immune system again. But as HIV multiplies, it can change. It knows the ARVs we used to control it, and may change so that it is no longer harmed by them. This is called *drug resistance*. If our HIV becomes resistant to the ARVs we were using, our doctors will need to try and find other ARVs that can control our HIV. These may be hard to find.

2. Remind participants of the game we played in Exercise 12.2, when they acted as CD4 cells, HIV, and ARVs. Ask them to replay the game to show what happens when we take ARV pills correctly, when we need them.

3. Invite them to show what happens if we stop taking the ARVs. (The people pretending to be HIV will wake up, and attack the people playing the CD4 cells.)

4. Lastly, invite them to show what can happen when we start taking ARVs again after stopping taking them. (The people playing ARVs can try to cover the people playing HIV, but the HIV can dodge out of the way because it has changed.)

For all peer groups in their separate groups

1. Ask participants to form groups of three, and to share experiences of taking any medicines (not just ARVs), or helping someone else to take medicines.

Ask: 'What made it difficult to take the medicines correctly every day? Why was it difficult? Please draw the difficulties on a mind map.'

Next, ask: 'How did you overcome the difficulties? Add any solutions to your mind map.'

Next, ask: 'What made it easier to take or give the medicine correctly? How did that help? Add any helpful tips to your mind map.'

2. Invite participants to come together again, and share the solutions and the things that help people to take their medicine correctly. Add ideas as necessary from Table 14.1.

Table 14.1 Helpful ideas for taking medicines correctly

What helps?	How does it help?
Understanding why it is so important to take the medicine	Now I know how the medicine works and what could happen if I stop, I am motivated to do it well for my future.
Getting praise from my auntie	It makes me feel strong, and that I'm practising my virtues.
My brother is taking pills too	We are partners in remembering to take them; we remind each other and take them at the same time.
Linking each time I should take pills to an action, so it has become a habit to take them	The actions fit with when I should take pills: getting out of bed, getting back from school, and brushing teeth before going to bed. To begin with we put pictures out to remind me – one was by my toothbrush – but now it is a habit.
Setting an alarm on my mobile phone	The alarm reminds me every time. I just have to remember to keep my phone charged!
Making a chart and marking a tick every time I take my medicine, and a cross if I forget	I show my chart to my auntie and get hugs for the ticks, sometimes a treat. For the crosses, we talk about what happened and how we can prevent it next time.
Being able to take the medicine in private	We organize it so I can take my medicines privately at home. I've also learned to take them discreetly when I'm not at home.

SESSION 15   PARTNERS IN HEALTH CARE

Purpose: To support caregivers and children in recognizing and appreciating their central role in accessing health care; to build on their abilities to use available services; to work with health personnel to improve the services for children.

Contents	Materials required	Time required
Opening circle (see p.13)		15 mins
15.1 Partners in health – ability spotting		40 mins
15.2 What services do children affected by HIV need?	Picture of a child on flipchart paper	30 mins
15.3 The health journey		60 mins
15.4 The ideal clinic		30 mins
15.5 Supporting each other when we go to the clinic		40 mins
15.6 Playing in the queue		30 mins
15.7 Having a blood test or injection		30 mins
15.8 Working together to support our children		90 mins
Closing circle (see p.14)		15 mins

About 6.5 hrs

Preparation

This session supports the participants in linking up with local providers of HIV services by having health workers as a fourth peer group in the session. Working in peer groups and together, the participants and health workers can become partners in strengthening HIV-related health services for children.

Talk to health providers to identify people interested in participating – people who are likely to benefit from the session, contribute to strengthening services for children, and act on ideas for improvements. For example, you might invite counsellors, clinic providers, home-based health workers, and a health committee member, to form a health-provider peer group in this session.

Box 15.a Information for facilitators

Many children and caregivers struggle to access health services and do not find them friendly to children. At the same time, health providers struggle to provide a good service with limited resources and human support. They too are affected by HIV, and are doing their work with the best intentions. Facilitate the groups in an appreciative way, by spotting abilities and listening to the reasons why providing services for children is challenging. We are aiming to build a strong and positive partnership between caregivers, children, and health providers to develop child-friendly services.

Opening circle

1. Bring all the peer groups together and welcome the health workers.

Explain that in this session we aim to build strong partnerships between caregivers, children, and health workers, so that we can work together to better support our children affected by HIV.

2. Invite the health workers to introduce themselves and their work, and help them choose a *Stepping Stones* name.

3. Invite everyone to move around in an interesting way, such as skipping, or flying like a bird. When you clap, ask them to introduce themselves to the person standing next to them. Repeat three times.

4. Split into four peer groups.

 ## EXERCISE 15.1 PARTNERS IN HEALTH – ABILITY SPOTTING

AIMS: To share our abilities in using or providing HIV-related child health services. To create images of caring, respectful health workers interacting with children.

DESCRIPTION: In pairs, participants interview each other and spot abilities. They create songs and drawings inspired by their ideas of caring, respectful health workers.

Directions

1. Ask participants to pair up, and to interview each other using the relevant question below. The interviewers ask questions to find out more about what happened and to spot abilities. They add new abilities to their partner's necklace.

Explain ability-spotting to the health providers and give them the materials to make their own necklaces.

Caregivers. 'Tell me about a time when you visited the health service with your child and felt proud of the way you were supporting your child in keeping as healthy as possible.'

Children. 'Tell me about a time when you visited the health service and felt proud about what you were doing to stay as healthy as possible.'

Health providers. 'Tell me about a time when you provided services to a child aged between 5 and 14 years, and felt proud about how you were making your services child-friendly and helping the child stay healthy.'

2. Invite the peer groups to draw or make up stories, poems, songs, and role plays about health workers who help children stay healthy or get better from an illness. Ask the participants to make up believable situations, recognizing that although children are sometimes dealt with badly in clinics and hospitals, there are also instances of them being treated in a kind and friendly way.

3. Bring all four peer groups together to share their art and drama.

EXERCISE 15.2 WHAT SERVICES DO CHILDREN AFFECTED BY HIV NEED?

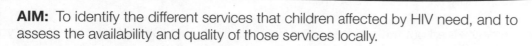

AIM: To identify the different services that children affected by HIV need, and to assess the availability and quality of those services locally.

DESCRIPTION: Each peer group creates a drawing of a child affected by HIV, surrounded by all the services that they might need.

Directions

1. Show participants a picture of a child on flipchart paper (you should have drawn this in advance). Ask participants to form groups of three and to discuss, for three minutes, 'What are all the services that this child might need related to HIV?'

2. Ask each group in turn to suggest a service, and draw or write it around the child. Continue until everyone has run out of ideas. As needed, add services from Box 15.b.

Box 15.b HIV-related services for children aged 5–14 years

- HIV counselling and testing;
- counselling for caregivers on talking about HIV with a child;
- ARV treatment;
- treatment for prevention of infections;
- early treatment of infections;
- nutritional counselling and vitamin supplements;
- ongoing counselling and support services.

---

3. Now invite everyone to discuss each service for children with and affected by HIV. Ask:

'Is the service designed specially for children or do children have to use the adult service?'

'At what age do children start to use the adult service?'

'What are the good points about the way the services are arranged for children at this time? What would we like to change?'

 4. Ask participants to score each service for children as follows:

Not available at all	0
Sometimes available	1
Always available but needs improvement	2
Good service	3

Ask participants to cover their eyes or form an outward-facing circle. Using Box 15.b, read out each service which is available and, for each one, say: 'Please put up your fingers and thumbs to show how many times you have used this service for yourself (about your own health) in the past three months. Use both hands if you need to. For answers higher than 10, please show all 10 fingers but with your hands crossed.'

If participants identified a service which is not in Box 15.b, ask them to give a score to it too. Record the scores in your Facilitator's Journal.

For caregivers only. Read out the services again, but this time, ask: 'Show how many times you have used each service in relation to your child's health in the past three months.'

Each time, record the number of fingers shown by each person (from zero to 10+) in your Facilitator's Journal.

5. Explain that in the next exercise we will return to the picture and scores to see how we can work together to improve them.

 EXERCISE 15.3 THE HEALTH JOURNEY

AIMS: To identify positive and challenging factors in seeking help for a health problem. To identify ways of improving services together.

DESCRIPTION: Participants draw or role play an imaginary journey to seek health; discuss what was good about the journey and what was difficult; and add ways of improving the service to the drawing or role play.

Box 15.c Information for facilitators

 Participants may become upset in this exercise, when they think about their own distressing experiences in trying to access or provide health care. Support them by appreciating the strengths that we all use in adversity, so that they can lay down more positive memories. Encourage participants not to judge or blame caregivers, children, or health workers, but to look for positive ways forward.

Directions[49]

1. Explain to the peer group that we are going to make up a story about a child who has HIV and lives in a community like ours. The child is trying to stay healthy, and the caregiver and health workers are trying to support the child in staying healthy. We tell what happens on their journey to get support and treatment. The story should include: asking advice from different people; the journeys they make; the places they visit, including the clinic or hospital; and the help they get. Because the story and the character are made up, we can add ideas based on our own experiences without feeling uncomfortable about sharing private information.

2. Encourage everyone to take part in telling the story. You could work around the circle, asking each person in turn to add to the story.

Ask questions to help participants continue adding to the story. For example: 'Who is our story going to be about? A girl, what shall we call her? Now, let's say Mary is falling sick a lot. Her caregiver is called … Martha? OK, who does Martha talk to about Mary being ill? What does that person do or say? How do they get to the clinic?'

3. Ask one or two participants to draw the steps of the journey, and ask others, if they wish, to role play particular points to make things clear.

4. When the story comes to an end, ask participants to divide into as many groups as there are characters in the story and give each group a character. The people in each group imagine that they are this character. Explain that you will act as a news reporter with a microphone, and interview a representative from each group. This representative will stay in role, and answer the questions from their character's point of view.

5. Invite a participant to tell the story from the start, using the picture of the journey. Every time the story mentions a character, you, acting as the news reporter, interview that character, asking:
- 'How do you feel about this part of the journey?'
- 'What do you like about this part of the journey?'
- 'What do you find difficult about this part of the journey?'
- 'What would you like to be different at this step of the journey?'

6. Record the changes that people would like to see from their answers to the last question on the picture of the journey.

7. Look at these changes together with the diagram and scores from Exercise 15.2.

8. Keep these diagrams to use in Exercise 15.8, when you will plan ways of improving HIV services for children with health workers and participants.

EXERCISE 15.4 THE IDEAL CLINIC

AIM: To dream and imagine an ideal, friendly health service for children affected by HIV.

DESCRIPTION: Participants dream of a perfect clinic and share this with a partner; the whole group then draws or acts a combination of their ideas to build a group vision of an ideal, child-friendly clinic.

Directions

1. Ask participants to close their eyes and imagine:
- *(for children)* that they have to go to the health clinic;
- *(for caregivers)* that they are taking their child to the clinic;
- *(for health workers)* that they are working in the clinic.

Ask them to dream of their ideal child-friendly clinic, for example: What is the waiting area like? How long is the wait? How do the staff interact with patients? How do you feel?

2. After a couple of minutes, ask everyone to open their eyes and talk with the person next to them about their ideal clinic.

3. Divide the group into two. Facilitate one group to draw a picture of the ideal clinic.

4. Facilitate the other group to use role play to show the ideal ways in which caregivers, patients, and staff interact in the dream.

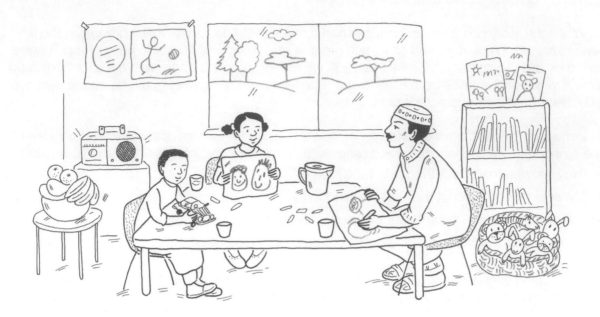

 EXERCISE 15.5 SUPPORTING EACH OTHER WHEN WE GO TO THE CLINIC

AIMS: To support children in the way they would like when they visit the clinic: before, during, and after the visit.

DESCRIPTION: Each peer group uses role plays to show how they would like to support children, or be supported, when visiting the clinic.

Box 15.d Tips for supporting children when going to the clinic

Information to share as appropriate with participants.

Before the visit

Prepare children by:
- explaining why they are going, how it will help them, and what is likely to happen;
- telling them the truth in a simple way that they can understand;
- explaining if you will need to be separated;
- exploring any fears they have and answering their questions.

During the visit

Try to make it as pleasant as you can. To help make waiting more fun, take food and drink, books to read, paper and crayons, or toys. Be ready to play some games too!

- Try to role model being positive and assertive when you communicate with health workers.

- Try to include the child; if a health worker talks to you and ignores the child, repeat what they've said to the child and ask the child to respond.

- Encourage the child to interact and give them praise.

If you need to be separated:

- Give the child something of yours to hold onto, for example, a face cloth or scarf.

- Tell them when the visiting hours are and when you will come. Keep your promises!

- Assure them that when they are better you will bring them home.

- When it comes to saying goodbye, go calmly and quite quickly. Prolonged goodbyes can make children more upset.

- Be compassionate if the child is upset when you visit. Explore their feelings and talk about the virtues they have to give them strength.

After the visit

Talk about the visit with the child. For example:

- 'How did you feel when …?'

- 'Was there anything that made you feel anxious or scared?'

- 'What could we do next time to make it easier?'

- 'How has the visit helped us?'

Directions

1. Remind participants of Exercise 15.1, which showed their abilities in using and providing child-friendly services, and their images, songs or role plays portraying health workers being kind and caring.

2. In separate peer groups:

Children. Explore what happens before, during, and after visiting the clinic and what they would like to happen. Create three statements (before, during, and after the visit) to present to the caregivers. Create one or two statements (during the visit) to present to the health workers.

Caregivers. Discuss how they help their children before, during, and after clinic visits. Look for what they can do to improve the situation in any way, even in small ways, before, during, and after visits.

Health workers. Explore the issues, reflect on whether they themselves behave like the kind people portrayed in Exercise 15.1, and look for what they can do to improve the situation for children during visits.

3. Bring the three peer groups together. Invite the children to present their statements to the caregivers and to the health workers. Then ask the caregivers and health workers to present their ideas on improving children's experience of the services.

Ask each group to say after the presentation, 'This is what we are thinking of; what do you think about it?'

Record the children's statements to the health workers and their caregivers in your Facilitator's Journal. Record the ideas from the caregivers and health workers on how to improve services for children. Make short notes on each group's response to the statements and ideas.

If you are running behind time at this point, you might want to prioritize Exercise 15.8, and just describe Exercises 15.6 and 15.7 for participants to try outside the workshop, by themselves.

 EXERCISE 15.6 PLAYING IN THE QUEUE

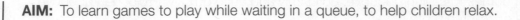

AIM: To learn games to play while waiting in a queue, to help children relax.

DESCRIPTION: Games for pairs, which caregivers can play with their child in a queue; a discussion on ways of helping children relax while waiting in the queue.

Directions

1. Explain: 'Waiting in clinics can be boring, and if we are anxious it can make us feel worse. It's good to have something fun to do to keep us on our hubs. What tips can you share about how to make waiting more fun?'

2. Here are some games that can be played while waiting in a clinic. Invite participants to play games from this list, to see which ones they like.

Game 1. In pairs, one person says: 'I can see something!' The other replies: 'What can you see?' The first person replies: 'I can see something [red]', for example. The other person guesses what the [red] thing might be. When they guess correctly, it is their turn to choose a colour and say: 'I can see something […]'.

Game 2. You can play 'I can see something […]' in other ways, too, for example: 'I see something starting with the letter [A]', or 'I see something that makes me feel [happy]'.

Game 3. Think of a category (for example: animals, cities, countries, foods), and take it in turns to try to find something belonging to that category for every letter in the alphabet (for animals: ant, bee, cat, …).

Game 4. One person says: 'I packed my bag and in it I put a [chicken]', for example. The next person adds an item, and also has to remember yours: 'I packed my bag and in it I put a [tree] and a chicken!'

Game 5. Try to say the alphabet backwards!

Game 6. Say a word, for example 'foot'; the next person then says a word which somehow connects to it, for example 'ball'; the next follows with another connecting word, for example, 'round'; and so on. When someone makes a mistake, start the game again.

3. If you are short of time, you could show the participants how to play these games, and ask them to try them at home with friends or family. Point out that these games support children in developing their brains and memories.

4. Ask: 'Is there anything the clinic can do to make waiting with children easier?'

EXERCISE 15.7 HAVING A BLOOD TEST OR INJECTION

AIMS: To find ways of making it easier to have blood tests or injections. To practise using a strategy for coping with big feelings.

DESCRIPTION: Participants use role play to demonstrate and practise using the Connect and Redirect strategy to cope with blood tests and clinical procedures that may frighten children.

Directions[50]

1. Explain that many of us can get anxious or frightened about things such as blood tests and injections. Children may be overwhelmed by big feelings, and even run away from the clinic. But sometimes doctors need to look at our blood to see what germs are making us sick or might make us sick in the future. They also use regular blood tests to check our health, for example, how our immune system is working.

2. *Children*. Ask: 'How many of us have had blood taken?'

Then, invite the children to pair up and ask each other: 'What gave you the patience and calmness to accept having the blood taken?'

'What else could help us to accept it and stay on our hubs?'

Caregivers. Ask: 'What did you do to support your child in staying calm and being patient when they have had an injection or blood test?'

Health workers. Ask: 'What did you do to help children stay calm and cope with blood tests and injections?'

3. Ask each peer group to draw a mind map of what helps them stay on their hubs during blood tests, or how they support children in staying calm, as appropriate. As needed, add information from Box 15.e.

Box 15.e Tips for coping with having blood taken

- Explain why it is happening: how the needle is going to help us get well, and how we will have plenty of blood left.

- Sit in a chair and relax our muscles all over our body, so nothing is feeling tight.

- Use our breathing exercises to breathe slowly and deeply, and to think of something enjoyable.

- Look at a lovely picture, or at the smiling face of our caregiver, while the blood is being taken.

- Ask for anaesthetic cream to stop it hurting.

- Reassure that we usually only feel a sharp scratch at the start, and that it's over quickly.

- Distract ourselves while the nurse is taking blood by counting down from 100, listening to songs or stories, or chatting.

- Build confidence by talking about using virtues of courage, and use the wheel of awareness to stay on our hub.

---

4. Remind participants of the Connect and Redirect strategy, as set out in Box 15.f. See whether this strategy is on the mind map.

Box 15.f Connect and Redirect

The caregiver *connects* with and acknowledges the child's feelings. They use non-verbal signals like touch, empathetic facial expressions, a nurturing tone of voice, and non-judgemental listening.

The child calms down and becomes more open to listening to what the caregiver has to say next. The upper brain reconnects with the lower brain.

The caregiver *redirects* the child's focus towards ways of improving things, communicating with words and empathy so the child becomes more balanced.

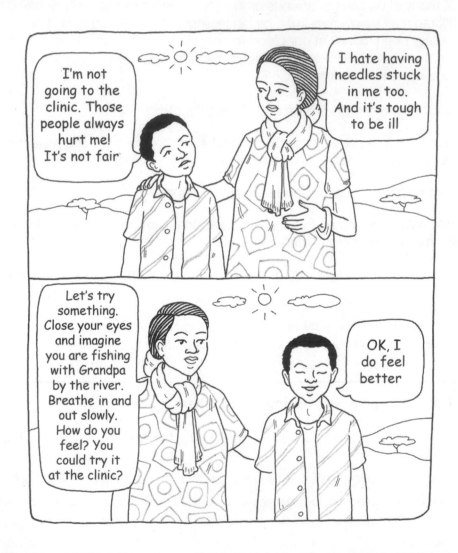

5. Ask participants to think of times when they have used this strategy.

EXERCISE 15.8 WORKING TOGETHER TO SUPPORT OUR CHILDREN

AIMS: To show and discuss the pictures, mind maps, role plays, and ideas that the caregivers, children, and health workers have produced throughout Session 15. To discuss actions participants and health workers can take together to develop child-friendly HIV services and homes. To understand children's rights to high-quality health services and good treatment.

DESCRIPTION: All four peer groups come together to share their pictures, mind maps and role plays. They use them to make a plan of next steps through which to create more child-friendly HIV services.

Box 15.g Information for facilitators

Remember to encourage appreciative and positive thinking, and virtues. If any group feels shamed or blamed by the other, they will find it difficult to work together to improve things.

Directions

1. Welcome all the peer groups and acknowledge the work they have done. Say: 'This exercise aims to begin or strengthen an ongoing partnership to improve services for children affected by HIV. We will look at all our ideas and suggestions, and make a "first steps" action plan for how we will move forward. Let's all think positively and appreciatively of each other, practising our virtues so that we achieve a lot.'

2. Display or review the products from the exercises: the mind maps; pictures and songs of the best health workers; the health journeys; the ideal clinic; role plays of good interactions between caregivers, children, and health workers; and suggestions for improvements in health care for children affected by HIV.

3. Explain that we all – providers, caregivers, and children – have certain rights to good health care. Do children have the same rights as adults? Invite everyone to call out the rights that they know and write them on a flipchart, adding information from Box 15.h if necessary.

Box 15.h Rights related to health services

Everyone in the world has the right to good quality, non-judgemental health information and services. It makes no difference whether we are children or adults, men or women, rich or poor, single or married. It makes no difference where we live, or whether or not we have HIV.

Explain that in many countries, policies exist to protect these rights, and national laws reinforce them. Caregivers and health staff have a responsibility to advocate for services and encourage people, including children, to access voluntary HIV testing and medication because it is their right.

---

4. Ask: 'In what ways do our health services uphold our children's rights to health care? In what ways could they improve?'

'How can we work together and strengthen the services in order to meet children's rights to good health services?'

5. Draw a mind map of all the positive points about the health services. See how different parts of the mind map link up. Add the challenges that people would like to see overcome. In a different colour, change the challenges into solutions. For each solution, suggest actions to help achieve it.

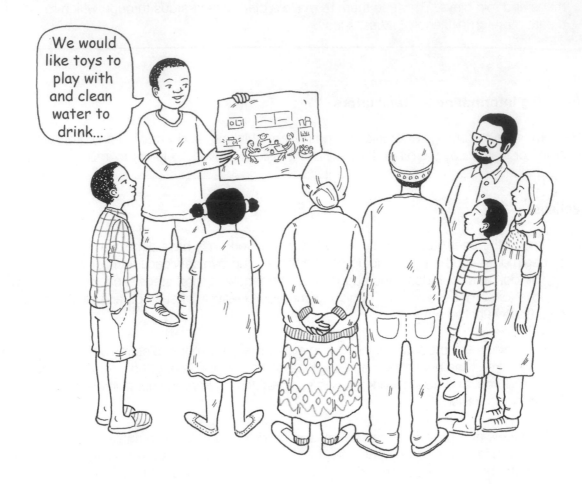

6. Make a list of things that participants and health staff can do together to begin change. Encourage people to think of small, achievable changes.

 Record the actions and changes that participants and health staff plan to do and help each other achieve in your Facilitator's Journal.

SESSION 16 FRIENDSHIP

Purpose: To understand the importance of friendship and how to be a good friend; to use skills to solve problems with friends; to learn to enjoy the good things about friendship groups, avoid problems, and create a more friendly environment for everyone. The caregivers use the exercises to see how they can help their children make lasting friends and join supportive friendship groups, and how they can promote a friendly environment.

Contents	Materials required	Time required
Opening circle (see p.13)		15 mins
16.1 What makes a good friend?	Ability necklaces	45 mins
16.2 Dragons	A tie or piece of cloth, or paper and tape	20 mins
16.3 Responding to challenges in relations between friends		45 mins
16.4 Friendship groups		30 mins
16.5 Making our environment friendlier		30 mins
Closing circle (see p.14)		15 mins

About 3.5 hrs

 EXERCISE 16.1 WHAT MAKES A GOOD FRIEND?

AIM: To discover and affirm the qualities and behaviours that nurture friendship.

DESCRIPTION: Participants do ability-spotting in pairs, followed by mind mapping. They share poems and songs.

Directions

1. Ask participants to pair up and say: 'Today we are thinking about friendship. Tell a story or draw a picture about a time when you did something that showed that you were a good friend. The person listening should spot abilities and virtues, and add any new ones to the teller's necklace.'

2. Back with the whole group, ask each pair to stand up in turn and introduce each other to the group, highlighting all the person's abilities or virtues. For instance: 'This is Musa, and his abilities as a friend are kindness, helpfulness, good listening, making people laugh, sharing tasks, and loyalty.'

3. When everyone has had their turn, ask: 'How do you feel, hearing about all your virtues? How are you going to make more use of them now?'

4. Jointly create a mind map of all the abilities that have been mentioned that relate to friendship. As needed, add points from Box 16.a.

Box 16.a How good friends behave towards each other

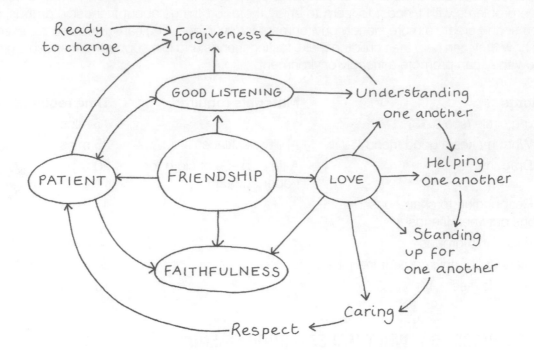

- We share our ideas, feelings and dreams with our friend.
- We listen to our friend with all our heart and mind.
- We respect and value each other.
- We love our friend.
- We are loyal and stand by our friend when others are against us.
- We are dependable and trustworthy.
- We keep our promises and know right from wrong.
- We don't push each other into doing things that we don't want to do.
- We are willing to change if we see that we are doing wrong.
- We imagine how it feels to be our friend, and see things from their point of view.
- We share our things with our friend.
- We want good things for our friend.
- We help and protect our friend.
- We forgive and forget quarrels.
- We spend time with our friend.
- We talk openly and honestly.
- We find solutions to problems together.
- We show understanding.
- We move from 'me' to 'you' to 'we'.
- We support one another in staying on our hubs.
- We can make use of the virtues within us all to support one another.

5. *Caregivers.* Ask: 'How do you teach your child to be a good friend?' Share examples in small groups.

Children. Read this poem, then ask participants to get into pairs and act out the poem as you read it.[51]

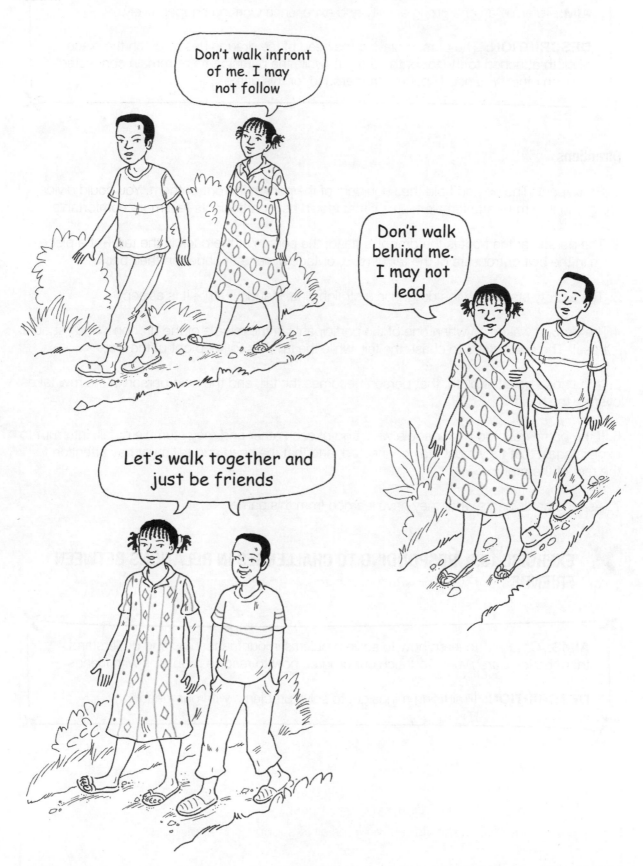

EXERCISE 16.2 DRAGONS

AIM: To enjoy an energizing activity and experience working cooperatively.

DESCRIPTION: The person playing the head of the dragon has to catch the piece of cloth attached to the tail of the dragon, while the participants all remain connected to each other. You need space to run around for this game.

Directions

1. Participants line up and hold the shoulders of the person in front of them. You could divide the group into male and female teams if that would help participants feel more comfortable.

2. The person at the front is the dragon's head; the person at the back is the tail. Put a piece of cloth in the belt or trousers of the tail person, or tape a piece of paper on their back.

3. The activity starts with the dragon in a straight line, standing still – it is asleep.

4 The dragon wakes up when one of the participants in the middle of the dragon's body shouts: 'Chase!' The head starts to chase the tail, while the tail tries to keep out of the way.

5. If the head gets the cloth, that person becomes the tail, and the next person in the row takes over as the head.

6. If the game gets too wild, people will let go of each other and may stumble or fall. Interrupt to explain again that they must stay connected, and that the head and tail must pay attention to the rest of the group.

7. Ask the participants what they have learned from this game.

EXERCISE 16.3 RESPONDING TO CHALLENGES IN RELATIONS BETWEEN FRIENDS

AIMS: *Children*. To learn how to solve problems in our friendships and understand them better. *Caregivers*. To teach our children how to resolve problems with friends.

DESCRIPTION: Practising mindsight to solve problems with our friends.

Box 16.b Information for facilitators

Information to share with participants

Trustworthiness, caring, and honesty are all important virtues in friendship.

Sometimes friends do not understand each other well and get angry or upset. If we listen carefully and imagine ourselves in our friend's place, we can see how they are feeling and how to talk in a caring way and solve the problem together.

If we are feeling hurt or confused in a friendship, it is best to tell our friend how we feel and what we would like. This is where 'I' statements are so helpful. Then our friend can say how they feel and what they would like, and we can discuss and agree. So we move from 'me' to 'you' to 'we', together.

Directions

1. Show everyone the picture of mindsight from Session 2, page 47.

Ask: 'Who can explain what *mindsight* means?'

Remind everyone that mindsight means 'seeing with our mind'. *Insight* means looking inside our own mind to see what's going on in there. It is about *me*.

Explain that the second part of mindsight is seeing someone else's mind and trying to look at things the way they do. This is about *you*. If we use mindsight with our friends, we can understand them better and we'll all feel happier.

The third part of mindsight is *connecting between us*: moving from me, to you, to we.

2. *Children*. Ask your peer group to divide into smaller groups of males or females.

Say: 'Let's think of some problems that can happen in a friendship to people like us. The problem needs to be a problem within the friendship. For example, a boy tells his friend a secret, but the friend tells other people. Or a girl wants to spend time studying with her friend, but the friend wants to go to town and socialize. Discuss in your group, and then choose an important problem to work with.'

Caregivers. Ask caregivers to divide into four groups according to the age and sex of their children. Ask each group to think of a problem situation that could happen between children of this age and sex.

3. Invite each group to prepare a role play, in which two people show their problem situation and how those two people handled it. Caregivers handle the situation as they would like to see their children handle it.

4. Bring the pairs together and ask one pair to show how they solved the problem.

Ask: 'What did they do that worked well?'

5. Explain the steps in using 'I' statements to solve the situation, as set out in Table 16.1. Invite two participants to act them out as you explain them.

6. Ask participants to return to their small groups, and to try using 'I' statements in their role play situation.

Table 16.1 Steps for using 'I' statements to discuss a problem

1. One person explains what has upset them and why. The other person responds with their feelings and reasons for these.	'I felt […] when […] happened, because […].'
2. Each person says what they heard the other person say about their feelings and reasons.	'I now realize that you felt […] because […]. Is that right?'
3. Each person says what they would like to change in future.	'In future I would be glad if we could […].'
4. Both people agree on what changes they will make.	'Yes, from now on, we will […].'

7. If there is time, ask one or two groups to show their role plays to the rest of the peer group.

8. Ask the caregivers how they will teach their children to use what they have learned in this exercise.

 ## EXERCISE 16.4 FRIENDSHIP GROUPS

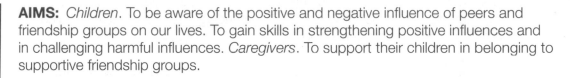

AIMS: *Children*. To be aware of the positive and negative influence of peers and friendship groups on our lives. To gain skills in strengthening positive influences and in challenging harmful influences. *Caregivers*. To support their children in belonging to supportive friendship groups.

DESCRIPTION: Participants reflect on the good things about being in a friendship group, and use role plays to practise coping with challenges. Be aware that some children may not have a group of friends. Talk about a friend or friends.

Directions

1. Say the following, with pauses to allow people time to reflect: 'Let's close our eyes and breathe deeply. (…) Now, imagine you are sitting with your friends. (…) See their faces. (…) Think of the things you like about them. (…) What do you like to do together? (…) What are the good things about having these friends? (…) OK, let's say goodbye to them now, and open our eyes.'

Ask: 'How does it make you feel to think about friends?'

2. Explain that having friends, and belonging to a friendship group, can be very supportive for us, whatever age we are. Friends give each other practical and emotional support; they help us feel brave and good about ourselves. Friends help each other do new things and can protect each other from bullying and abuse. Working together and encouraging each other helps us do better and become independent. But sometimes friends influence us to do harmful things. It is not easy to resist negative peer pressure, to be different and stand by our values and ideas.

3. Divide into separate peer groups.

Children. Ask them to form single gender groups of four, and to prepare a role play about dealing with a challenge that might happen to people like them in a friendship group. For example, problems due to being excluded (for example, being left out, not allowed to use a toy), or pressured to do something harmful (for example, drinking alcohol, taking drugs, having unsafe sex, stealing). They can use strategies such as 'I' statements, being assertive, leaving the group, or convincing the group to change.

Caregivers. Ask them to form small groups and prepare a role play about supporting their child in choosing a good friendship group or in resisting negative peer pressure.

4. Come back together as a big group. Ask one or two groups to show their role play and invite comments.

5. If there is time, go around the circle asking each person to say one way in which friendship groups use their virtues to have a positive influence on their members. For example, they show compassion by making sure that everyone feels they belong.

 EXERCISE 16.5. MAKING OUR ENVIRONMENT FRIENDLIER

AIM: To understand the importance of friendliness and how to practise it.

DESCRIPTION: Peer groups role play being inside and outside a friendship group (option A) or, in smaller groups, role play different situations showing unfriendly behaviour and what they would do to make the environment friendlier (option B).

Directions for option A

1. Call out two or three feelings and ask participants to show them through their body language. (This is something we did in Exercise 1.6 'Our feelings'.)

2. Ask two or three people to step to one side, while the rest of the group plays a simple game together, or does any other group activity from which someone might be excluded, such as chatting or dancing together.

3. Shout: 'Stop!' Ask those watching the group activity to show with their body language how they feel about being outside the activity.

4. Ask those in the activity to think about what those outside are feeling, and check whether they are correct. Ask why people might be outside the group.

5. Invite someone inside the group to talk to one of the outsiders. For example, by saying: 'I will feel happy if you come and talk with us', or 'Do you want to join in?' If the person agrees, they join the group. If they disagree, they stay where they are. Those inside ask them to explain why, and try inviting them in a different way.

6. Repeat with the outsiders taking it in turns to try and join the group, and different insiders talking to them. What happens and why?

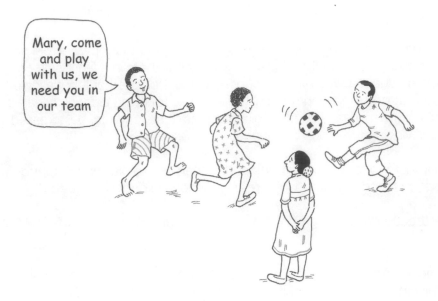

7. Ask the *caregivers*: 'How can you support your children in being friendly to people outside their friendship group?'

'How can you support your children in joining a friendship group?'

Directions for option B

1. Divide your peer group into groups of four males or females.

Children. Give each group one of the situations in Box 16.c, or others that your group is concerned about.

Box 16.c Challenging friendship situations

- A person in your class, home or community is being bullied.
- One of your friends looks like she or he has been crying.
- You walk past someone who looks strange and dresses differently.
- You see two boys harassing a girl on the way to the market.
- Your sibling or friend wishes they had more friends.
- Your friend's mother won't allow her to play with you because your mother has HIV.
- Your friend is missing schoolwork owing to caring for a sick parent.

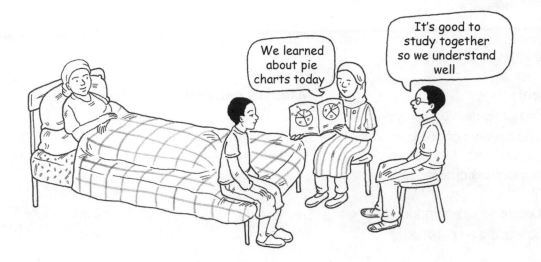

Caregivers. Give out the situations in Box 16.c, and ask each group to role play how they would like their child to respond.

Ask them to discuss how they would teach their child to be friendly in this situation, and how they would support their child in this.

2. Show as many role plays as you have time for, and invite comments on the friendliness shown and the outcome. Invite people to come up and be friendly in a different way.

3. Ask participants to call out the key points they have learned about friendliness from the activity.

Closing circle

Tell participants to bring to the next session any drawings they created about their dreams in Exercise 1.5 'Our dreams'.

Purpose: To support caregivers in helping children to attend school, and children in attending and performing well at school.[52]

Contents	Materials required	Time required
Opening circle (see p.13)		15 mins
17.1 The benefits of going to school	Drawings from Exercise 1.5, lots of pieces of paper	45 mins
17.2 Supporting children in attending school		90 mins
17.3 Dreaming of a supportive school		60 mins
Closing circle (see p.14)		15 mins

About 4 hrs

Preparation

Participants should have brought any drawings they created about their dreams in Exercise 1.5 'Our dreams', page 26.

If participants have a good relationship with staff from local primary schools and they are eager to develop their school, ask them if they want to invite a head teacher, teacher, or guidance counsellor from each school to come to this session. They can form their own peer group and participate in the activities from their point of view. Invite them to use diagrams and mind maps to share their ideas with the other peer groups during the session and in follow-up meetings.

If, on the other hand, you are not sure how teachers might react to requests for improvement by caregivers and children, it might be best to run the session without them. You could then invite the teachers to join a follow-up session, by which time caregivers and children will have a clear idea about the changes they want to see at school and how they could support them. You could also invite local NGOs that are engaging with the schools.

EXERCISE 17.1 THE BENEFITS OF GOING TO SCHOOL

AIM: To increase or reinforce understanding of the benefits for vulnerable children of going to school, so that families and communities support them in doing so.

DESCRIPTION: Participants interview each other in pairs, and draw or write benefits on pieces of paper to position around a picture of a school.

Directions

1. Explain that in this exercise we will focus on the benefits of going to school. We will look at the challenges of going to school in a later exercise, and find ways of overcoming them.

2. Ask the participants in your peer group to pair up and interview each other about the role of school in fulfilling their dreams of the future. (Remind them of the exercise they did in Exercise 1.5 'Our dreams'.)

Children. Ask each other: 'What do you plan to achieve at school, and why is this important on your life journey and in fulfilling your dreams?'

Caregivers. Ask each other: 'What do we hope our children will achieve at school, and why is this important for their life journey and in fulfilling their dreams?'

Teachers: Ask each other: 'What do we hope the children we teach will achieve at school, and why is this important for their life journey and in fulfilling their dreams?'

3. Invite a participant to draw a picture of a school in the middle of flipchart paper, and place it on the floor in the middle of the circle.

4. Ask people to draw or write down the benefits of school, in relation to children's life journey and future, marking each benefit on a different piece of paper.

5. Ask: 'What are the other benefits of going to school, or sending our children to school?'

Ask them to draw or write each of these other benefits on a different piece of paper.

6. Take it in turns to position one piece of paper around the picture of the school and explain the benefit. If ideas are similar, put them together.

7. If needed, add any information from Box 17.a.

Box 17.a Some benefits for children of going to school

Going to school can provide all children, and particularly vulnerable children, with:
- a safe and structured environment;
- a routine, which gives stability in times of change;
- adult supervision and emotional support;
- friendships that last into adulthood.

The learning gained from going to school can give children:
- improved thinking processes, which help them whether they remain in their village or not;
- more and better opportunities for different types of work and further learning, and to fulfil their dreams;
- reduced vulnerability to early pregnancy, early marriage, and sexual health problems (including HIV), due to better knowledge, confidence, life-skills, and opportunities;
- when these children have grown up, better health and opportunities for *their* children.

---

8. Discuss the benefits and summarize.

EXERCISE 17.2 SUPPORTING CHILDREN IN ATTENDING SCHOOL

AIMS: To identify barriers to school attendance. To share and affirm the ways that caregivers and teachers support children in going to school, and that children contribute towards their own school attendance. To identify, jointly, ways of overcoming barriers and increasing support to children in going to school and achieving their best.

DESCRIPTION: In separate peer groups, participants draw or write down barriers to school attendance on paper 'bricks'. Caregivers and teachers interview each other in pairs to identify ways that they support children in attending school and achieving their best. Children interview each other to identify ways that they contribute towards their own school attendance. The pairs then come together and make mind maps to share learning and identify ways of getting over the barriers to going to school.

Directions

1. Divide the participants into peer groups.

2. Ask everyone to call out things that get in the way of children attending, and getting the most out of, school.

3. Ask participants to write or draw each idea on a different piece of paper. As the paper ideas are done, lay them on the floor or stick them on the wall, as if they were bricks forming a wall. Explain that this wall prevents children from attending school regularly and from fully benefiting from it.

4. Ask participants to interview each other in pairs:

Children. 'Tell me about a time when you did something that helped you get to school on time, or do well in class.'

'What other things have you done to attend school regularly and do well?'

Caregivers. 'Tell me about a time when you did something that supported your child in attending school or in doing well at school.'

'What other things have you done to support your child in staying at school and doing well?'

Teachers: 'Tell me about a time when you did something that supported your learners to attend school or to do well at school?'

'What other things have you done to support your learners in staying at school and doing well?'

5. Ask the pairs to share their supportive actions with their whole peer group, using a mind map, drawings, or key words. Write in the middle bubble 'girls supported in attending school'. Key words around this might be 'menstruation', 'school fees', and 'praise learning'.

6. Bring all the peer groups together to share their ideas of support. Spread out the mind maps, drawings, or words, and ask: 'What have we learned from each other? What more can we do?'

7. Share the bricks out among participants and invite them to work in fours to find ways around the barriers, building on the ideas they developed in points 4–6. Ask them to draw or write their ideas on the back of the bricks. As you listen in on each group's discussion, add ideas from Box 17.b if appropriate.

Box 17.b Ways of supporting children in attending school and achieving their best

For caregivers

- Pack food for children to take to school.

- Praise and encourage children's learning, and take an interest in it.

- Help them understand the long-term benefits of education for their life journey.

- Try to be involved with the school, and work with other caregivers to develop the school or advocate for changes.

- Support children in making good choices regarding sex, contraception, drugs, alcohol, and early marriage.

- Support children in avoiding unwanted sex, in delaying sex, and in protecting themselves and others from harassment and sexual abuse.

- Support girls in coping with the challenges that arise from menstruation.

- Teach boys appropriate, respectful behaviour towards girls.

- Encourage children to be active at school, and to join clubs where they can spend time having fun and build practical as well as academic skills.

- Support older children in being motivated to attend school, and in delaying competing roles, such as that of mother or wage earner.

- Remind children how gender roles can change: girls can excel in all subjects, and fulfil dreams of working in jobs or businesses that interest them; boys can gain respect through their virtues and achievements.

- Listen to children's concerns about school and find ways of acting on them together, for example, if they are being bullied or beaten by teachers.

- Support grieving children in coping with their feelings.

To prevent children from dropping out of school owing to lack of money or time:

- Find ways of paying school fees: plan and save in advance; negotiate reduced fees or agreement to pay them 'in kind' with labour or farm produce; or seek contributions from elsewhere, such as a faith-based organization or HIV-support group.

- Prioritize investing in education over expenditure on things that give short-term pleasure (e.g. alcohol, costly clothes).

- Look after all family members' health (this may include HIV testing), so that children are not needlessly sick, or caring for others who are sick, instead of going to school.

- Share domestic and other work, and caring for the sick, among males and females in the household.

- Set up shared child care with others, to look after young siblings.

- Ask relatives or friends for help.

Ways children can contribute

- Be diligent in studying and doing homework.
- Remind yourself about why you want to do well at school and keep your dreams alive.
- Work together with siblings and friends who also want to do well at school.
- Talk with your caregiver about what happens at school and ask for their support.

8. Ask each group of four to explain their ideas and to lay their bricks, with the solutions showing, in a path of stepping stones heading roughly towards the school.

9. Ask each caregiver and their child to chat and agree on one thing each of them will do next week to support the child in going to school and doing well.

 ## EXERCISE 17.3 DREAMING OF A SUPPORTIVE SCHOOL

AIMS: To identify ways in which local schools could improve their support to children and caregivers in coping with HIV and other illnesses or disabilities.

DESCRIPTION: Participants dream of a supportive school and think of the actions needed to move towards that ideal.

Directions

1. Ask participants to shut their eyes and imagine that they are walking along the stepping stones they just created to an ideal school. Encourage them to think of a school which supports children who face challenges such as HIV to feel safe, happy, and healthy, and which enables them to benefit fully from attending. If you are working with a children's peer group, ask them to imagine they are in the school. What happens in the school, and how does it feel?

2. Ask participants to pair up and interview each other to find out what happens in their imaginary school to make it so good.

3. Ask them to draw a picture to show what is happening in the school.

4. Bring the group back together to share their pictures.

5. Now ask everyone to think backwards, to work out what steps would need to have been taken to make the school so good. For example, if the ideal school is very friendly, with no bullying, what steps were taken to achieve this?

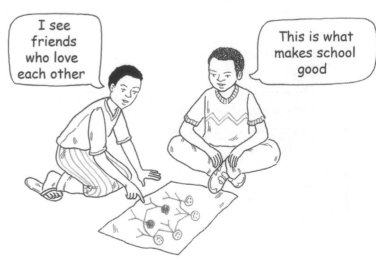

Draw or write down the steps.

6. Try to identify steps that participants can do, and other steps that the school could do. Encourage people to think of plausible steps: things that can actually be done.

7. Bring all the peer groups together to present and discuss the steps they have identified. Agree what to do next. Contribute ideas from Box 17.c if appropriate, but focus on ideas from groups.

Box 17.c Ideas for creating a more supportive school

Use the learning and ideas generated by participants in this session to advocate for and support specific actions. For example, you might:

- train one teacher or person in the school in counselling;
- offer to run a session for all teachers about HIV, ways of supporting children, and the importance of confidentiality;
- provide a space for children who feel unwell to rest while at school;
- provide different toilets for girls and boys, bins for sanitary materials, and water and soap for washing hands;
- keep a stock of menstrual pads and spare uniforms for girls who need them;
- make food available (snacks or a meal);
- teach all age groups about health, how people get sick, and how to stay healthy, with HIV as one condition among many;
- give training to specific teachers whose knowledge or behaviour is problematic (e.g. they discriminate on the basis of gender or HIV, or use corporal punishment or verbal abuse);
- develop actions to prevent teasing, abuse, and bullying in school;
- teach about virtues such as respect, kindness, caring, appreciation of strengths and difference, justice, and friendliness;
- stop the use of corporal punishment and name-calling by teachers;
- train teachers how to use positive discipline;
- teach children their rights and set up a system to report and act on abuse;
- teach all staff members that they must not touch children inappropriately, nor have any form of sexual contact with a child;
- ensure sanctions are in place to check teacher's inappropriate actions.

Members of the *Stepping Stones* group could advocate for specific actions by meeting key people from the school and Ministry of Education. Or they could work in partnership with others, such as the parent–teachers' association or a local NGO, to try to improve things.

---

8. Suggest that the *Stepping Stones* groups and your organization may wish to set up a follow-up meeting with district education officers, school heads, teachers, parent teachers' association, caregivers, and children. The learning and ideas from this session could contribute to an action plan aimed at supporting children affected by challenges such as HIV. People at the meeting could look at drawings and listen to presentations by caregivers and children, then identify resources available.

Box 17.d Information for facilitators

Many teachers are also living with HIV, or have family members with HIV. They have many challenges and few resources, and actions need to be feasible. The film *Courage and Hope. African teachers living positively with HIV* [https://www.youtube.com/watch?v=OmjlNea7u64] shows how some teachers with HIV have been wonderful role models to their learners. We can show this film at the start of the session and at the meeting and get inspiration from this, and the teachers in our local schools.

Closing circle

Remind participants to bring their ability necklaces with them to Session 18 'Managing alcohol and other drugs'.

Purpose: To understand what substances people use locally to change their mood; why people use them; what effects these can have on their health, lives, and families; and how to use our skills to take control and support others.

Contents	Materials required	Time required
Opening circle, (see p.13)		15 mins
18.1 Exploring drug use		60 mins
18.2 Do what I do, not what I say		15 mins
18.3 Supporting ourselves in taking control	Ability necklaces	30 mins
18.4 Supporting others in taking control		75 mins
Closing circle, (see p.14)		15 mins
Additional exercise		60 mins
18.5 Drug use in the household		

About 4.5 hrs

Preparation

Our focus in this session is on the mood-changing drugs used in the community. If you don't know much about those drugs and their effects, please find out about them. Please also take time to reflect on your own attitudes to drug use. Remember: people all over the world use substances that change their mood. There is no need to blame people for taking drugs, or make them feel ashamed. We need to accept this usage, and support ourselves and others in taking control by either not starting using them, stopping using them, or using them safely. Some drugs are illegal.

Today you will be asking participants to focus on the virtue of *self-discipline*.

EXERCISE 18.1 EXPLORING DRUG USE

AIMS: To know what drugs adults and children use in our area to change their mood. To know the reasons why people use drugs. To explore the positive and negative consequences of using drugs and of not using them.

DESCRIPTION: Participants learn about different types of drugs, identify the ones most used by people like them, and explore the positive and negative consequences of using specific drugs and of not using them.

Directions

1. Explain that in this session we are going to explore the positive and negative consequences of using alcohol and other drugs, and how we can support each other in taking control of the use of them, rather than them being in charge of us.

Ask: 'What is a "drug"?'

If necessary, explain that a drug is a substance that has effects on the body. Drugs may be:

medicinal: they treat or prevent illness (for example, aspirin, ARV, Septrin);

mood altering: they change how we feel (for example, alcohol, cannabis, heroin, glue);

performance-enhancing: they increase strength in sports or sex, keep us alert, increase our confidence, or free our imagination (for example, coffee, steroids, cola, cannabis, tobacco, snuff).

Some drugs can do all these things. For example, cannabis can relieve pain, change our mood, and free our imagination.

2. Ask participants, in small groups, to think of as many drugs as possible and draw or write them on pieces of paper. Come together and arrange the paper slips on the floor in the three groups: medicines, mood-altering substances, and performance-enhancing substances.

3. Focus on the medicines, and ask: 'How do we use medicines properly?'

If needed, explain that we always take them as prescribed, in the right dose, and ensure we finish the course of medicine. Otherwise, the sickness in our bodies can build up resistance to them, and next time they will no longer work for us.

4. Focus on the performance-enhancing drugs, and ask: 'How can we use performance-enhancing drugs properly?' If needed, explain that we do not use any of these until we are fully grown. Adults take them as prescribed, or in moderation. Some are illegal.

5. Explain that for the rest of this session we are going to focus on the mood-altering substances.

Put aside all the pieces of paper marked with medicine and performance-enhancing drugs, and ask participants to consider those marked with mood-altering drugs. Some medicines also alter mood, for example, they make people feel more relaxed (Valium) or happier (Prozac). Say: 'Of all these mood-altering drugs, including alcohol, which are used in our community?'

Then ask: 'Of these mood-altering drugs that are used in our community, which are used by people of our age?'

'Does use differ between males and females of our age?'

6. For the following peer groups:

Children aged 9–14 years and caregivers in separate peer groups. Ask the peer group to divide into enough small groups so that each group has one drug to think about.

Children aged 5–8 years. Choose the two most commonly used drugs, or the ones most used by older children. Split the group into two, so that the facilitator and the assistant each guide one group's discussion.

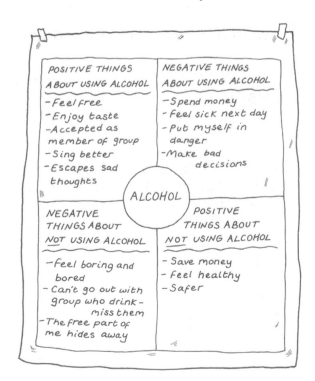

POSITIVE THINGS ABOUT USING ALCOHOL
- Feel free
- Enjoy taste
- Accepted as member of group
- Sing better
- Escapes sad thoughts

NEGATIVE THINGS ABOUT USING ALCOHOL
- Spend money
- Feel sick next day
- Put myself in danger
- Make bad decisions

ALCOHOL

NEGATIVE THINGS ABOUT NOT USING ALCOHOL
- Feel boring and bored
- Can't go out with group who drink – miss them
- The free part of me hides away

POSITIVE THINGS ABOUT NOT USING ALCOHOL
- Save money
- Feel healthy
- Safer

7. Give each group a sheet of flipchart paper and two coloured pens. Ask them to write the name of their drug in the middle, and then divide the sheet into four quadrants. The top quarters are for their thoughts about the positive and negative things about using the drug. The bottom quarters are for the positive and negative things about not using the drug (see picture previous page).

Ask the groups to discuss each quarter and to add their thoughts using words or symbols.

Note. They can talk in general about how the drug is used by people like them; they don't have to mention personal experiences. It is OK to leave a quarter blank if participants cannot think of anything to write there.

As needed, add information from Box 18.a.

Box 18.a Information about mood-altering drugs

Reasons why people use mood-altering drugs

- They like the feeling that using the drug gives them.
- They feel the drug helps them cope with challenges in their life.
- They are curious to try the drug.
- They are copying what they see others, including older people, doing.
- They want to fit in with what others are doing.
- They think that using the drug makes them look good in some way.
- There is a social expectation that they will use the drug.
- They haven't thought carefully about the effects of the drug and whether it is a good choice to use it.
- They have tried to stop using the drug but didn't succeed.
- They are addicted to the drug and need help to stop taking it.
- Alcohol and some drugs are used for spiritual rituals; for example, blessings, holy communion, and pouring libation to the ancestors.

Consequences of using mood-altering drugs

Alcohol. Drinking too much alcohol causes people to fall down, think or talk unclearly, react slowly to situations, and make poor decisions. People are more likely to have an accident, be violent, or have sex which they do not want. Over time, drinking too much alcohol causes liver problems, reduced fertility, high blood pressure, and increased risk of various cancers and heart attack. Drinking a lot of alcohol while pregnant seriously affects the baby's development.

Cigarettes, pipe tobacco, and chewing tobacco. These contain a drug called nicotine, which narrows blood vessels and causes high blood pressure and heart disease. Tobacco also contains tar, which increases lung infections and causes cancer of the lungs and throat. Smoking also harms people, including unborn babies, who don't smoke but who breathe in poisons in the smoke.

Cannabis. This is a leaf that can be smoked or eaten. People who use it a lot can find it difficult to think and do well at school or work, and may have accidents. Some people get violent or have serious mental health problems after using strong cannabis regularly. Users who mix tobacco with cannabis to smoke face the same problems as tobacco users. As growing, possessing, selling, or smoking cannabis is against the law in most countries, using it can result in prison or a large fine.

Sniffing e.g. glue, paint, solvent, petrol, gas, or turpentine. This causes problems with seeing, thinking, and remembering. It can lead to violent behaviour, loss of judgement and body control, and death. It is easy to become addicted to sniffing these substances.

Heroin and cocaine. It is very easy to get physically addicted to these illegal drugs. Once addicted, users' bodies need the drug so badly that they will do anything to get money to buy more. This makes people who are addicted vulnerable, and leads to other criminal acts such as stealing. If injected using unsterilized needles, their use can spread illnesses such as HIV and hepatitis, which damage the liver. Users can die from using supplies that are contaminated with other substances, or from accidently taking too much.

Drinking a lot of alcohol, smoking cigarettes, or using drugs during pregnancy. This can cause children to be born with disabilities.

Alcohol and drug use among children. This is more harmful than among adults because children's brains and bodies are still developing. Selling or giving children alcohol, tobacco, or other drugs is against the law in many countries and can be a form of abuse. Children also need protection from the harmful effects of drugs and alcohol on the behaviour of the adults they live with.

Interference with ARVs. Taking drugs can prevent users from taking ARVs regularly and lead to the ARVs not working so well, or causing dangerous side effects.

Benefits of not using mood-altering drugs

- We are better able to make good decisions about sex and safety.
- We avoid suffering a 'hangover' the next day (headache, vomiting, dizziness, regret, lack of self-respect).
- We are able to have a good conversation with people and remember it the next day.
- People may prefer how we are when we are not intoxicated.
- We are able to perform well at school or work, and in sports.
- We feel and look better.
- We save money.

EXERCISE 18.2 DO WHAT I DO, NOT WHAT I SAY

AIMS: To have fun and practise active listening and observation. To learn about how we copy people's behaviour.

DESCRIPTION: A copying game adapted from the game 'Simon Says', where players follow what Simon *does,* not what he *says* they should do.

Directions

1. Say: 'I am the leader and I want you to follow my actions. If I say, "Don't smoke a cigarette", but I mime smoking a cigarette, you must mime smoking a cigarette. If I say, "You must smoke cigarettes", but I don't mime it, then you must stay still.'

2. To get participants used to the idea, call out other types of local drugs and alcohol, sometimes miming the opposite to what you are saying, and sometimes saying an instruction but not miming it.

3. Play this as a game. The participants who have done what you did, rather than what you said they should do, get to stay in the game, while the others have to sit out. Everyone is allowed to get it wrong twice in the first round. People who are sitting out should watch those who are still playing, and think about whether to mime or stay still.

4. Discuss how hard the game is, and how you have to listen, watch, and think closely (be *mindful*) to get it right. Ask what we can learn from this in terms of real life. Do we listen to what people say, or copy what they do? Ask caregivers whether we 'practise what we preach'.

 ## EXERCISE 18.3 SUPPORTING OURSELVES IN TAKING CONTROL

AIMS: To identify ways of avoiding alcohol and drug use, or taking control of it. To understand the virtue of self-discipline.

DESCRIPTION: Participants pair up and spot abilities in relation to controlling use of drugs or other substances, such as food; they discuss the virtue of self-discipline.

Directions

1. Ask participants to pair up and take it in turns to tell a story about a time that they felt proud of themselves, about: (a) their own alcohol or drug use, or supporting someone else regarding drug use; (b) not eating too much of something, or resisting eating something; or (c) doing something right although they really wanted to do something else.

The listener asks questions to learn more about the story, spots and feeds back abilities, and adds to the teller's necklace.

Then invite participants to ask each other: 'How will you use these abilities to control your alcohol or drug use, or to do the right thing in the future?'

2. Back in a big group, draw the abilities and virtues that participants have used on a mind map. The central phrase is 'abilities used to control drug use'. Self-discipline is likely to be one of the most important virtues.

3. Ask: 'What do we mean by self-discipline?' As needed, add information from Box 18.b.

Box 18.b The virtue of self-discipline

Self-discipline means being in control of ourselves, rather than letting other people or other things be in control of us. It is getting ourselves to do what we really want to do rather than being tossed around by our feelings. With self-discipline, we take charge of ourselves. We observe our thoughts and feelings and then decide how we are going to behave. It is our choice – no one else's. We can set limits for ourselves, and create routines in our day, which help us reach our goals. This can help us in studying at school or getting daily jobs done – a whole range of different things.

---

4. Ask participants for examples of using self-discipline to stay in control. What tips can they share with each other?

 EXERCISE 18.4 SUPPORTING OTHERS IN TAKING CONTROL

AIMS: To practise using our abilities to support our children, peers, or friends in staying safe around alcohol and drugs.

DESCRIPTION: Participants hear a story and answer questions about how we can support each other in making good decisions about drug use, then work in groups of three to practise skills in doing this.

Box 18.c Information for facilitators

Younger children's experience of drugs and alcohol may be less about their own use of these substances, and more about the consequences of substance use among adults they live with. They may need protection, and will have limited ability to support others. The activities for 5–8 year olds in this exercise focus on thinking about resisting pressure to start using drugs or alcohol.

Directions

1. Divide into separate peer groups: caregivers, children aged 9–14 years, and children aged 5–8 years.

2. Follow the directions below with the relevant group.

Caregivers and children aged 9–14 years. Read or act out Nina's story.

Box 18.d The story of Nina

Nina is 13 years old. She cared for her sick mother until she died and is now caring for her sick father. She also has HIV. She thinks to herself, 'I am so lonely. I am different from everybody. I just want to get drunk and forget. I can take care of myself, I don't need anyone else.'

A group of boys are at the bar. They notice Nina buying two bottles of beer to take home. One of them says loudly, 'There's the walking dead coming to get drunk again.' The others laugh. But Joshua, a friend of Nina's, interrupts, saying, 'Oh be quiet! You get drunk for no reason at all. Nina is a brave girl who is looking after her dad. You should admire her, not tease her.' A man goes over to Nina saying, 'Let me pay for those beers; you look as if you need cheering up! Let's go to my place where we can relax, and you can forget how hard life is for a while. You're too pretty to look so sad.' Nina smiles. She likes the idea of drinking and forgetting, and the man says she's pretty, which makes her feel warm inside.

Joshua and his girlfriend Florence have heard what the man said, and feel worried for their friend. Florence goes over to Nina and puts her arm through Nina's, saying, 'It's beautiful by the sea now, why don't we three go for a stroll along the beach and see the sunset? You don't have to talk, we don't mind. We just like being with you.'

Nina sees that Florence is being sincere, and together they leave and go to the beach. She cries and they hug and comfort her and she feels a bit better. They agree that, Joshua and Florence will come round to Nina's house and play draughts with her dad, eat fried chicken, and help Nina clean the house.

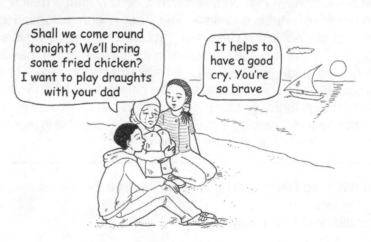

Discuss the story by asking questions such as:
- What happened in the story?
- Why did Nina want to get drunk?
- What might have happened if she had got drunk with the man?
- How did her friends help her?
- Does this happen in our community?
- How can we use our virtues to support one another when we have problems, like Nina, with drink or drugs?
- What can we say to each other about drinking or using drugs?
- Who else could support Nina in living with her situation and managing her alcohol use?

As appropriate, add information from Box 18.e.

Children aged 5–8 years. Read out Daliso's story.

Box 18.f The story of Daliso

Daliso is an eight year old boy who is very good at sport. He often plays with older boys, who like to have him on their team. One day after a match, some of the older boys begin to smoke cannabis and drink beer. They offer him some. He feels nervous; he thinks he should say no, but he also feels proud that the older boys are including him. It makes him feel grown up. He smokes some cannabis, but it makes him cough, which makes everyone laugh and he feels a bit silly. But the boys give him a cheer every time he takes a big gulp of beer. He begins to feel different. To begin with, he feels more confident and finds things funny, but then he begins to feel ill. He makes an excuse to leave. On the way home he feels terrible, and is sick on his shoes. He is worried about what will happen if his caregiver finds out what he has been doing.

Ask: 'Why did Daliso feel he shouldn't smoke the cannabis and drink the beer?'

'Why did he do it anyway?'

'How did he feel while he was taking the drugs?'

'How did he feel afterwards?'

'What do we learn from this story?'

What do we learn from this story?

Ask the children to form small groups and think of ways in which Daliso could have avoided taking the drugs. If necessary, prompt them to think of key strategies of: avoiding the situation, leaving the situation, and staying but resisting peer pressure to take the drugs.

3. *For all separate peer groups*. Ask participants to form groups of three. Each group is going to make up three five-minute role plays.

Caregivers and children aged 9–14 years in separate groups. Give each small group one of these situations to act out:

- A person who wants to try a drug for the first time.
- A person who wants to take control of their drug use and use drugs safely.
- A person who wants to stop taking drugs altogether.

In each role play, one group member should play the character facing the drug challenge, while the two members do their best to support the character to stay safe from harm. The character should be someone like them, or like their child. Ask each person to get into their character privately, by imagining their background story, why they want to use or are using drugs, and why they want to control their drug use.

Ask the groups to perform their first role play. Explain that when they finish, the character facing the drug challenge should say what they liked and didn't like about what the supporters did, and the supporters can add their comments.

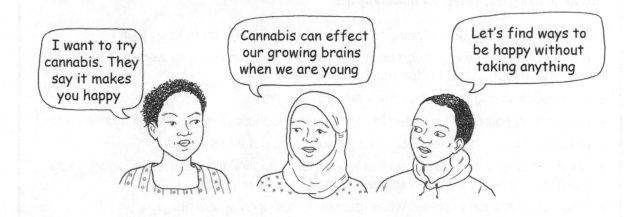

Repeat the process for the other two role plays, so that each group member has a turn at playing the character, and two turns at playing a supporter.

Children aged 5–8 years. Ask the children in their groups of three to make up role plays about these situations:

- A child who is resisting pressure to try a drug for the first time.
- A child who wants to try a drug for the first time.

Ask the children to swap roles, so each group member has a chance to pretend to be a child like them, who is either resisting pressure to take a drug or tempted to try a drug; one of the participants is putting pressure on the child to take a drug; and the other is supporting the child who wants to try taking drugs. The third person observes the interaction and comments on the strategies used to resist pressure or to support the child.

Ask a few groups to show one of their role plays. Make sure that both of the situations are shown.

4. *For all peer groups*. After each role play, invite the audience to give feedback on the strategy used to support the character facing the drug challenge. If people have another idea, they can go in the middle and act out their idea for feedback. As appropriate, add information from Box 18.g.

Box 18.g Tips for being in control of alcohol and drug use

Watch out for people putting drugs or strong drink into your drink. Some people think that this is funny but it can be very dangerous.

To avoid using the substance at all:

- practise saying 'no'.
- Be ready to use your courage and self-respect to protect yourself.
- Say that your religion does not allow you to drink.
- Say you have something really important to do the next day.
- Say you don't like the taste of alcohol.
- Say it's not good for your brain at your age to use alcohol or other drugs.
- Say it's against the law to drink at your age.

Tips for drinking less (adapt for other drug use)

- Decide how much you are going to drink in an evening and try to keep to it.
- Keep a note of how much you drink, when you drink, and who you were with. Can you see what makes you drink too much and why?
- Drink fewer strong drinks and mix them with soft drinks.
- Have a long soft drink (or water) between every alcoholic drink, to fill your stomach up.
- Drink slowly, and don't let people fill up your glass; put a mat over it.
- Drink soft drinks on a day when you would normally drink alcohol. Use the money you would have spent on alcohol to treat yourself or someone else.
- Relax and have fun in places where people do not drink or use drugs.

Steps to take to overcome a drink or drug problem

1. Accept that you have a problem and decide that you want to stop.
2. Decide to do something today, not tomorrow.
3. Tell at least one other person what you are doing. Ask for their support.
4. Stop – or use less, and then stop.
5. If you start again, don't blame yourself. Try to stop again right away.
6. Try to increase the support you have. Meet with friends who are also trying not to get drunk, or have decided not to use drugs. If a group of friends decide to stop together, you can give each other strength. Go to services that support people to address their dependency on alcohol or drugs.

---

5. Ask what participants have learned from this exercise, and sum up abilities used and suggestions made.

6. Say: 'Using our virtues to support our friends regarding drugs and alcohol use is important. However, people who use these substances may also need support from counsellors, services, and support groups.'

Closing circle

Bring the peer groups together to imagine how they can control their use of alcohol or other drugs so that these do not interfere with their dreams of a good future.

Explain: 'When we next meet for Session 19, we will talk about growing up and puberty, when we change from a girl or boy into a woman or man. It's an exciting time! Please write down (or tell us, privately if you like) questions that you have about puberty; for example, about periods or wet dreams. Put them in the question box and we will answer them over the next six sessions.'

If you are going to do Exercise 19.7, you'll need to find a young man and a young woman who were born with HIV, and who are willing to share their experiences of growing up with HIV and their lives now. Invite the caregivers and children to write down or tell you their questions about growing up with HIV to put in the question box. Explain that you will give these to the visitors before the meeting, so they can select the questions they are comfortable with and prepare their answers. Ask participants to think about how they would feel about answering these questions, and to ask the questions in a friendly way.

 ### ADDITIONAL EXERCISE 18.5 DRUG USE IN THE HOUSEHOLD

AIMS: To understand the consequences of household members drinking too much or using drugs. To find strategies to support people with drug problems in changing. To find strategies to protect caregivers and children.

DESCRIPTION: Participants draw a picture or act out role plays to show what can happen if a household member drinks too much or uses drugs. They dream of a family with no alcohol or other drug problems. They try to find ways of staying safe and supporting the person in changing, including linking them to support services.

Box 18.h Information for facilitators

Participants may not wish to share that they have problems with alcohol or drugs in their household, so the discussion here is about an imagined household. Encourage participants to talk about their personal experiences as if they relate to someone else. Invite participants to talk with you, a counsellor, or a community worker, about household alcohol or drug problems after the workshop. If several households have a problem, they might want to start a support group.

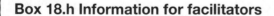

Directions

1. Divide into separate peer groups. Explain that we are going to talk about living in a household where someone drinks too much alcohol or uses other drugs. This can be worrying, increase poverty, and make the house unsafe. We are going to look at what household members, local services, and the community can do to support each other in this situation.

2. Ask participants, in small groups, to draw a picture or act out scenarios to show what can happen in a family if a person drinks or uses drugs too much.

3. Form three groups, and give each group two of the questions below to discuss and record as pictures or key words.

Questions for children
- What can we do to protect ourselves?
- What would we like to ask our caregivers to do to protect us?
- What would we like to say to the person who uses alcohol or drugs inappropriately?
- What can we do to support other household members?
- Who else can we go to for help? How can we get support from the community?
- What can we do if we know our friend is going through this situation?

Questions for caregivers
- What can we and other adults do to protect our children and others in the household?
- What would we like to say to the person who uses alcohol or drugs inappropriately?
- What can we do to support ourselves and other household members in changing?
- Who else can we go to for help? How can we get support from the community?
- What can we do if we know our relative, neighbour, or friend is going through this?

4. Share and discuss the small group pictures or words drawn from the answers to the questions above.

Ask: 'How can we use our virtues together to support one another in taking control of drug and alcohol use?' Add any further ideas from Box 18.i.

Tell people about the services available to help households where someone has an alcohol or drug problem.

Box 18.i Tips for those living with someone who uses drugs or alcohol

Talking with the person who uses drugs or alcohol

1. Use *'I' statements* when the person is sober, so they have compassion for how the drink or drug problems affect the rest of the family. For example:

'Usually I am so happy to see you coming through the door because you are my good companion and husband. But yesterday you had drunk a lot and were angry. I felt afraid that you would harm us. The children ran and hid. I know that you are a loving person. What can we do together to support you in controlling your drinking?'

2. Use *questions* that help the person think about the effect of their drug use on other family members and how it would be if they stopped. For example:

'If you asked your children what would improve their lives, what do you think they would say?'

'When your wife or children see you, what do you think makes them feel happy?'

3. Use virtues and *ability spotting* to encourage the person to use their abilities to control their drug use. For example:

'I know you like to drink, but you have managed to control your drinking before. How did you do that? Who supported you? How could you use that experience to take control of it now?'

4. Encourage *self-compassion* and *forgiveness*. For example:

'I feel that you are suffering. Many people take alcohol or drugs to reduce their suffering. What might soothe your suffering in a better way? How can we support you?'

'I know that you feel bad about the effect of your drug use on your children. Forgiving yourself and asking others to forgive you can be healing. Shall we say words of forgiveness to each other?'

Other tips

Have a family meeting, ideally including the person who uses drugs or alcohol, to plan how you will protect yourselves when they are intoxicated (for example, not allowing them to drive) and if they become aggressive and violent (for example, identifying a safe place you can go to, but not telling the person who uses alcohol or drugs where this is).

Ask for support from neighbours and friends, and from service providers such as counsellors, health workers, social workers, faith organizations, and NGOs. It does not help to try to keep the problem a secret. Many people have these problems and it is not helpful to feel shame or blame them.

Do not blame yourselves either. You can't 'rescue' the person; they have to decide to change themselves if they want to resolve the situation. No one else can do this for them.

Purpose: To understand the changes in our bodies as we grow up; to support ourselves or our children in feeling positive about growing up, and in managing the changes and challenges safely and happily.

Contents	Materials required	Time required
Opening circle (see p.13)		15 mins
19.1 Physical changes in puberty		30 mins
19.2 Our sexual and reproductive organs	Pictures on pages 243, 244 and 246 and Annex	90 mins
19.3 Social and behavioural changes in puberty		45 mins
19.4 Finding and giving support during puberty		45 mins
19.5 Managing menstruation	Picture on page 250 and Annex and samples of locally used ways of absorbing menstrual blood	60 mins
19.6 All about wet dreams		30 mins
Closing circle (see p.14)		15 mins
Additional exercises		
19.7 Growing up with HIV	Visitors who have grown up with HIV	60 mins
19.8 Male circumcision		60 mins
19.9 Female genital cutting		60 mins

About 5.5 hrs

Preparation

You asked people to put their questions about puberty in the question box at the end of Session 18. Read and sort them into themes to use during relevant exercises in this session.

Exercise 19.5. Find out what methods women use locally to absorb menstrual blood, and get a sample of each to show, for example: cloths, reusable cloth pads, disposable pads, and tampons. If reusable cups are available in your country (for example, Miacups and Mpower cups), buy a sample of those too. Sort the questions on periods and answer them in this exercise.

Exercise 19.7. If you are going to do this exercise, arrange the time for the visitors to come and ensure that they have the participants' questions from the box.

Exercises 19.8 and 19.9. To decide whether or not to do these exercises, find out the situation regarding male circumcision and female genital cutting (FGC) in the peer groups and local communities before this session. Male circumcision and FGC are often carried out between the ages of five and fourteen years; it is important that children and caregivers have correct information about these practices and explore what they can do to protect children from harm caused by them. As part of preparation for Exercise 19.8, find out where males can access safe, voluntary male circumcision locally.

Box 19.a Information for facilitators

Many of the 9–14-year-old participants will have started puberty. A few older girls in the 5–8-year-old group may have reached puberty, and the others will do so in the next few years. This session aims to provide the 5–8 year olds with simple information, positive attitudes, and support at a time when most of them are not emotionally engaged with sexual matters. This will enable them to manage puberty comfortably when they start it.

 ## EXERCISE 19.1 PHYSICAL CHANGES IN PUBERTY

AIMS: To understand the physical changes that take place during puberty.

DESCRIPTION: Participants learn about and discuss physical changes and challenges associated with puberty.

Directions

1. Explain: 'In this exercise we will talk about an important time in our lives called puberty. We will answer the questions about puberty in the question box, and you can add more questions to the box today, or ask questions during the exercises.'

Ask: 'What do we mean by the term "puberty"? What different words are used in our languages for "puberty"?'

Explain that puberty is the gradual process by which our bodies change from those of children to those of adults. Girls start from around eight years to twelve years, and boys usually between twelve and fourteen years. The changes happen because our bodies start to produce 'hormones', which are chemical messengers that tell our bodies and organs to change. We all change at different times and speeds during puberty, but eventually we will become adults.

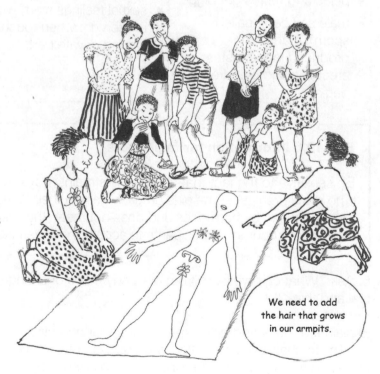

We need to add the hair that grows in our armpits.

During puberty we experience changes in our physical bodies, our thinking and emotions, our social lives, and our behaviour. Our culture expects us to behave differently as we grow up into adults.

In this exercise, we will look at the physical changes that occur during puberty.

2. Divide your peer group into males and females. In each group, draw the outline of a body of the same sex as the participants.

3. Ask participants to mark on the body all the changes that happen to the bodies of people of their sex as they grow up.

4. Bring the male and female groups together to share their body maps.

Note: Each drawing belongs to the group that made it; the group should not make changes to a drawing that isn't theirs without permission from the artists.

Ask: 'Which changes happen to both boys and girls? Put a coloured tick against these changes.'

'Which changes happen only to girls? Which changes happen only to boys?'

As needed, add information from Table 19.1.

Table 19.1 Physical changes in puberty

Boys	Boys and girls	Girls
• hair on the face starts to grow • voice gets deeper and goes squeaky for a while (voice 'breaks') • shoulders and chest get broader • penis and testes get bigger • male sex cells, called sperm, start being produced in the testes; erections and wet dreams begin	• height increases suddenly • pimples develop on skin • hair starts to grow under arms • pubic hair starts to grow • sweat smells different and need to wash more • sexual feelings start, with excitement when touched around private parts	• breasts develop and hips widen • ovaries get bigger and develop • female sex cells, called ova or egg cells in the ovaries, start to develop • periods start, usually about a year after breasts develop

---

Box 19.b Information for facilitators

Be sensitive to the fact that although it is mainly boys who get facial hair, and mainly girls who grow breasts, some girls do grow hair on their faces and some boys grow breasts. This is caused by hormones and does not mean that the girl is masculine or the boy feminine. Encourage participants to accept these variations in body changes as normal.

---

5. Ask: 'What can we learn from our body maps of changes in puberty? What do they make us feel and think?'

Explain that boys and girls experience similar and different changes in their bodies as they grow up. These changes are exciting and positive but sometimes challenging as well. Boys and girls are going through the same experience of change, and can support each other in managing it comfortably.

6. Ask the relevant peer groups:

Caregivers. 'What do you remember about puberty? What were the challenges? How would you like your children's puberty to be the same, and different, from your own?'

Children aged 9–14 years. 'What challenges may we experience with the changes? What are the good things about these physical changes? Let's celebrate them!'

Explain that we will talk more about the challenges in the next exercises. If there are challenges that are not covered in this session, say that we will discuss them in a later session. For example, one challenge of puberty is that older people may start to show unwanted sexual interest in boys and girls at this time and try to abuse them. We will deal with that in Sessions 26 and 27 on sexual abuse.

Children 5–8 years. 'What are you looking forward to about growing up and puberty? Is there anything that you feel concerned about?'

Say that you will talk together about their concerns later.

EXERCISE 19.2 OUR SEXUAL AND REPRODUCTIVE ORGANS

AIMS: To talk and learn about our sexual and reproductive organs and how they work. To agree on what names to call the sexual and reproductive organs. To have positive feelings about, and value, our sexual and reproductive organs.

DESCRIPTION: *Children aged 5–8 years.* Participants draw body maps and some of the organs in the body, before talking about the sexual and reproductive organs. They learn their names and, in a simple way, what they do. *Caregivers and children aged 9–14 years.* Participants draw the external and internal sexual and reproductive organs on body maps, learn how they work and decide what to name them.

Directions[53]

1. Explain: 'Now we are going to look at sexual and reproductive organs and how they work in more detail. We need to understand our organs and how they work so we can grow up happy, healthy, and safe in this aspect of our lives.

'We don't need to feel shy about talking about these organs because we all have them. They are a natural part of our lives. They are not dirty or funny; they are beautiful and amazing. We are not using the words as an insult, just as a fact of life. We can call each organ a name that we feel happy with, as long as we all understand what we mean. It's also useful to learn the "official" names so that we can talk with a health worker if we need to.

Children aged 5–8 years

2. Draw an outline of a woman, and explain that we are going to look at the organs that women use when they have sex and make babies.

3. Ask: 'Who can tell us what we have inside our bodies?' If necessary, say: 'Organs!' Point to the woman's chest and say: 'Who can tell us the name of an organ which sits in here?' Draw the organs that people mention, for example, the heart. Ask: 'What does the heart do?' You

might explain that it pumps blood around our bodies to give us energy. Repeat this with a few more organs.

4. Say: 'We also have organs for making babies. Who can tell us about a part or organ that women use for having sex and making babies?'

With each organ they mention, ask: 'Is this organ inside or outside the body?' Draw the organ or part on the picture of the woman.

5. Explain the biological name for the organ, and agree on what they would like to call it.

6. Continue to add drawings of sexual and reproductive parts and organs until participants run out of ideas. Add any organs they have not mentioned.

7. Ask people for their ideas on what the parts and organs do. Give simple explanations to add to their knowledge. For example, females have three openings between their legs: a tube for passing urine in the front; a hole for monthly periods, having sex, and giving birth, in the middle; and the anus at the back, for getting rid of waste.

Caregivers and children aged 9–14 years in separate peer groups

2. Split into male and female participants. Explain that we are going to start with the female organs. Invite the groups to look at the female body map and draw on any parts *outside* the body that are to do with sexuality and making babies.

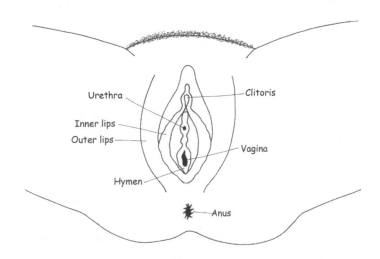

Urethra
Clitoris
Inner lips
Outer lips
Vagina
Hymen
Anus

Box 19.c Information for facilitators

Depending on the group's level of knowledge, you may find it helpful to draw at least some of the parts yourself and name them. If people in the group want to do this themselves, encourage them to do so, and provide the correct information when necessary.

3. Divide into groups of three and give each group one or two of the sexual or reproductive parts they have drawn. Ask them to write down all the names that people use for this organ. Invite them to put a circle around those they are comfortable using, and cross out those they don't like. Ask each group to choose one word they want to use on the body map. If a group chooses a word that is offensive or degrading to females or males, ask them to select a more respectful word. Explain that it is also good to know the biological name that is used by, for example, health workers.

4. Ask each small group to share the name they want to use with the rest of the peer group and, if there is agreement, label the part.

5. Now ask people to draw the parts *inside* the body used for making and growing babies, and to name them – again agreeing on what they want to call each part.

6. Show picture below and explain as appropriate. Talk about the different names for the *female reproductive organs* shown in the picture.

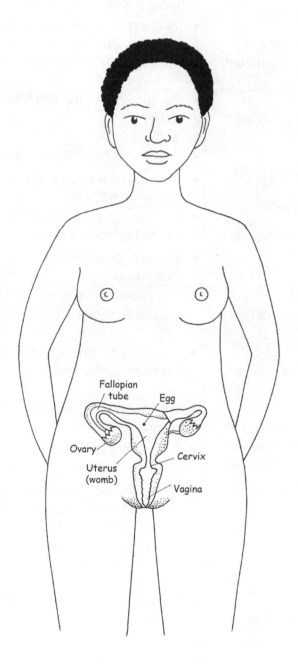

7. Have a question and answer session about what each part does in expressing sexuality and/or making a baby. As appropriate, use information from Table 19.2.

Table 19.2 Names and functions of female reproductive organs

Organ name and what it is	What it does
Urethra. Tube with a valve, which opens when we urinate. It is the first hole in the front of the vulva. Further back are the vagina and then the anus.	• This allows urine to pass from the bladder (where urine is stored) to the outside when females urinate.
Vagina. A tube inside the body that connects to the uterus, and has an open end between the legs.	• During sex, the penis goes inside the vagina and puts sperm into it. • Babies come out through it at birth. • Menstrual blood leaves the body through it. • The vagina is separate from the anus, the hole through which faeces pass.
Clitoris. Small 'bean' inside the inner lips around the vagina entrance, in front of the urine tube.	• Touching the clitoris gently increases sexual feelings and pleasure. This helps women be satisfied sexually and have an orgasm.
Labia or lips. Folds of skin around the entrance to the vagina.	• The lips protect the entrance to the vagina and the urethra.
Hymen. Piece of skin that covers the vaginal opening in girls.	• The hymen protects the vagina. • It can be broken by exercise, using tampons, and sexual intercourse.
Eggs. Tiny cells inside the woman's ovaries.	• The female's eggs carry half of the ingredients needed to make a baby. • If an egg joins with sperm, together they begin to make a baby.
Ovaries. Two little sacs on each side of the womb.	• The ovaries store about 300,000 eggs, and take it in turns to send one each month to the womb.
Fallopian tubes. Two tubes connecting the ovaries to the womb.	• Every month, one egg travels along the tube from the ovary to the womb.
Uterus or womb. Bag at the top end of the vagina. There is a small opening between the uterus and the vagina called the cervix.	• The uterus is where a baby grows during pregnancy. • Every month the womb prepares itself for a baby by making a thick lining. o If the woman or girl has sex and sperm join with the egg, then they stay in the womb and grow into a baby. o If the egg is not fertilized, the womb throws away the lining. This is the blood which comes out when a woman or girl has her period.
Anus. Hole at the end of the digestive system.	• When females go to the toilet, faeces (food waste) come out through the anus.

8. Now repeat steps 2–7, but for the *male reproductive organs*. As with the female organs, discuss and agree on what names participants want to call the organs.

Show picture below If needed, draw the male sexual and reproductive parts, and add information from Table 19.3 as needed.

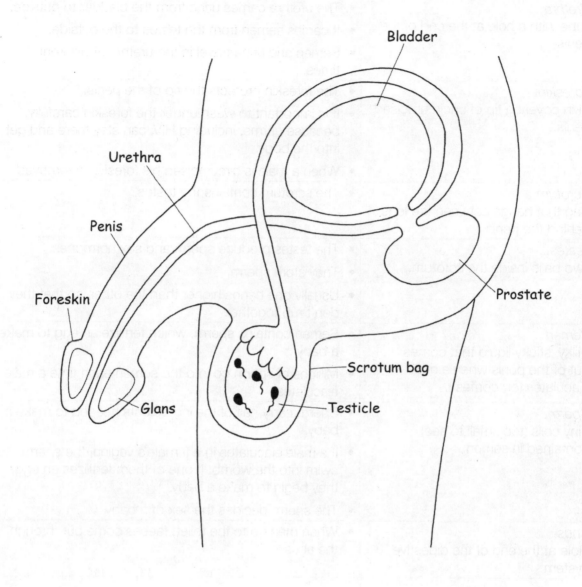

Table 19.3 Names and functions of male sexual and reproductive organs

Organ name and what it is	What it does
Penis. Tube which contains the urethra, which carries semen and urine.	• The penis can become stiff, which enables it to be placed in the vagina during sexual intercourse. • At orgasm the male ejaculates and semen spurts out.
Urethra. Tube with a hole at the end of the penis.	• The urethra carries urine from the bladder to outside. • It carries semen from the testes to the outside. • Semen and urine travel in the urethra at different times.
Foreskin. Skin covering tip of uncircumcised penis.	• The foreskin protects the tip of the penis. • It is important to wash under the foreskin carefully because germs, including HIV, can stay there and get into the body. • When a male is circumcised his foreskin is removed.
Scrotum. Bag that hangs between the legs behind the penis.	• The scrotum contains the testes.
Testes. Two balls inside the scrotum.	• The testes produce sperm and sex hormones. • They store sperm. • Usually one hangs higher than the other, so that they don't rub together.
Semen. Milky, sticky liquid that comes out of the penis when a male ejaculates (or 'comes').	• Semen contains sperm, which fertilize an egg to make a baby. • Millions of sperm go into the semen each time a male ejaculates.
Sperm. Tiny cells (too small to see) contained in semen.	• Sperm carry half of the ingredients needed to make a baby. • If a male ejaculates in a female's vagina, the sperm swim into the womb. If one of them fertilizes an egg, they begin to make a baby. • The sperm decides the sex of a baby.
Anus. Hole at the end of the digestive system.	• When men go to the toilet, faeces come out through the anus.

 EXERCISE 19.3 SOCIAL AND BEHAVIOURAL CHANGES DURING PUBERTY

AIM: To explore other changes that take place during puberty.

DESCRIPTION: Participants engage in a question and answer session about social and behavioural changes during puberty. They work in small groups on cultural expectations, adult and peer support for boys and girls during puberty, and requesting support.

Directions

1. Say: 'We have talked about physical changes in puberty. In this exercise we will think about mental, emotional, social, and behavioural changes.

'In Session 2, we learned that we are gaining new *mental* skills as our brains develop, for example: imagining and analysing future situations, making good decisions, and developing our virtues.

'In Sessions 1 and 2 we learned about our *emotions*, and how to manage our big feelings and empathize with others. During puberty, we may experience unexpected mood swings, until the levels of different hormones settle down. We establish a sense of identity, and of how we see and feel about ourselves: our qualities, gender, sexuality, ethnicity, roles, goals, interests, and values.'

2. Split into male and female groups, each with a facilitator.

Ask: 'What changes do we (or our children) experience in our *social* lives during puberty? That is, relating to the people we form relationships with, and how we interact with family and friends.'

If necessary, explain that socially, at this time in our lives, we are learning how to be independent from our families, and our peers become very important to us. By identifying with our peers, we develop our own identity and see how we differ from our families. We may argue with our caregivers as we reach for independence. This is normal, but we should still show respect and listen to their ideas. As we get older, we start to have closer one-to-one friendships, and we may get sexually attracted to people of our sex or the other sex. We become more able to accept difference in ourselves and other people.

3. Ask: 'What changes do we experience in our *behaviour* as we grow up?'

As we grow up, we use our developing skills and drive to experiment with new behaviours. This is normal, and helps us shape our identities, try out new skills, assess ourselves, and gain peer acceptance and respect. The part of our brain that drives us to try new things and excites us develops before our skills in decision-making, so we are more likely to take risks. We can support each other in finding positive ways to satisfy our need to try new things. We can put our new skills, energy, and creativity to good use in our communities.

4. Ask: 'How do adults in our society support us when we reach puberty? What and how does our *culture* teach us how to behave as males and females? What changes does it expect us to make in how we dress, behave, interact with others, and contribute to meeting our and our family's needs?'

Our culture has ways of guiding and protecting us over this period, for example: initiation courses and ceremonies; setting new rules and expectations, which are intended to keep us on a good path; and monitoring our progress. Our society may also change how they behave towards us, for example: expecting us to have sex, make more contributions to our upkeep, leave home, or cover ourselves up.

Ask: 'What do we like and not like about these changes?'

'What requests would we like to make to our caregivers about the support we would like during puberty?'

5. Ask: 'How do our male and female peers support us during puberty?'

'What requests would we like to make to our peers about the support we would like during puberty?'

 ## EXERCISE 19.4 FINDING AND GIVING SUPPORT DURING PUBERTY

AIMS: To make requests to caregivers and peers about how we would like to be supported during puberty. To identify people who are easy to talk to about personal matters during puberty. To practise asking questions and seeking support during puberty.

DESCRIPTION: Participants make requests to caregivers and peers; identify people who can support children during puberty; and create role plays to practise talking to a trusted person about puberty.

Directions

1. Bring together all the participants. Ask the children to sit in their peer groups, each in a semicircle, with boys sitting together and girls together. Ask the caregivers to sit in a semicircle opposite their children. Explain that the children are now going to make their requests for support during puberty to their peers and their caregivers.

2. Invite the girls in each peer group to make their requests to the boys as to how they would like the boys to support them during puberty. Invite the boys to make requests in turn to the girls.

3. Next, invite the girls and boys in each peer group to make their requests to the caregivers as to how they would like the caregivers to support them during puberty.

4. Remind participants of the supporters they identified in Exercise 1.8 'Supporting each other in being strong' (who would support them across the river) and Exercise 10.5 'Who is there for me?' (when they made a bracelet to remember their helpers). Ask them to think about these people for a moment.

Ask participants: 'Who would you talk to if you had a problem about growing up and puberty? What are your reasons for choosing that person?'

5. Direct the relevant peer groups as follows:

Children. Invite them to form groups of three and create role plays to practise asking these trusted people for help with different puberty problems.

Caregivers. Ask them to role play giving their children opportunities to talk and ask questions about puberty, and then giving them support.

6. Give the relevant peer groups this homework:

Children. Ask them to talk about one aspect of growing up with their caregiver or trusted person during the next week.

Caregivers. Ask them to give their children opportunities to talk about growing up during the next week.

EXERCISE 19.5 MANAGING MENSTRUATION

AIMS: To learn what menstruation is and why it happens. To have positive attitudes towards menstruation. To support girls in managing menstruation happily at home and at school. To support boys and caregivers in supporting girls during menstruation.

DESCRIPTION: Participants create drawings, answer questions, and have group discussion about periods. They look at sanitary materials and fluid absorption. They make a mind map of things that support comfortable menstruation, and challenges.

Directions

1. Divide your peer group into males and females.

2. Explain that we are now going to learn about the monthly 'periods' that girls and women have. Adults often feel shy about talking to their daughters about periods, and children get the wrong ideas about them. Today we are going to talk openly about them and learn the truth, so that we can manage them comfortably.

3. Divide participants into smaller groups and ask them to discuss the following questions:
- What have you heard, or what do you know, about periods?
- What do you think is happening in a girl's body during her monthly cycle?
- Encourage them to draw what they know on pieces of paper.

4. In the whole peer group, put all the papers on the ground and encourage participants to share and discuss the ideas. Provide correct information if people have misinformation about periods. Summarize, adding correct information from Box 19.d as needed. Keep it simple and reassuring.

Ask: 'What is "menstruation"?' Show picture here and from Annex and, if needed, add information from Box 19.d.

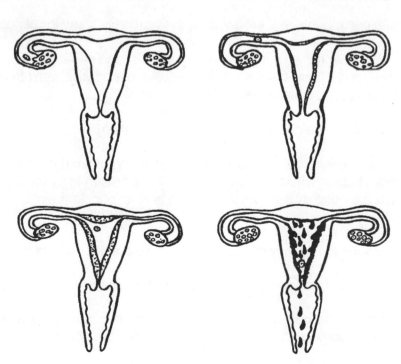

Box 19.d Information about menstruation

Note: For children aged 5–8 years, simplify the information, and encourage positive attitudes.

- Menstruation is a normal monthly bleeding from the vagina that happens to all females from puberty (from about nine years old) to menopause (at about 50 years old). It is normal and healthy.
- 'Ovulation' happens once a month: it is when one egg leaves its ovary and travels down the fallopian tube to the womb. The womb wall becomes thick like a nest, ready to house a baby.
- If the egg is not fertilized, the lining of the womb breaks down and leaves the body through the vagina as menstrual blood. This happens about 14 days after ovulation.
- Menstrual bleeding usually lasts four to six days. If the period lasts more than eight days, or is very heavy with thick blood, the girl should see a doctor.
- Periods do not come regularly at first, but they usually settle down to a regular pattern.
- If a girl or woman has sexual intercourse, and the egg meets sperm and becomes fertilized, it embeds itself into the wall of the womb where it begins to grow into a baby.
- A girl can get pregnant before she starts her periods, because her first ovulation is before her first period.
- If a young woman has not started her monthly period by the age of 16 years, she should see a doctor.
- Some girls have pain during menstruation, as the muscles of the womb push out blood. This is normal. Exercises, resting, and painkillers can reduce or stop the pain.
- It is normal for some girls to feel moody and down just before their periods begin.
- Girls need to use something to absorb or catch blood during their period, and to replace this when needed. They should also wash between their legs at least once, or ideally twice, a day.
- Girls should eat foods such as dark green leafy vegetables and meat, which contain a lot of iron, to replace the iron lost in blood.

5. Invite participants to think about all the words we know for periods in all our languages.

Ask: 'Which words sound positive and which sound negative?' For example, 'the curse' is negative, and 'moon-time' is positive. Agree on a positive word to use in the session, with which participants are comfortable.

Ask: 'What are the good things about menstruation?'

You might explain that menstruation shows that girls are growing up to become women who can have babies when they are ready to. It is a time to feel proud of our bodies and abilities. Periods are not dirty if we wash properly, and we should never be made to feel unclean at this time.

Invite groups to sing any songs in their culture about girls becoming women and menstruation.

Ask: 'How do these songs make you feel about menstruation?' What makes you feel that way?'

If the songs have negative points, say that we will look at these again at the end of the exercise to see if we agree with them. Emphasize the positive points.

6. Lay out all available sanitary materials, such as towels, cloths, or tampons.

Ask: 'How do girls and women manage menstruation in our communities?'

Invite participants to draw the methods they know, or to pick one sample up and explain how to use it. Pass the materials around and invite questions and answers.

Ask: 'Which ones are available in our neighbourhood, how much do they cost, and how easy are they to use and dispose of?' Explain how to use them safely.

7. Try putting a teaspoon of water or coloured liquid (for example, coke) onto a sanitary towel, a cloth, and a tampon to see how well it is absorbed.

8. Ask: 'What are the challenges that girls here face in managing their periods?'

Put participants' ideas on a mind map. See how different parts of the mind map join up.

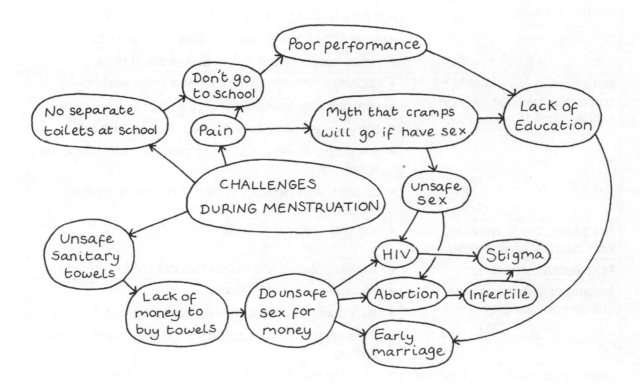

Ask: 'What are the things that support us, and make it easier for girls to manage their periods?'

Add the support mentioned in Exercise 19.3 related to periods, and any others participants can think of. See if they can identify forms of support to tackle challenges. Encourage everyone, including boys and male caregivers, to think of things they can do. As needed, add information from Table 19.4.

Table 19.4 Challenges and support in managing menstruation

Challenges	Support
Shortage of materials to absorb menstrual blood	• make reusable pads from scrap material • prioritize purchase of pads or tampons • ask school to supply pads and tampons
How to wash and dry pads at home and at school privately	• create more openness in the household so that privacy is less important • make a private place at home and school
How to dispose of pads and tampons privately	• put them in a pit latrine • if it's a flushing toilet, provide a bin beside it • empty this bin regularly and bury the contents • make sure the toilet is lit to use safely at night
Not knowing when period might come, and getting blood on clothes outside home	• understand fertility cycle (covered in Session 25) • carry pads or towels just in case • carry a waterproof bag for used, reusable pads • ask school to keep a stock of sanitary pads and some spare clothes • be open with friends, in order to borrow or lend as needed
Not being able to wash regularly with clean water and soap	• find ways to access soap and water
No toilets at school	• organize community to build school toilets
Teasing or bullying by other children or teachers	• educate to change attitudes • use courage to challenge bullying behaviour • show empathy and support if a girl gets blood on her clothes
Getting grumpy before a period starts, and having pain during the period	• be understanding and supportive: hormone changes make some girls and women moody before each period • carry or provide painkillers • show love and support

 ## EXERCISE 19.6 ALL ABOUT WET DREAMS

AIMS: To understand what wet dreams are, and have positive attitudes towards them. To know that wet dreams do not mean that boys and girls should have sex.

DESCRIPTION: Participants engage in storytelling and group discussion.

Directions

1. Explain that in this exercise we are going to talk about a sign that boys have started puberty and are growing into men.

2. Read the story of Juma (Box 19.e), or an adaptation of it.

Box 19.e The story of Juma

Juma is 12 years old. Last week he woke up with wet patches on his bed. It smelled funny, and he noticed that the liquid was on his penis too. He remembered that he had had a sexy dream about a girl in his class. He wanted to touch her body.

His older brother noticed the wet patches and laughed at him. He said the only way Juma could stop this happening was to get a girl to have sex with him. Now Juma is afraid. Please advise him.

---

3. In small, separate groups of males or females, discuss and agree on what advice to offer Juma.

4. Back with the whole group, invite participants to share their advice, and role play giving it to Juma. As needed, provide additional information from Box 19.f.

Box 19.f Information about wet dreams

- When a boy reaches the age of about 12, the testes start producing sperm.
- A 'wet dream' is when a boy becomes sexually excited during a dream and ejaculates in his sleep. He finds sticky wetness in his bed. This is natural and healthy, and not a sin.
- Some boys may have wet dreams regularly and others hardly ever have them. Both are normal. Wet dreams can continue into adulthood.
- Wet dreams do not mean that a boy should start to have sexual intercourse. It is safer to let wet dreams take care of sperm production until boys are mature enough to have a safe, caring sexual relationship.
- Ejaculation means that a boy is capable of making a girl pregnant. It does not mean that he is ready to become a father.
- Girls can also have sexy dreams, and some might find that they are wet between their legs at these times. This wetness is good and normal – it is made in the vagina and protects it during sex.

---

5. Ask if anyone has further questions about wet dreams. Turn them into statements, then ask participants to vote on whether they are true or false and explain why. Clarify with correct information as needed.

Here are some examples:
- If a boy ejaculates in wet dreams, he is not 'abstaining'.   False
- Wet dreams mean that you have had sex with a ghost.   False
- Wet dreams mean that you are being unfaithful to your girlfriend.   False

6. Summarize the correct information about wet dreams. Emphasize that wet dreams are the normal and healthy way in which the male body gets ready for adulthood, sexual activities, and

making babies. At this time, the body is growing faster than the mind. Boys at puberty are not ready to have sex safely, nor to make and raise children.

Closing circle

Ask participants to bring their mind maps on words and actions showing love (from Exercise 8.2) to Session 20, which is all about relationships, love, and sexuality.

 ## ADDITIONAL EXERCISE 19.7 GROWING UP WITH HIV

This extra exercise could take place as part of Session 19, as a separate activity, or at the start of Session 21.

AIMS: To reassure caregivers and children that children with HIV can grow up in the same way as children who do not have HIV, in terms of their sexuality, relationships, and ability to have babies. They can take control of HIV in their lives rather than allowing HIV to control them. To understand and practise the main points about living positively during puberty.

DESCRIPTION: A visit from a young man and woman with HIV, who are comfortable talking with children and their caregivers about the questions asked by participants at the end of Session 18. They may also be happy to answer additional questions from the participants during this exercise. Box 19.h gives some examples of questions asked by participants at other workshops. Invite the visitors to talk about any that have not been asked and they feel are important.

Box 19.g Information for facilitators

Participants put questions about growing up with HIV in the anonymous question box at the end of Session 18. You gave the questions to the young man and woman with HIV and asked them to sort and select the questions they were comfortable answering. Participants may have asked questions that express their fears and anxieties about the future for themselves or their children. This is fine, because the answers can make them feel less anxious. Help them ask some more positive questions as well.

Directions

1. With all the peer groups together, introduce and welcome the visitors and thank them for coming to talk with your groups about their lives with HIV.

2. Divide participants into males and females.

Invite the male visitor to sit in the middle of the male group, and the female visitor to sit with the female group, with their facilitators. Invite the visitors to read out the questions from participants one by one, and answer them. Invite participants to ask questions for clarification or share ideas with the visitors.

Box 19.h Growing up with HIV: examples of topics and questions

About coping

- What made us feel better about having HIV?

- Who supported us at different times, and how did they support us?

- What are the challenges about having HIV? How did we overcome them?

- What advice would we give to children and young people who have HIV? What would we say to their friends? To their caregivers?

About friendships and sexual activity

- Did we tell our friends that we have HIV? How did they respond?

- What effect did HIV have on the games we play(ed)? Did we do anything to stay safe?

- Do/did we have a boy- or girlfriend? Does/did HIV affect our friendship? In what way?

- What did we do and say if someone was unkind to us because we have HIV?

About the future

- How do we think we will know that someone loves us when they know we have HIV?

- How can we decide on a good enough person to marry us?

- Do we plan to have children? How many? How can we keep them free from HIV?

About health

- What are we doing to stay healthy and live a long time?

- What helps us take our medicines on time?

About work

- What work do we do and how does having HIV affect it?

 ## ADDITIONAL EXERCISE 19.8 MALE CIRCUMCISION

This extra exercise may be useful if male circumcision happens in the participants' communities, and if there are health programmes encouraging boys and men to get circumcised in your country.

AIMS: To understand male circumcision, what it does and doesn't do, and how to do it safely. To support caregivers and their children in making safe and healthy decisions about male circumcision. To support families in acting on these decisions.

DESCRIPTION: Participants engage in a question and answer session and discussion, and draw mind maps.

Directions

1. Explain that in this exercise we are going to talk about male circumcision. You may wish to divide your peer group into males and females.

Ask: 'What is male circumcision? What is done to the penis?'

'What is the difference in looks between a circumcised and uncircumcised penis?'

If necessary, explain that male circumcision is cutting the foreskin off the penis, leaving the glans at the head of the penis exposed. When an uncircumcised male does not have an erection, the end of his penis is covered by the foreskin, whereas for a circumcised man the end of the penis is not covered.

Explain that some boys in our peer group may have been circumcised, and others not. Invite anyone who is circumcised, and happy for group members to know this, to help the other participants understand it better.

Note: Encourage boys not to tease each other about differences in how their penises look. Explain that whether circumcised or not, a man can make love, ejaculate sperm, and make healthy babies.

2. Ask: 'Are any boys and men circumcised in our communities? Which groups are circumcised, and why those in particular?'

'Why do people circumcise males? What do they see as the benefits? What are the challenges for the male and his partner?' As needed, add information from Box 19.i.

Draw a mind map to show benefits and disadvantages. The first circle in the middle reads 'Male circumcision'. Add a circle labelled 'Benefits' to the right, and one labelled 'Challenges' to the left. Add all the benefits on the right side of the paper, and all the challenges on the left side.

Box 19.i Information about male circumcision

Male circumcision is cutting the foreskin off the penis, leaving the glans at the head of the penis exposed. It is a traditional practice in some communities.

Recently, governments have started to promote voluntary medical male circumcision, because it reduces the chance of males getting HIV from females through intercourse. Removing the foreskin makes it harder for HIV to enter the body, as HIV uses the cells under the foreskin as a route for transmission.

Male circumcision:
✓ reduces the likelihood of HIV transmission from female to male by 40–70%
✗ does not reduce the likelihood of HIV transmission from male to female;
✓ gives lifelong reduction in risk from a single operation;
✗ is not as effective as using a condom, which reduces the likelihood of transmission to both male and female by around 90%;
✗ does not protect against pregnancy;
✗ does not mean males are 'protected' or 'cured' from HIV, if they already have it, nor that it is safe for them to have more sexual partners;
✓ reduces the risk of males getting some STIs, including herpes and chancroid, and penile cancer.

It is important that uncircumcised boys and men have good hygiene; they should pull the foreskin back and wash underneath it every day. Otherwise, germs can grow and a secretion called smegma will smell.

---

3. Ask: 'At what age is male circumcision done in this community? Where is the circumcision done? Is it available in health facilities?'

If participants are not aware of local services, explain what is available.

'Who carries out the circumcision, and how is it done?'

'What is done to ensure that it is safe, at the time and later? What are the risks of being circumcised?'

Add information from Box 19.j as needed. During the discussion, encourage participants to talk about circumcision with their family and children, and refer them to local services, counselling, and more information.

Box 19.j Making male circumcision safe

Complications of male circumcision can result in infection, bleeding, damage to the penis and, in rare cases, death. Good training, sterile equipment, and a clean environment with support afterwards, minimizes these problems.

Many families are deciding to have voluntary medical male circumcision, meaning it is done in sterile conditions in a health facility, by trained staff. This is the safest way to do it, providing proper standards of hygiene and training are met.

Males wishing to be circumcised in a health facility should be offered an HIV test. Those who have HIV should be counselled on the advantages and risks of being circumcised, for them and their partners. Some may already have HIV, but it doesn't yet show in their blood test (see Session 13). Male circumcision does not reduce male-to-female transmission of HIV. However, it may reduce the transmission of other STIs to both the male and the female.

For safer circumcision in the community on groups of boys, a new razor should be used or a knife (which should be sharp) must be sterilized between use *on each boy* to avoid passing HIV and other STIs from one boy to the next. After cutting, the wound must be kept clean to prevent infections that could damage the penis.

Caregivers, children, and facilitators could meet with circumcisers and support them in providing a safer service. Initiation counsellors could refer boys to the health service for medical circumcision, but still teach the boys how to be good men; practise safer sex, including using condoms; and to respect, care, and love sexual partners.

After circumcision – whether or not it takes place in a health facility – males must not masturbate or have sex for four to six weeks. This is to give the wound time to heal, and eliminates the relatively high risk of getting or passing on infections (including HIV) caused by the wound. After this time it is safe to have sex, but they must use a condom each time for six months, to protect the wound and prevent them from getting or sharing infection. After that, condom use is recommended to prevent getting or sharing STIs (including HIV), and unwanted pregnancy.

---

4. Ask: 'How are child rights realized if children are circumcised before the age of consent? What happens in our country? Should boys be able to refuse circumcision until they reach the age of consent?'

Add information from Box 19.k if needed.

Box 19.k Male circumcision and boys' rights

In most countries, caregivers are asked to sign the consent form for surgical procedures, such as circumcision, on boys in their care. However, children's rights also demand that children are given full information and participate in decisions that affect their lives. Children are able to understand and take part in decision-making about circumcision, just as they can about HIV testing. Caregivers need to start discussing the issue with boys some time before they are due to be circumcised, to give them time to think about and agree (or not) to circumcision.

 ADDITIONAL EXERCISE 19.9 FEMALE GENITAL CUTTING

This extra exercise should only be used if female genital cutting happens in the participants' communities.

AIMS: To understand female genital cutting (FGC) in girls, and its perceived benefits and negative consequences. To support caregivers and children in upholding the rights of all children by finding new ways of making safe and healthy decisions about cutting.

DESCRIPTION: Participants discuss the reasons for FGC, its perceived benefits and its negative consequences.

Box 19.l Views on FGC

 We believe that FGC is a practice that violates the following: a female's right to life; her protection from harmful practices; her health; safe child-bearing; and her sexual pleasure. We believe that we have a duty to protect girls from this practice, and to support survivors in ways that bring them the most good and the least harm.

People who don't cut are often, rightly, very negative about the practice of FGC because of the violence and pain it causes, and the negative consequences it has for physical and mental wellbeing. However, people who cut often believe that the practice benefits girls and women, and is an important part of their culture. We need to acknowledge these ideas as well as talking about the damage caused by the practice if we are to contribute to change. Caregivers, male peers, and females who have been cut or are at risk of cutting need an opportunity to weigh up the perceived benefits against the negative consequences, and find new ways of supporting girls in becoming women. It can be hard for females who have been cut to accept that their rights have been violated. They may cope with the trauma later by believing in the perceived benefits and having their own daughters cut. Talking about their experiences, and focussing on their courage and survival, can support them in changing their attitudes towards the practice.

Directions

1. Explain: 'In this exercise, we are going to talk about female genital cutting, which is practised in some of our cultures.'

2. Ask: 'What type of female genital cutting is done in your culture? Is it removal of the clitoris and hood? Are the labia removed? Is the vulva sewn up, leaving a small hole for urine and menstrual blood?'

If children in the peer groups do not know, explain to them.

3. Ask: 'Why do some families cut (and re-cut) their daughters?'

'Why do some girls ask to be cut?'

'Why do some women ask to be cut before marriage or childbirth?'

'What do males generally think about female genital cutting?'

Ask: 'What benefits do you think come from cutting?'

'What harmful effects may come from cutting?'

Use participants' ideas to draw a mind map of perceived benefits and harmful effects. Write or draw 'Female genital cutting' in the first circle in the middle. Add a bubble labelled 'Benefits' on the right side of the paper, and a bubble labelled 'Challenges' on the left side of the paper. Add further words or drawings related to each bubble. Use Box 19.m to add any harmful effects that participants have not included. See how different parts of the mind map link up.

Box 19.m Perceived benefits and harmful effects of FGC

Perceived benefits (things people may believe, but which may not be true)
* The genitals look more beautiful.
* Girls who are cut together remain close friends throughout their lives.
* Girls who are brave are celebrated and gain confidence in being able to cope with pain, for example, in childbirth.
* Males and females approve of the way girls who have been cut look, so cutting allows girls to make good marriages.
* Females are more chaste and faithful without a clitoris, because they feel less sexy.
* Females become more womanly without a 'male' part (the clitoris).
* During initiation, girls learn how to be good women and good wives.

Harmful effects
Genital cutting can:
* cause severe bleeding and shock from pain when it is done; this can in turn cause death;
* cause severe infection (including HIV) when it is done, if knives or blades are shared;

- make it difficult for women to enjoy sexual relations and pleasure, and fearful of sex if it is painful; this weakens marital bonds and may make it more difficult to stay with one partner;
- make it difficult to pass urine and menstrual blood, causing serious infection and pain;
- cause obstructed labour, and associated death of the mother and child;
- cause mental ill health in females, both when undergoing the cutting and as a result of its effects during the rest of their lives.

4. Put a sign in one corner of the room saying 'agree'; one in another corner saying 'disagree'; and one in another place saying 'don't know'.

Read out one of the perceived benefits, and ask participants to go to the place that represents their opinion. Invite people in the different corners to say why they chose that corner. Encourage participants to listen to each other and really try to understand their views.

Ask if anyone would like to move to another corner as a result of the discussion. If so, ask them to give their reasons.

When all the benefits have been discussed, ask participants to vote on whether they think the benefits of FGC are worth the negative consequences.

5. Remind participants about Session 4 on children's rights.

Ask: 'Which of children's rights does female genital cutting violate?'

Explain that FGC is a violation of the following: a girl's human rights to life; her health; safe child-bearing; protection from harmful practices; participation in decisions which affect her; and sexual pleasure.

6. Ask: 'What does the law say about female genital cutting in our country?'

Say that many countries have made FGC illegal because of the harm it does and because it violates girls' human rights.

7. Ask: 'What happens when a girl does not want to be cut? How do we feel about that?'

Work with the relevant peer groups as follows:

Children. Support the girls in identifying who they will tell if they think they or a friend is to be cut. Support boys in doing the same, in relation to their female siblings and friends.

Ask: 'What support will you ask for from that person?'

Caregivers. Ask: 'How do you feel about supporting a girl who does not want to be cut, or a friend or relative who is trying to protect their child from cutting? What could you do?'

Ask people to think about:
- how to keep the child safe;
- who could support us – perhaps our peer group, family, community group or leaders, or certain services;
- how we could change community ideas about female genital cutting.

8. Read and discuss the story in Box 19.n, or invite stories from participants about the cutting that happens in their community, from the perspective of girls and women.

Box 19.n FGC story – perspectives as a girl and a woman[54]

I was circumcised when I was 10 years old at my initiation ceremony. Even now, if I think of the pain, tears come into my eyes. I remember bleeding for three days until I was certain I was dying – all my blood had drained away. I heard my mother calling for the spirits to save me. Well, I lived to marry when I was 20 years old. My husband was a good man, but we could not enjoy our sexual life because it caused me such pain. I have never had the blessing of sexual happiness throughout my whole marriage. I have lost my 'pleasure button', as those fortunate enough to have a clitoris call it. I wish there were a shop where I could buy one. Eventually I became pregnant. The delivery nearly killed me. I had to be cut again and re-sewn. I shall never have another child. Now my daughter is nine years old. I shall never allow her to be cut. I keep her with me in town. I never visit my family in the village with her, in case she is snatched away and cut. If I travel anywhere without her, my sister cares for her.

---

9. Bring male and female participants together to share ideas about alternative ways of achieving the same purpose as FGC. You may want to read out the story in Box 19.o.

Box 19.o FGC story – a circumciser's perspective

I used to be a circumciser, but I always feared cutting too deep, and every year one or two mothers' daughters would not return home. I shut my ears to their pain, because I convinced myself that cutting was good. After all, it had been done to me. Now I think it's right to call it mutilation. I was robbed of my birthright: to have pleasure in sex. Now, I still teach the girls in the initiation ceremony, it is still a private, special time just for them, but I teach them new things about health and love as well as the best of our traditions. I don't do any cutting, but I teach them to treat sex with respect and caution – it is not a game. They behave well and receive the respect they used to get from cutting. And I still have my power and rewards in the community.

Explain that in many communities people are stopping the harm caused by FGC and adapting their rituals. The new methods allow former cutters to keep their status and still teach the educational aspects of initiation ceremonies. The new generation of girls are free from the fear of cutting and the health problems that it causes. When they grow up, their sexual relationships are happier and childbirth is safer.

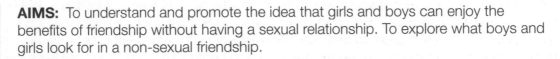

SESSION 20 RELATIONSHIPS, LOVE, AND SEXUALITY

Purpose: To appreciate the value of non-sexual friendships between boys and girls; to think about the relationship between love and having sex; to explore sexual identities, the challenges of early marriage, and steps towards an ideal long-term loving relationship.

Contents	Materials required	Time required
Opening circle (see p.13)		15 mins
20.1 Friendships between boys and girls		40 mins
20.2 The pairing game		10 mins
20.3 Love, sexual feelings, and having sex	Mind maps from Session 8.2	60 mins
Closing circle (see p.14)		15 mins
Additional exercises for children aged 9–14 years and caregivers only		
20.4 Early marriage	Picture on page 271 and in Annex	60 mins
20.5 An ideal long-term, loving relationship		30 mins
20.6 Love between people of the same sex		30 mins

About 2.5 hrs

 EXERCISE 20.1 FRIENDSHIPS BETWEEN BOYS AND GIRLS

AIMS: To understand and promote the idea that girls and boys can enjoy the benefits of friendship without having a sexual relationship. To explore what boys and girls look for in a non-sexual friendship.

DESCRIPTION: *Children.* Participants discuss friendships between girls and boys and create role plays about them. *Caregivers.* Participants discuss friendships between girls and boys and create mind maps about them.

Directions

Children

1. Divide into groups of four, with boys and girls in different groups. Explain that we are going to explore friendships between girls and boys.

2. Ask half the groups to discuss the negative aspects using the questions below:
• What are the things you do not like in friendships between girls and boys?
• What makes it difficult to have a good friendship between a girl and a boy?

Prepare a role play to show the things that get in the way of a good friendship.

Ask the other half of the groups to discuss the positive aspects using the questions below:

• What are the things you do like in a friendship between a girl and a boy?

• What behaviours would show a good friendship between a girl and a boy?

Prepare a role play to show some of the behaviours that make a good friendship.

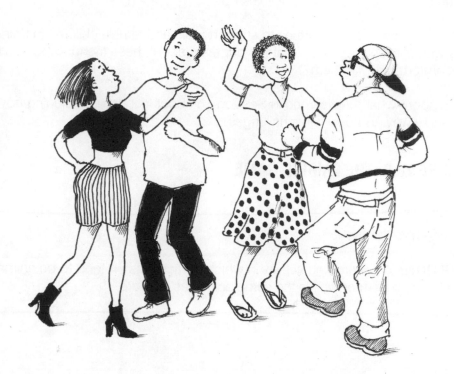

3. Invite each group to present their role play to the other, followed by discussion using the questions below.

For role plays showing what does not make a good friendship:

• What things show that this is not a good friendship?

• What might be making it difficult for them to have a good friendship?

• What would you like to change to make it a good friendship?

• How can we use our virtues to support all of us in being good friends to each other?

For role plays showing what makes a good friendship, ask:

• What shows that the friendship is going well?

• What things show that the two people care for each other?

• Is each character a good friend to the other? Why, or why not?

4. At the end, ask participants what they have learned from the activity.

5. Invite each person to think of one way that they will show care to someone else over the coming week.

Caregivers

1. Ask participants to form small groups, and to discuss changes in friendships between boys and girls from the time when they were growing up. What are the good and challenging points about these changes?

2. Ask the whole group to make a mind map to show what they have learned from the discussion. See how the different parts of it link up.

3. Discuss how we can all use our virtues to support male and female children in being friends and in dealing with challenges. Ask: 'What are our fears about these friendships, and how can we feel more comfortable with them?'

Remind people about what they learned in Session 16 about friendship, including how to behave in a friendly way and deal with challenges.

 ## EXERCISE 20.2 THE PAIRING GAME

AIM: To energize the group.

DESCRIPTION: An energizing activity in which participants pretend to be animals and have to find a partner who is the same animal as they are.

Directions

1. Ask the participants to stand in a circle. Explain that you are going to go round the group giving each person a male or female animal to act out. The animal can be a different sex to the participant. There can be two males or two females of the same animal, or one of each. Ask them to remember the sex and the animal.

2. Go round the group whispering to each participant so no one else can hear (for example, Mr Hare, Mrs Elephant, Mrs Mouse, Mr Chicken) until you have been all the way around. Alternatively, write the names on slips of paper in advance. Make sure there are no more than two of each animal in the group.

3. Now explain that participants are not allowed to speak, but they can act and make noises as the appropriate animal would. Then ask them to move around and find their same animal partner. Stop the game when everyone has found their partner.

 ## EXERCISE 20.3 LOVE, SEXUAL FEELINGS, AND HAVING SEX

AIMS: To think about the meaning of love as a virtue, and different types of love in relationships. To think about how we practise the virtue of love in non-sexual and sexual relationships.

DESCRIPTION: Participants read and discuss a letter, explore scenarios, and discuss questions about these.

Box 20.a Information for facilitators

 This exercise is sensitive because it is about sexual feelings. Some children may already have had sex, while others may not. Encourage them to talk about 'people like themselves', rather than talking about their own personal experience.

Directions

1. Explain that we are going to return to the virtue of *love*. Ask participants to remind each other of Exercise 8.2, when we looked at the love between caregivers and children. Bring out the mind maps that participants drew in that exercise, showing different words for love.

Say: 'Today we are going to focus on love in connection with sexual feelings and relationships. This session helps children prepare for the future, by thinking about sexual feelings, and how they can practise the virtue of love and make good decisions about sex when they are older.'

Invite participants to think of any other words for love that we might use in talking about love with sexual feelings.

2. Split the peer group into males and females.

3. Ask for a volunteer to read the letter to Uncle Nelson (see Box 20.b) aloud to the group. (If you are working with a girls' group, adapt the story so it is about a girl who loves two boys.)

Box 20.b Letter to Uncle Nelson

Dear Uncle Nelson

My friend Rebecca and I have been going around together since primary school. We are now 14 years old. I really love her. We can talk about anything, relax together, and be ourselves. We are interested in each other's problems, and we laugh and cry together. We enjoy challenging each other at school work, and at the weekend we sing in the school choir. Now I have met this girl called Rosie, and I think I have fallen in love with her. I think about her all the time. I want to be with her, hear her voice, kiss and cuddle her – and yet sometimes I can't think of one word to say when we are together. She has left school and works as a hairdresser.

I often do not have time to see Rebecca now. I know that she feels sad, but I have to be at home in case Rosie comes by. Is it possible to love two people? Is there more than one kind of love and, if so, which one is best?

Jacob

4. Ask the questions below to the separate peer groups of caregivers and children aged 9–14 years.

Note: With 5–8 year olds, adapt the questions so they are looking to the future, or talking about people who are older than the children.

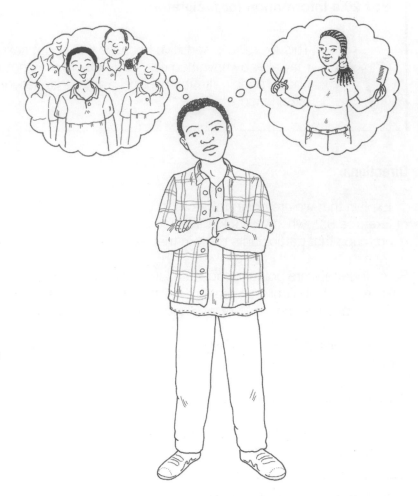

'What would you say to Jacob?'

'Are there different kinds of love?'

'What words do you have in your language for love that involves sexual feelings?'

'How do we know that we love someone, or that they love us, in a sexual way?'

'How do we behave towards someone we love in a sexual way, and how do we expect a person who loves us in a sexual way to behave?'

'What are the most important qualities and behaviour that you expect from a boyfriend or girlfriend?'

5. Now ask each participant to consider what they think are the most important virtues in a loving friendship with sexual feelings, and how their girlfriend or boyfriend would show these virtues. Ask them to share these ideas with the group.

For example:
• 'I expect to be treated with kindness. Someone is kind to me when they understand my feelings and comfort me if I am sad.'
• 'I expect someone to be faithful to promises we have made to care for each other.'

Ask one member of the group to write the virtues down, as they are being stated.

6. Now bring the whole peer group back together. Ask them to read out the virtues, with everyone listening carefully. Ask participants to identify the similarities between the two lists, and then the differences.

7. Ask: 'Do love and sex always go together?' As needed, add information from Box 20.c.

> ### Box 20.c Combinations of love and sex
>
> *Love without sex.* It's normal to love our family members and our friends, and to hug and touch them, without having sexual feelings.
>
> People can also love someone they are sexually attracted to, without having sexual intercourse with them. They find other ways to show their love (see Exercise 21.4).
>
> Delaying or postponing sex does not harm our sexual organs, or prevent us from making love well when we are ready.
>
> *Sex without love.* Sometimes people say 'I love you' when they only mean 'I want to have sex with you'. People may also have sex with someone without loving them because they are forced to, because it is expected, because they want to please the person, or in exchange for money or favours.
>
> *Love and sex.* People may love the person they have sex with. Having sex is an expression of their love, and more enjoyable because both people love and care for each other.

8. Ask participants to form groups of two or three with others of the same sex. Give each small group one of the following scenarios to think about, or ask them to come up with their own scenarios. Ask them to make up a short story about the relationship they are thinking of, to explain the situation.

Love without sex. When two people love each other in a romantic way but don't have sex together.
- Luke and Suzanna are 14 years old, and they love each other; they feel happy when they kiss and cuddle. But they have decided that it is best to wait until they are mature in mind and body, and are ready to marry. Then they can show their love freely and fully.
- Ernest and Fred are 14 years old and they have been good friends since primary school. They study and run together. They feel nice in a new exciting way when they hug and hold hands. They pretend to like girls, but when they are alone, they say they love each other.

Sex without love. A boy or girl who has sex with someone they don't love.
- Twelve-year-old Joseph has sex with 20-year-old Freda because she gives him money, and shows him how to have sex like the people in porn films.
- Thirteen-year-old Rhoda has sex with James, a school mate, because he is good at sport and people admire her for having James as her boyfriend. She doesn't enjoy being with him very much.

Love with sex. A boy or girl who loves someone who loves them, and they have sex together.
- Edward and Edna are 15 years old and they love each other. They want to be closer, and feel that they are ready to have proper sex. They use condoms, but even if Edna gets pregnant they believe that their families will want them to marry.

9. Ask each small group to share their story with the rest of the peer group.

For each story ask: 'What would you say to the boy or girl if they were your friend?'

'What does the relationship tell us about love and sex?'

'What virtues are the pair in the story practising?'

'What virtues do you think would support them in making good decisions?'

Closing circle

In preparation for Session 21 'Our sexual feelings and sexual safety', ask participants to think of all their questions about sexual feelings and put them in the question box. Before you lead that session, sort the questions into themes so you can integrate them into the session.

 ADDITIONAL EXERCISE 20.4 EARLY MARRIAGE

We suggest that this extra exercise is not done by children aged 5–8 years. Caregivers and children aged 9-14 are in their separate peer groups.

AIMS: To understand our rights concerning marriage, and the causes and consequences of early marriage, and to identify strategies to prevent forced early marriage.

DESCRIPTION: Participants discuss a picture of early forced marriage, and perform role plays of action to prevent early marriage.

Box 20.d Information for facilitators

 Some children in the group may be at risk of forced early marriage. Make a plan with your team about how you will handle this as safely as possible before you run this exercise.

Find out about the statutory and customary laws in your country concerning marriage.

Directions

1. Ask participants to split into males and females. Facilitate a discussion among the females about the positive and negative consequences of getting married and not getting married, for a young girl from a poor household. Facilitate a similar discussion among the males in relation to a young boy. You might want to structure their discussion using a flow chart, with early marriage in the centre, positive consequences on one side, and negative consequences on the other. As needed, add information on consequences from Box 20.e.

2. Ask the groups to put their flow charts on the wall or floor, and invite participants to comment on them or ask questions.

Box 20.e Reasons and consequences of early marriage and the law

Reasons for early marriage. A girl may be married to an older man because: her family feels they need the dowry; they fear that the girl will get pregnant before marriage; they want to save the expense of catering for the girl's needs.

Boys may be forced to marry early and leave school because they made a girl pregnant.

Consequences of early marriage. For girls these include: unsafe early pregnancy with higher risk of obstructed labour, fistulas, infertility, and death of the mother and baby; and leaving school and being dependent on her husband with reduced opportunities to do paid work. Where early marriage is to an older man, consequences include: higher risk of STIs, including HIV; very unequal power relations between husband and wife; and a higher rate of divorce.

For boys the consequences relate to leaving school early, and having reduced opportunities to make a good living.

Laws about early marriage. In some countries the statutory law of the state differs from customary laws of ethnic groups.

The statutory law in many countries gives women and men the same right to choose a spouse freely and enter into marriage only with free and full consent. Marriage under the age of 16 years is not allowed and is regarded as sexual abuse. Betrothal and marriage of a child is not legal. No dowry is required to establish marriage. However, the enforcement of these laws is often weak. Customary law may allow marriages to be arranged by families when children are thought to be physically mature, and may involve dowry.

Many countries have also signed up to rights agreements, including the Convention on the Rights of the Child, and the Convention on the Elimination of all forms of Discrimination against Women. These promise to uphold the rights of children to own their bodies, to make decisions that affect their lives, and to be educated.

3. Bring the group back together and show them the picture of a girl given in marriage. See Annex. Ask the participants what the picture shows.

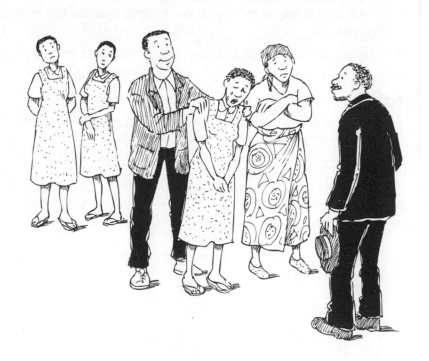

4. Ask some participants to act out the scenario.

5. At the end, ask the actors to stay in character, and invite the spectators to ask them questions.

6. Ask everyone: 'How do you feel about the marriage?'

'What do you think about the marriage?'

'Does this happen in many families in our community?'

'What does the state law of our country say about marriage?'

'Are the girl's rights being met?'

'What would you like to happen next?'

7. Divide into groups of three or four, and ask people to imagine that their friend or a friend's daughter is in this situation. Ask each group to role play one of the following scenarios, as the family prepare for the marriage:
- The girl's teacher finds out that the family plan to make her student get married – what does the teacher do?
- The girl tells her friends – what do her friends say and do?
- The girl talks to her caregivers or relatives – what does she say, and what do they say and do?
- The Community Development Committee meets with community members to discuss forced early marriage. What do they say?

8. Encourage discussion and, as needed, add information from Box 20.f.

Box 20.f Strategies to prevent early marriage

- Educate the community on rights and the benefits of later marriage with consent, including through advocacy by community leaders, law enforcers, and health committees.
- Keep an eye out for girls at risk of early marriage, and take action.
- Teach girls to be assertive and seek support if their families try to marry them early.
- Create community dramas to show the benefits of later marriage.
- Plan actions which address the reasons for early forced marriage, and support girls who are already married early.

ADDITIONAL EXERCISE 20.5 AN IDEAL LONG-TERM, LOVING RELATIONSHIP

We suggest that this extra exercise is not done by children aged 5–8 years.

AIMS: To dream about our vision of a good long-term, loving relationship.

DESCRIPTION: Participants imagine advertising for a long-term loving partner, and dream of their life together.

Directions

1. Explain that we are going to dream about our vision of a good, loving, long-term sexual relationship. It is good to think about what good things we want in a partner, and how we want to live together. If we have a vision about our future life, we can start to act now in a way that supports us in reaching our vision. And, if we meet someone we like, we can talk about our ideas on how we want to live together. This is better than finding out later that we have very different dreams.

For caregivers, it is useful to have dreams for our children, to talk about our dreams and their dreams, and to work together in trying to achieve them.

2. Ask participants to form single-sex pairs. Invite them to relax, close their eyes, and focus on their breathing.

3. Say: 'Now imagine you are putting a notice in a newspaper, or online, to find a long-term loving partner, or a partner for your child.'

Ask: 'What good things do you look for, and what would you love about this person?'

Invite participants to open their eyes and make a drawing of the person, and to draw or write all the good things about them around the drawing.

4. Invite the pairs to spend five minutes sharing their pictures with each other.

5. Ask males and females to put their pictures on the wall or floor, and invite people to look at them. Ask: 'What are the similarities and differences between our pictures?'

6. Suggest that children and caregivers might like to share their pictures and their dreams, to see how much they coincide.

7. *Homework*. Suggest that, if people are interested, they do their breathing at home, and imagine that they are living together with their partner. They could think about these questions:
- How do you show your love for each other?
- How do you feel when you are together? How does your body feel?
- What makes you laugh together?
- What do you like to do together?
- How are you sharing housework, child care, and economic work between you?
- How are you making, sharing, and using money and resources, like food?

- How many children do you want? Who is taking care of the children?
- If you are sick, who is looking after you?

 ADDITIONAL EXERCISE 20.6 LOVE BETWEEN PEOPLE OF THE SAME SEX

We suggest that this extra exercise is not done by children aged 5–8 years.

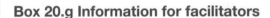

AIMS: To understand that some people in all societies are naturally sexually attracted to people of the same sex. To think about how we can support those of us who love people of the same sex in having a safe, healthy, and happy sexual life.

DESCRIPTION: Participants read a story and discuss it using questions.

Box 20.g Information for facilitators

Before running this session please carefully consider the laws in your country about sex between males and sex between females. Discuss the situation with your team and with managers in your organization. All adults have the right to be able to have a loving sexual relationship with another adult. However, some countries have laws which criminalize some sexual activities between people of the same sex, and which criminalize anyone 'promoting' same-sex relationships. This session can be used legally in some settings (e.g. South Africa) and not in others (e.g. Uganda).

In this manual, we are not 'promoting' or trying to persuade people to have sex with someone of their own sex. We are providing information on sexual health, rights, and virtues in sexual relationships, and how people can have sex safely with someone of either sex. Most sexual activities can be engaged in by people who have sex with someone of either sex (see Session 21 'Our sexual feelings and sexual safety'). However, your organization needs to look at what the law says and the reality of how it is enforced, and weigh this against the benefits of running this session with people who are attracted to the same sex as themselves.

Directions[55]

1. Explain: 'In this exercise we are going to think about whom people are attracted to, and whom they get close to. This is called our sexual identity. In most societies, males are expected to be attracted to females, and females are expected to be attracted to males. People who feel like this are known as *heterosexuals*. Some males are only attracted to males, and some females are only attracted to females. Their sexual identity is *homosexual*. But a larger number of people may be attracted to people of either sex during their lives. We are not so fixed in our feelings as many believe.

'Many societies disapprove of homosexuals, and in some countries they are seen as criminals. This is against their human rights, and results in great suffering for them and their families.'

2. Invite participants to form small groups. Read out Ernest's story (see Box 20.h), or adapt it to be a story about two girls. Say that we will talk about it afterwards.

Box 20.h The story of Ernest

'I've always felt different from other boys. I like playing football with my friends, but now that we are older I get bored when they keep talking about girls and how sweet they are. I like being with girls but I don't get sexy feelings about them at all. Now I've realized that I am falling in love with a boy that I meet at school. I think about him so much, and want to touch him and get close to him. I'm worried that I might be what they call "gay". I don't know who to talk to about it, because in our society gay people are not accepted.'

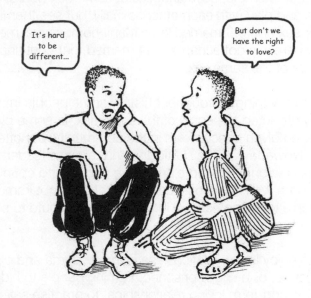

3. Ask participants in their small groups to discuss the story, using the questions below.
- What is Ernest worried about?
- Do any girls or boys have these feelings in our community?
- What do you feel when you hear Ernest's story?
- What would you say to him if he was your friend?
- Who do you think might help him?
- How could we make it easier for him at our school?

4. Bring the groups together and go through the questions one by one. Invite each group to answer one question and invite others to add different views. As needed, contribute information from Box 20.i to the group's discussion.

Box 20.i Information about same-sex relationships

As we grow up we often form close relationships with people of the same sex. We feel love for them, which we may show by hugging and kissing. We may keep these close friends throughout our life.

When we get older, most people become interested sexually in people of the other sex. Some people find that they love people of the same sex as themselves. In some countries, people like this call themselves 'gay' to show that they are happy to be the way they are. A woman who has sexual feelings for another woman is called a lesbian.

People may have loving sexual feelings for a person of the same sex at certain times, or throughout their lives. For example, boys and girls at same-sex boarding schools may have close friendships and play with each other sexually, but see themselves as people who will love the other sex and get married later. Many homosexual men and women who live in countries where it is not accepted get married, but continue to have secret relationships with others of the same sex.

Homosexuality is not a new thing. Throughout history some people in all societies have been naturally sexually attracted to people of the same sex. In some places they have been accepted, and even given special roles in the community, but often they have been discriminated against. Nowadays some politicians and religious leaders may tell us that that being homosexual is wrong. But more and more people and countries are accepting that some people are born with a homosexual identity. This is not immoral, or dangerous, or frightening, and people with homosexual identity can contribute to society and have loving relationships just like everyone else.

We all have the right to enjoy loving relationships without stigma and discrimination, feelings of shame, violence, or being imprisoned. Forcing people to hide their love makes it hard for them to enjoy long-term loving relationships, to practise safer sex, or to get medical services to ensure their sexual health.

SESSION 21 OUR SEXUAL FEELINGS AND SEXUAL SAFETY

Purpose: To understand sexual feelings and know that they are natural and good if we respond to them in a way that doesn't harm ourselves or others; to learn how to respond to sexual feelings safely.

Contents	Materials required	Time required
Opening circle (see p.13)		15 mins
21.1 Managing sexual feelings		30 mins
21.2 Masturbation		45 mins
21.3 Safe and unsafe ways of showing sexual love	Picture of 'HIV transmission chain' page 154, plastic bag	45 mins
21.4 *For older children and caregivers only* Setting boundaries		45 mins
Closing circle (see p.14)		15 mins

About 3.5 hrs

Preparation

Read the questions that participants put in the question box at the end of Session 20, and make sure that all their queries will be answered within today's session.

Box 21.a Information for facilitators

Encourage young participants to talk about sexual feelings and experiences as if they were happening to 'people like them' or an anonymous friend, rather than as personal experience. Children often feel safer doing this, and prefer to keep their own experiences private.

Remember that many children, maybe all of those in the 5–8-year group, may not have experienced sexual feelings in relation to another person, and this is fine. We do not want them to feel that they should be having sexual feelings, nor encourage them to think that they are struggling with intense sexual desire.

If children or caregivers have been abused, they may associate feelings about sex with pain and distress. Keep an eye out for participants who are distressed and who need support. They may also be more knowledgeable, interested, and open about sexual matters than one would expect at their age. See Sessions 26 and 27.

 EXERCISE 21.1 MANAGING SEXUAL FEELINGS

AIMS: To understand that sexual feelings are a normal part of growing up, and to find ways of managing sexual feelings.

DESCRIPTION: Participants engage in pair work and group discussion about sexual feelings and ways of managing them.

Directions

1. Split the peer group into males and females. Ask participants to pair up with someone of a similar age to discuss these questions:

Children aged 5–8 years. 'How does our body feel when we love someone (for example, our caregivers, siblings, or friend) and we hug or hold hands? What are our favourite ways of showing that we love someone?'

Children aged 9–14 years. 'What sexual feelings might people like us experience? How would they know that they are having sexual feelings?'

Caregivers. 'What do you remember about beginning to experience sexual feelings?'

2. Invite pairs to share their ideas with others of their own sex in their peer group.

3. Explain that during puberty, our bodies produce sex hormones. These change our bodies, and also cause us to have sexual feelings. When boys feel sexy, the penis gets bigger and stands up. When girls feel sexy, they may notice wetness and warmth in their genitals.

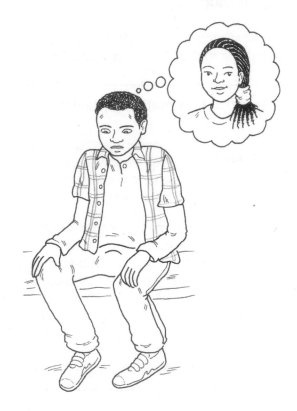

We can feel happy about sexual feelings during puberty, as they show us that we are growing well. As with puberty generally, some people start to experience sexual feelings earlier and more strongly than others. This is all normal.

4. Ask: 'What are the things that might make us feel sexy?'

Participants might say:
- touching, hugging, or kissing someone we find attractive;
- touching our genitals or breasts, or someone else touching them;
- the sight of an attractive person, or thinking about them;
- dancing or doing other physical activities with a person who attracts us;
- reading a love story, looking at sexy pictures, or watching a sexy film;
- tension, anxiety, or stress;
- no reason at all.

5. Ask participants to go back into their pairs. Ask:

Children aged 5–8 years. 'How do we feel about developing sexual feelings? When we get them, what may we do to manage them?'

Children aged 9–14 years. 'What do children like you do to manage their sexual feelings?'

Caregivers. 'How did you manage your sexual feelings during puberty? What and who supported you? What can you do to support your child in managing their sexual feelings?'

6. Bring the peer groups back together in their single-sex groups and draw a mind map, starting with 'Ways of managing our sexual feelings' in the middle, to show how people might manage their sexual feelings, or how they might support their children in coping with their sexual feelings. Add information as needed from Box 21.b.

Box 21.b Managing sexual feelings

Sexual feelings are a natural part of growing up. They start at different times for different people.

Sexual feelings do not mean that you need to have sex. They cannot damage your body.

Sexual feelings come from the lower part of our brains; we may take less notice of our thinking, upper brains when we are feeling sexy. This is more so for children, because their upper brains are not yet fully developed.

We can manage our sexual feelings; we are in charge of our bodies. For example, we can:
- seek advice and support (from friends, health workers, our religion);
- think about the benefits of delaying sex to achieve our future dreams;
- consider the problems that having sex can cause ourselves and others;
- distract our minds or tire our bodies (pray, sing, play sports, ride a bike, dig);
- avoid encouraging our sexual feelings (avoid porn movies, sexy books, and being alone with someone you are attracted to);
- avoid alcohol, cannabis, and other drugs, as they reduce our self-control;
- release our sexual feelings in a safe way (see Exercise 21.4).

If we decide to act on our sexual feelings and have sexual intercourse, we must make sure it is wanted by both partners, and use a condom.

It is never right for adults to have sex with children, even if the child has sexual feelings for the adult (see Session 26 'Protecting each other from sexual abuse').

 EXERCISE 21.2 MASTURBATION

AIMS: To talk about our feelings and beliefs about masturbation; to learn correct information about masturbation, and to feel more comfortable with masturbation as a personal choice.

DESCRIPTION: Participants discuss masturbation; with information inputs as appropriate.

Directions[56]

1. Ask participants to sit in a circle. Go around the circle asking people to finish this sentence: 'The thing I like most about my body is [...].'

Additional question for children. Ask them to finish the following sentence as well:

'The thing that makes me happiest about growing up is [...].'

2. Explain that one way of managing sexual feelings safely is masturbation. We are now going to talk about the good things about masturbation, and some of the concerns that people have about it.

Ask: 'What is masturbation? How do people do it?'

As needed, add information from Box 21.c.

Box 21.c What is masturbation?

From before puberty certain parts of our bodies can become very exciting to touch, especially our genitals. For boys, this area is the penis and testicles. For girls, it is the area around the breasts and around the vagina (especially the clitoris), and inside the vagina.

Some people enjoy massaging or rubbing these areas. This is called masturbating. It is something they do to themselves, in private. If they do this for a while, they may reach a moment when it is very exciting and have an orgasm.

The penis and vagina often produce fluids during masturbation. Semen comes out of the penis, and vaginal fluid comes out of the vagina. This is normal.

People may also masturbate each other. This is safe as long as they do not get vaginal fluid or semen on each other's genitals.

Ask: 'What words do we have in our country for masturbation?'

'Do we like these words? Which words do we want to use?'

3. Ask: 'What have you heard about masturbation? What are the good things people say about it, and what are the negative things? What worries do you have about masturbation?' As needed, add information from Box 21.d.

Box 21.d Information about masturbation

Most people – males and females – masturbate at some time in their lives. Even babies touch their genitals.

We are all normal: if we masturbate; if we think about it but don't do it; or if we never think about it.

Masturbation is a natural and very safe way of coping with sexual feelings. It has no risks for us or for others. We cannot get or pass on any diseases by masturbating, or get pregnant or make someone pregnant, because it does not involve any exchange of fluids.

Masturbation can teach people how their bodies work, and what gives them pleasure. When they decide to have sex, they can use this understanding to help each other enjoy sex more.

Sometimes boys masturbate in a friendship group, and have competitions or play games. This may be part of learning about puberty and supporting each other.

Myths about masturbation

It does not:
- cause harm to our private parts,* or any other part of our bodies;
- cause harm to our minds;*
- make us less attracted to others;
- waste semen or vaginal fluids – our bodies are always producing more;
- stop us from marrying;
- mean we are no longer a virgin;
- cause infertility.

* Masturbation is only a problem (and then only temporarily) if we do it so often that it makes our penis or vagina painful, or disturbs our daily routines. Then we need to reduce how often we do it; there is no need to masturbate every time we get sexual feelings.

Many people, including religious leaders, believe that masturbation is a more responsible way of coping with sexual feelings than having sex. But sometimes caregivers, teachers, or religious leaders may say that masturbation is wrong, and this can make us feel guilty. There is no need to feel guilty about it. It is a private matter and a personal choice. If it feels wrong to us, we don't need to do it.

How to masturbate safely
- Find a private place and time. In most cultures masturbation is something to be done privately.
- Wash your hands. Rub yourself gently. Stop if you feel any discomfort, and do not masturbate again until it clears up. The discomfort may be caused by an infection.
- *For males*: It is safest to use your hands. Do not insert things into your penis, or insert your penis into anything.
- *For females*: It is safest to use your fingers. If do you use an object, make sure that it is very clean, and cannot cut, bruise, or break inside you.
- Some people use sex toys such as vibrators; wash these in hot soapy water and bleach, especially if they are shared.

4. Do not advise children to masturbate. Simply provide them with accurate information in a positive way, and make it clear that how they handle their sexual feelings safely is their choice.

EXERCISE 21.3 SAFE AND UNSAFE WAYS OF SHOWING SEXUAL LOVE

AIMS: To learn which sexual activities are safe, mostly safe, and unsafe; and to feel positive about safe alternatives to sexual intercourse.

DESCRIPTION: Participants identify ways of expressing sexual feelings, and decide whether they are safe, mostly safe, or unsafe in relation to HIV, other STIs, and pregnancy.

Directions

1. Show participants the picture of the HIV chain, to remind them about whether an activity is safe or not in relation to HIV transmission.

Ask: 'What are the three things that HIV needs to be shared between two people?' If necessary, remind them about the quantity and quality of the virus, and transmission routes.

2. Remind participants of the game in Exercise 12.3, where they shook hands and tried different ways of stopping HIV from being shared between two people. Ask: 'Who can remember the four ways we shook hands? What did each way represent?'

If needed, remind them using Table 21.1.

Table 21.1 Ways of avoiding sexual transmission of HIV

In the game, we can avoid getting/sharing HIV by:	In real life, we can avoid getting/sharing HIV by:
Putting a bag on our hand	using a condom
Shaking hands with same person	Only having sex with one person
Using fingertips only	Engaging in (other) safer sexual activities
Refusing to shake hands	Abstaining from sex

3. Divide into males and females. Ask each group to draw a line on the wall, chalk board, or floor. Label one end of the line 'safe', the middle 'mostly safe', and the other end 'unsafe'.

4. Work with the relevant peer groups as follows:

Caregivers. Divide into two groups: females and males. Ask each group to think of all the ways that two adults might express their sexual feelings and to draw or write them on pieces of paper. Bring them together to discuss the safety of each activity.

Children aged 9–14 years. Divide this group again by age, into two groups of 9–11 years and 12–14 years. Ask each group to think of all the ways that two people of their age or a bit older might express their sexual feelings, and to draw or write them on pieces of paper. For example: kissing, dancing together, hugging, holding hands, touching breasts or sexual organs, or having sexual intercourse.

Children aged 5–8 years. Give this group a list of non-sexual activities that people might do to express love and affection, such as hugging, kissing, holding hands, and dancing, as well as one or two unsafe sexual activities.

5. Ask the groups to discuss each activity and place each piece of paper along their line according to whether it is safe, mostly safe, or unsafe, in terms of sharing HIV – provided that either of the people has enough quantity of HIV to share it. (Remind them that if a person with HIV is taking ARVs correctly, they will probably have very little HIV in their body fluids.)

Listen to their discussion and, as needed, add information from Box 21.e.

Box 21.e Safe, mostly safe, and unsafe sexual activities for sharing HIV

For HIV to be passed during sexual activities it needs:
- to have enough quantity and quality: if someone has HIV and is not taking ARVs correctly, they can share it through their blood and semen or vaginal fluid;
- to have a route of transmission: HIV can pass through a cut or break (for example, a sore) in the skin, and through wet skin found in the vulva, labia and vagina, inside the foreskin and tip of the penis, and in the anus. Our mouths also contain wet skin, but it is unusual for HIV to be passed through oral sex because saliva contains enzymes which inhibit HIV. HIV is shared more easily if there are sores or infections in the mouth or gums.

The safety of sexual activities is the same whether they are engaged in by people of different sexes or the same sex. For example, anal sex using a condom is mostly safe for everyone.

Safe activities. Holding hands; hugging; putting arms round each other; saying nice things to each other; stroking hair, face or other parts of the body; closed-mouth kissing or massage; caressing; cuddling; dancing; moving against each other with clothes on; stroking nipples, buttocks and other hotspots; oral sex with a condom.

Mostly safe activities. Open-mouth kissing; masturbating each other; sexual intercourse (vaginal or, anal) using a condom; oral sex without a condom.

Unsafe activities. Vaginal or anal sex without a condom.

Notes
- For activities to be safe or mostly safe, partners must be careful that semen, vaginal fluid, or blood from one does not get onto the wet skin of the other. This might happen via hands or by touching genitals.
- To prevent safe activities turning into unsafe ones, it is good to be prepared by having a condom ready in case the desire for intercourse is overwhelming.

---

6. Bring the whole peer group back together, asking the groups to bring with them the pieces of paper marked with activities that are safe and mostly safe. Emphasize the number of safe activities that people can enjoy without having sexual intercourse. Explain that some people use the term 'outercourse' for activities that do not involve putting the penis inside the vagina or rectum.

7. Ask: 'What about other STIs? Is the safety of the activities the same as with HIV?'

If necessary, explain that condoms protect us from other STIs as long as the condom covers any rashes or sores. For example, condoms do not protect us from herpes or chancroid if the sores or rashes are not covered by the condom, and if these rub against the other person.

Some STIs, such as gonorrhoea, are more easily transmitted through oral sex than HIV. Oral sex can be made safer by using a condom for oral sex on a man, or an opened-out condom or latex glove for oral sex on a woman.

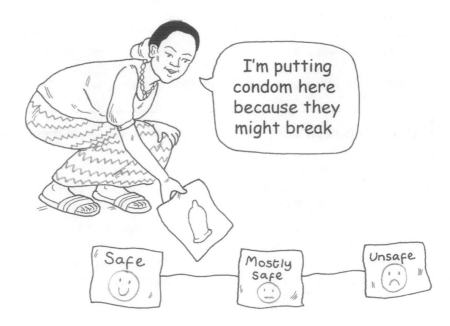

8. Ask: 'What about pregnancy? Is the safety of the activities the same as with HIV?'

If needed, explain that the only unsafe activities for pregnancy are ones where male semen, or the fluid which comes before ejaculation, touches female labia or the vagina. The sperm can then swim into the vagina and uterus and make the female pregnant.

9. Ask people to write down any questions they have about pregnancy and put them in the question box for Session 25, which is about fertility, pregnancy, and contraception.

 EXERCISE 21.4 SETTING BOUNDARIES

We suggest that this exercise is not done by children aged 5–8 years.

AIMS: To think about the advantages and challenges of engaging in sexual activities that do not involve sexual intercourse.

DESCRIPTION: Participants talk about setting boundaries, practise assertiveness, and make a group strategy to keep to boundaries.

Box 21.f Information for facilitators

Do not encourage 9–14 year olds to think that they should be involved in sexual activities. This exercise can help those who are not sexually active to think about their future, when they are ready to have a boyfriend or girlfriend.

Directions

1. Invite participants to look at all the activities at the safe end of the line they drew during Exercise 21.3.

Ask: 'Can people be satisfied with these sexual activities, without intercourse?'

'What are the good points about enjoying sexual activities without intercourse?'

'What are the challenges of enjoying sexual activities without intercourse?'

2. Split into males and females. Explain that people may touch us in ways that make us feel sexy, to persuade us to have sex with them. One way to handle this is to decide beforehand how far we will go.

Ask individuals or pairs to think about setting their own boundaries and sticking to them. They should be specific about what behaviours they will and will not do, for example: 'I will kiss and hug and rub with my clothes on, but I will not allow the other person to touch my private parts, or to undress me, and I won't touch their private parts, or undress them.'

3. Ask participants to form groups of three and to consider these questions:
• What will you do if the other person does something, or wants you to do something, that you don't want?
• What will you do if the other person doesn't want to do something that you want to do?

4. Explain that we are going to practise being assertive by choosing a situation where we are feeling sexy, but we don't want to go past our boundaries. The person with us does not seem to understand or care about our boundaries.

Ask: 'How are you going to use your assertiveness skills to stick to your boundaries in a positive way?'

For example, participants could use an 'I' statement, such as:'I can see that you are feeling very sexy and want me very much. I also feel sexy, but I don't feel ready to have full sex with you now. I have my own dreams, and I want to reach them without pregnancy or sickness. I would feel very happy if we could show our love without going the whole way. There are lots of ways we can have fun together – let me show you.'

5. Bring the males back together, and the females back together, and ask:

'What skills and strategies can we use to take control, and set boundaries for what we will and won't do sexually?'

'How can we as a group use our virtues to stay strong and safe, and keep to our boundaries?'

Ask the groups to create some rules and strategies for enjoying sexual activities without intercourse.

For example:
• Only engage in outercourse when you know each other well, trust, and respect each other.
• Only do outercourse when you are sober, without the influence of alcohol or drugs.
• Agree on a word or gesture which either of you will use if you feel that things are getting too hot.
• Be clear about the consequences if someone doesn't respect your boundaries, and stick to them.
• Only do outercourse in places where you can leave and go home safely if you feel unsafe.
• Have condoms with you, and know where you can get emergency contraception and other emergency advice and services if you do end up having intercourse.

Closing circle

Say that the next session (Session 22) is about pornography, for example, movies and magazines showing people having sex. Ask participants to put any questions they have about pornography in the question box.

SESSION 22 PORNOGRAPHY

Purpose: To understand that sex in pornorgraphy (porn) is fantasy, and not like sex in real life; to think about porn critically in relation to sexuality and virtues, and its effects on us and others; to discuss what participants can do to protect themselves and others from harm caused by porn.[57]

Contents	Materials required	Time required
Opening circle (see p.13)		15 mins
22.1 If I were …		20 mins
22.2 Asking questions about pornography	4 prepared flipcharts	45 mins
22.3 *For older children and caregivers only* Is it legal, is it right?	Knowledge of relevant national laws	45 mins
22.4 *For older children and caregivers only* Planet porn and planet earth	Prepared statements from Table 22.1	45 mins
22.5 The effects of pornography on children		30 mins
22.6 Protecting each other from the negative effects of pornography		45 mins
Closing circle (see p.14)		15 mins

About 4.5 hrs

Preparation

Learn about the laws regarding making and viewing pornography in your country.

At the end of Session 21 you asked participants to put their questions about pornography into the question box. Sort these into themes that you can answer in the relevant exercises. Use the questions to plan the exercises for your peer group.

Box 22.a Information for facilitators

In any group, some children will probably have seen pornographic images. Nowadays lots of children see porn in movies, on mobile phones, through the internet, and in magazines. If they don't have the opportunity to talk and think about porn critically, they can get confused and frightened, and imitate harmful gender and sexual behaviour.

Some children in the group may be shown porn by adults. This is sexual abuse, and illegal. The children may be traumatized by it. Watch out for children who are distressed by, or very knowledgeable about, porn. Make a plan before you run this session to provide support and protection to these children.

Caregivers may watch porn. This session can support them in thinking critically about their own use of porn, and what they think about their children watching it.

Ask children whether 'people like them' have seen porn (such as sexy movies), rather than asking whether they personally have seen it, and suggest that they talk about 'people like them'. Definitely do not introduce explicit sexual images to children, because this is illegal and can harm them.

Note: Children may also have seen people having real sex, for example, if they share a bedroom with their caregivers. They may misunderstand what they see.

Exercise 22.2. Prepare four sheets of flipchart paper, each one marked with one of the following sets of questions:

1. What do you think porn means? What kinds of porn are there?

2. Where do people see porn in your community? Who sees it, and from what source?

For this second question, draw a simple map of the community, which participants can use to indicate where people see porn, who sees it, and the source of the porn.

3. Why do people watch porn?

For this third question, write 'why' in a circle in the middle of the paper, so that participants can build a mind map around it.

4. What effects does seeing porn have on people? Are the effects different for children?

On the fourth flipchart, write 'effects of seeing porn' in a circle in the middle of the sheet; add a label 'positive effects' on one side of the circle, and another label 'negative effects' on the other.

Exercise 22.4. Select some of the 28 statements in Table 22.1. For the children aged 9–14 years, select statements depending on how much they already know about porn. Write 'Planet Porn', 'Planet Earth', and your chosen statements on separate pieces of paper.

Exercise 22.5. Decide whether to do option A or option B, and then prepare stories or letters to Dr Love about situations involving pornography which are relevant to your peer group.

 EXERCISE 22.1 IF I WERE …

> **AIM:** To think about the difference between reality and fantasy in a fun way.
>
> **DESCRIPTION:** Participants compare their fantasy futures with realistic futures that make the most of their talents and virtues.
>
> **GROUPS:** Use this activity either as an introduction to the session for all peer groups, or as an activity for 5–8 year olds while the other groups are doing Exercises 22.3 or 22.4.

Directions

1. Ask participants to form groups of three. Say: 'Please think of something you could be. Make it something extreme, such as the richest person in the world, or the best singer or footballer in Africa. Show each other what you would be like, and talk about these amazing fantasies and what they would enable you to do.'

2. Say: 'Now think about the reality of how things actually are for each of you, and what you can realistically achieve in your life. Help each other to think of how you can make the best of your opportunities.'

3. Ask each person to prepare a statement about the fantasy, the reality, and what they might achieve. For example:

- 'If I were the cleverest person in Africa I would invent amazing things and make lots of money. Actually, I am doing OK at school. I'm going to keep working hard to learn as much as I can, so I can get a good job when I'm older. Maybe I will invent something really useful!'

- 'If I were the most beautiful woman in the world, I would be a famous model and everyone would admire me. Actually, I am too short to be a model and the wrong shape. But I like my body and I'm good at acting. People will admire me for my acting ability and intelligence.'

4. Ask each group of three to announce and act out their statements with another group.

5. Summarize by noting that fantasies can be fun, but it's best to find ways of translating them into our real lives, and to think of dreams which are achievable.

 ## EXERCISE 22.2 ASKING QUESTIONS ABOUT PORNOGRAPHY

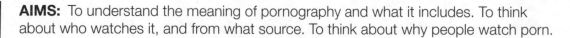

AIMS: To understand the meaning of pornography and what it includes. To think about who watches it, and from what source. To think about why people watch porn.

DESCRIPTION: Caregivers and older children in separate peer groups divide into small groups to draw or write answers to questions about pornography on 4 flipchart sheets. Younger boys and girls answer questions in separate groups with facilitators.

Directions

Children aged 9–14 years and caregivers in separate peer groups

1. Explain to your peer group that we are going to talk about porn, because many people have said that seeing sexy movies or pictures can arouse sexual feelings and make it more difficult to avoid having sex. Suggest that people talk about the experience of 'people like us', rather than their own experience.

2. Ask: 'What do you think porn means? What does it include?'

Put participants' ideas on sheet 1 (see 'Preparation', above), and add information from Box 22.b as needed. Agree that, in this session, you are going to focus on forms of porn used commonly in your local area.

Box 22.b What is porn?

'Porn' is short for 'pornography'. Porn is images of sexual organs or sexual activity, created with the purpose of causing sexual excitement in the people who see them.

Porn is intended as entertainment for adults, not children. In most countries the legal age for using porn is 18.

Porn is not sex education, because sex in porn is different from real sex. People who make porn do so to make money, not to educate.

Common forms of porn are:
- movies on DVD, or watched via the internet;
- photos available on internet sites and through phone apps;
- magazines.

 3. Explain that we are going to do our 'fingers up' activity so that we can measure later how helpful this session has been. Ask participants to sit in an outward-facing circle, and to close their eyes and lower their heads so they cannot see each other. Assure participants that you are not recording names.

For older children only. Ask: 'How many times have you watched porn in the past month?'

Say: 'If you have not watched porn, keep your hands in your lap. If you have watched it, put up your fingers and thumbs to show how many times. If you have watched it more than 10 times, put your hands up and cross your wrists.'

Record the numbers shown by each boy and girl in your Facilitator's Journal.

Then ask: 'On a scale of 1 to 5, how much does your caregiver do to try to protect you from porn?' Ask them to answer by raising a number of fingers, using the following scale:

1 – nothing at all; 2 – not very much; 3 – quite a bit; 4 – a lot; 5 – everything possible.

For caregivers only. Ask 'On a scale of 1 to 5, how much do you do to try to protect your child from porn?' Ask them to answer by raising a number of fingers, using the scale above.

For both peer groups. Now say: 'I'm going to make a statement and I want you to think about how you feel about it.

'Put your thumb up if you agree with the statement. Put your thumb down if you disagree. Keep your hand down if you are not sure what to think.

Ask people to shut their eyes and put their heads down again. Read out the statements one at a time and record the answers in your journal.
- 'There is nothing wrong with children watching porn because sex is a normal part of life.'
- 'It's impossible to stop children from watching porn because it's everywhere.'

4. Divide the peer group into three small groups, each made up of either males or females. Show them flipcharts 2–4 (see 'Preparation', above) and explain them. For flipchart 4 about effects, ask participants to underline the effects on children that are different to those on adults. Give each group one of the sheets, and explain that they have seven minutes to draw and write their answers to the questions.

5. Clap after seven minutes, and ask the groups to move round to the next flipchart and to add any new ideas to it. Repeat the process seven minutes later, so that everyone has had a chance to add to all the flipcharts.

6. Invite the whole group to review what they have jointly made. Explain that we will refer to these flipcharts as we work through the session.

Children aged 5–8 years

1. If the children have not already mentioned sexy films as a cause of sexual feelings, ask whether they have heard of people watching films of people having sex.

If they say 'no', explain that some companies make 'porn' movies and photos of sexual organs and people having sex. They make money by selling them to people who find them sexually exciting. But it is illegal for children to see them. They may find that adults or other children want to show them porn. We would like to talk about this a bit more, so that they have good information and can avoid watching porn until they are over 18 years.

If they say 'yes', simply explain that we would like to talk about this topic.

2. Divide into separate groups of boys and girls, and facilitate a conversation with the children using the questions below. If needed, add appropriate information from Box 22.b.

- What do you know about porn, such as sexy films and pictures?
- How do people see these?
- Who watches sexy films and pictures? Do children like us watch it? Where and with whom?
- How do you think seeing porn makes adults feel? How do you think it makes children feel?
- Why is it against the law for children under 18 years to watch sexy films?
- What are the bad things about children watching sexy films?
- Is there anything good about children watching sexy films?
- How can we all use our virtues to avoid watching pornography while we are under 18 years?

 ## EXERCISE 22.3 IS IT LEGAL, IS IT RIGHT?

We suggest that children aged 5–8 years do not do this exercise.

> **AIMS:** To understand the law regarding viewing and making pornography. To understand that just because pornography is available and legal, it is not necessarily right to watch it.
>
> **DESCRIPTION:** Participants learn about relevant laws regarding porn and discuss them.

Directions

1. Explain what laws exist in your country regarding making and viewing porn. Add information from Box 22.c as needed.

2. Invite participants to form groups of three or four. They may feel more comfortable in groups of only males or only females. Ask them to discuss the following questions:
- Are the laws in our country enforced?
- What are the outcomes of this?

Box 22.c Pornography and the law

In most countries it is illegal to make pornographic images of children, regardless of whether the child agrees or not.

In some countries, such as South Africa, the sale of certain kinds of porn to people over 18 years is legal, if done through registered shops. In countries where porn is legal it is usually illegal to show certain acts, such as sex with animals, or scenes of rape and torture.

In other countries, such as Zambia and Tanzania, making or viewing any pornography is illegal.

Without enforcement of laws there may be widespread access to pornography, by adults and children. In particular, it is difficult to prevent people accessing porn through the internet.

3. Explain that some countries allow porn to be watched by adults, but not by children aged under 18 years.

Ask: 'Why might adults be allowed to watch, but not children? Why is porn more harmful to children?'

'Do you think there should be an age limit on watching porn?'

As needed, add information from Box 22.d.

Box 22.d Why is porn more harmful for children than adults?

Children who see porn may:
- be confused and upset by what they see, making them scared of sex and affecting their future sexual lives;
- think that porn shows the right way to have sex, and imitate it;
- from an early age, learn harmful messages about sex – sex without virtues and outside respectful, equal sexual relationships – which shape their beliefs and behaviour;
- start to feel sexy and want sex when they are too young, making it more difficult for them to delay sex;
- be drawn into illegal and exploitative sexual relationships with adults by attending showings of porn movies or sexual parties.

4. Ask: 'If lots of people are watching porn, can it be so bad?'

'For a child, what kind of role model is an adult who watches porn? What if an adult shows porn to a child?'

'What is the link between pornography and our virtues?'

As needed, add information from Box 22.e.

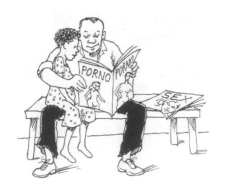

Box 22.e Pornography and virtues

We can think critically about porn in terms of our virtues. Just because it is available, does that mean it's right to watch it? There are several possible clashes with virtues:

- The people making porn may be being exploited; they may be forced to do the work, underpaid for the work, and/or put at risk of STIs, including HIV or other harms: for example, a porn actor took a drug so often to make his penis big that he had a painful erection all the time
- The acts shown may not promote virtues including respect, love, compassion, and responsibility.
- The acts shown may promote gender and sexual norms that harm women and children, such as male violence, aggression, and dominance; they may encourage women and children to behave passively and like servants rather than upholding equal rights.
- The acts shown are not honest, in that they are exaggerated fantasies.

 EXERCISE 22.4 PLANET PORN AND PLANET EARTH

We suggest that children aged 5–8 years do not do this exercise.

AIMS: To understand that:
- porn gives viewers a distorted picture of bodies and sexual activity, which affects male and female expectations and norms of how we should look, and what kind of sex we should have;
- porn is mainly made for men, and its content mainly promotes male power and unequal gender relationships. For example, men are in control of when, where, and how sex happens, and it is aimed at giving men pleasure rather than women.

DESCRIPTION: In same-sex pairs, participants consider whether statements refer to real-life sex ('Planet Earth') or porn sex ('Planet Porn').

Directions

1. Explain that the development of media technology means that people around the world get to see new images and ideas from many cultures. Some of these may be helpful and life-enriching, while others may cause harm. We can't stop technology, but we can learn how to think critically about what we see, discard negative ideas, and make choices, which help us reach our visions and enhance our wellbeing.

In this exercise we are going to look at the difference between porn sex and real-life sex. It is important to do this, because people may watch porn and believe that it teaches them how to have a good sex life.

2. Invite participants to pair up with someone of the same sex as themselves.

3. Place the signs for Planet Porn and Planet Earth on the floor. Give out the statements you have prepared from Table 22.1 (see 'Preparation') among the pairs. Ask them to discuss each statement and decide whether it comes from Planet Porn or Planet Earth.

Table 22.1 Planet Porn and Planet Earth statements

Planet Porn (a fantasy world)	Planet Earth (the real world)
Women exist to give men pleasure.	Women and men should both expect pleasure.
Sexual intercourse lasts for a long time.	Many men last for 2–4 minutes before ejaculation.
Women and men are all good looking, with really hot bodies.	Men and women come in all shapes and sizes, and still have good sex.
Men and women talk only about sex.	Men and women talk about feelings, what they like, and contraception.
Condoms are rarely used.	Condoms are used quite often.
The man is in control.	The man or woman can take control.
The lights are bright.	The lights are usually low or switched off.
There is no privacy.	There is privacy.
The people are acting; often they are not feeling sexy, nor enjoying it.	The people are in a relationship and mostly feel sexy.
The men all have big penises.	Most men have average-size penises.
Sex ends when the man has an orgasm.	Sexual play and love-making continues after the man has had an orgasm.
People make a lot of noise during sex.	People may be quiet or noisy during sex.
The focus is on vaginal, anal and oral intercourse only.	Love-making includes kissing, hugging, stroking, masturbating, intercourse, oral sex, laughing and talking.
Sex often involves more than two people.	Sex usually involves two people.

4. Invite a pair to read out a statement, place it next to Planet Porn or Planet Earth, and explain why they have put it there.

5. Invite comments from the rest of the group.

6. Repeat with the rest of the pairs, adding information from Box 22.f as needed to ensure you have covered all the differences between porn sex and real sex.

Box 22.f What is the difference between porn sex and real sex?

Porn bodies. Porn actors do not have average bodies like most people; they are chosen for their hot bodies. Actors may have operations, use drugs, and spend a lot of money to change their appearance. The film makers also use filming tricks to make the actors look more perfect. We should not compare our bodies with how theirs seem to be.

Porn sex. The purpose of porn is to make the viewer (particularly male viewers) feel sexy. This means that porn sex is all about performance and looking sexy, with a focus on intercourse. In real life, sex involves showing love and affection to each other, including stroking, hugging, and other less obviously sexy activities.

Sexy talk. Porn chat is all about sex, and it can be degrading and negative. There is often a lot more moaning and groaning in porn sex than in real-life sex. In real life people chat about what sex they like or dislike. They talk about contraception, condoms, feelings, themselves, have a laugh, and stop when they feel like it.

Porn stars are acting. Even though the actors do have sex in porn scenes, they are acting. It's all made up and, most of the time, the actors *pretend* to enjoy it. Porn films are edited to make it look as if the sex is very exciting and takes a long time – it's a show. Real sex may sometimes be like this, but often it is not.

Porn sexual activities may not be 'normal'. Some sexual activities are so common in porn that people begin to think that everyone enjoys them. Anal sex and ejaculating on someone are very popular in porn, but much less so in reality. People who watch porn may feel pressure to do activities that they don't want to do, or put pressure on others to do things they don't want to do.

Porn can be negative about women. Some porn is negative about women; it tends to show women with no intelligence, opinions or power. Some porn shows women being raped, beaten, or even killed. This can increase gender violence and other harmful gender norms.

Porn is mostly for men. Most porn is made for men, while male actors do not look at the camera (or their faces are not shown). Female actors often look into the camera, so that male viewers can imagine they are having sex with them. Watching porn can influence gender and sexual norms and practices, so that men are more dominant towards women.

Group sex. In porn, group sex is very popular because it means there is more activity in the film. In real life, most people prefer one-on-one sex, in a personal and intimate private space. They may feel pressured to have group sex by people who watch porn.

Condoms. Condoms are not often used in porn. Actors are supposed to have check-ups once a month for HIV and STIs. They are taking risks.

Sexual orientation. The same differences between porn sex and real-life sex apply whether the sex is between males and females, males, or females.

7. Invite participants to discuss the following questions:
- Does porn have an effect on how its viewers feel about their own bodies and how they work?
- Can people learn how to have sex from watching porn? Is this a good idea?
- What does porn teach us about how to be a man or woman?
- In general, do women like porn as much as men do?
- Why is there nothing about feelings or relationships in porn?

8. Summarize by saying that Planet Porn is a fantasy place, where fantasy sex takes place. We need to remember that it is very different from the real sex that happens on Planet Earth. Fantasies can be fun, but they can also be harmful if we believe them, compare ourselves with them, or expect them to come true.

EXERCISE 22.5 THE EFFECTS OF PORNOGRAPHY ON CHILDREN

AIMS: To explore possible benefits and harmful aspects of children watching porn.

DESCRIPTION: (Option A) Participants read stories and answer questions about them; (Option B) participants read letters and discuss how to respond to them.

Directions

1. If it would help the participants to talk comfortably, divide them into males and females, or into older and younger children within your peer group.

Option A

2. Read out the story of Idi, Chiku and Jahidi (see Box 22.g), or create a realistic story to suit your peer group.

Box 22.g The story of Idi, Chiku and Jahidi

Idi, aged 11 years, and his sister Chiku, aged eight years, came home from school to meet their older cousin Jahidi, aged 30 years, who was home from work. Jahidi was excited and said that he had found a new DVD in his uncle's drawer – they could watch it together. He said this would teach them about sex. He put the TV on and switched on the DVD. The film started by saying it was only to be shown to people over the age of 18 years. Jahidi told Idi and Chiku this didn't matter; he would explain it to them. Then a man and woman appeared on the screen, took their clothes off, and started to have sex. Idi looked at them wide-eyed, and Chiku started to cry and hid her face.

---

3. Ask questions along these lines and discuss the answers:

Does this happen in our community?
- Why did Jahidi show Idi and Chiku the sexy film? Do you agree or disagree with him?
- What was Idi feeling? What was he thinking?
- How might watching the sexy film affect Idi afterwards?
- How do you think Chiku felt?
- How might watching the film affect Chiku afterwards?
- What were the negative things about the children seeing the film?
- What were the positive things, if any?
- If you were Chiku and Idi's caregiver, would you allow them to watch the DVD? Why, or why not?
- If you would not allow them to watch, how would you make sure that they did not?

Option B

2. Read out either the letter to Dr Love (see Box 22.h) or the letter to Auntie Mary (see Box 22.i), or create a letter relevant to your peer group. Then ask participants the relevant follow-up questions and discuss.

Box 22.h Letter to Dr Love

Dear Dr Love,

I am a 13-year-old boy. I invited my classmate Mhima to watch a sexy movie with me. I thought he would enjoy it. The man in it was doing things that I have never seen before to the woman, and she was moaning. I was really turned on, and wanted to find a girl so I could do the same things with her. Mhima looked as if he was going to be sick and ran home. Now he won't talk to me; what went wrong? As his friend, growing up together, how can I help him to enjoy sexy movies?

Yours, Joseph

Questions

- Does this happen in our community?
- How did Joseph feel? What did he want to do?
- How did Mhima feel? What did he want to do?
- Is sex on films the same as sex in real life? What is different?
- If you were Dr Love, how would you reply to Joseph's letter?

For caregivers only

If Joseph were your child, what would you say to him?
- If Mhima were your child, what would you say to him?

Box 22.i Letter to Auntie Mary

Dear Auntie Mary,

I am an 11-year-old girl. Last week my big brother showed me a sexy movie while our mother was out. The woman was beautiful with big breasts. I don't think anyone will want me because I'm skinny and my chest is flat. There's something wrong with my private parts too. I didn't understand what they were doing, but it didn't seem like love, more like fighting, and the woman was screaming. Is there anything I can do to stop growing up?

Yours, Nina

Questions

- Does this happen in our community?
- How did Nina feel? Why does she feel like that?
- Why did her brother show her the movie?
- Is sex on films the same as sex in real life? What is different?
- If you were Auntie Mary, how would you reply to Nina's letter?

For caregivers only

If Nina were your child, what would you say to her?
- What would you say to her brother?

EXERCISE 22.6 PROTECTING EACH OTHER FROM THE NEGATIVE EFFECTS OF PORNOGRAPHY

AIMS: To find ways of protecting ourselves and our children from the negative effects of porn.

DESCRIPTION: Participants discuss how we can use our virtues to keep away from porn and protect each other from it. Then they draw or write means of protection on the relevant points of the map from Exercise 22.2 (question 2).

Directions

1. Show the map that the participants created in Exercise 22.2. Make sure all the places where children might see porn are included, such as in homes and cinemas, or on mobile devices.

Children aged 9–14 years and caregivers in separate peer groups

2. Divide into small groups and invite each group to choose one of the situations in which children like them/theirs might watch porn.

Ask: 'How can we use our virtues to support each other/our children in keeping away from porn?'

Invite them to brainstorm different ways of protecting each other or their children from this source of porn, and to draw or write their ideas on the relevant part of the map.

3. Invite the groups to share their ideas and agree on the first steps they will take. If needed, once the groups have shared their thoughts, add information from Box 22.j.

Children aged 5–8 years

2. Talk together about the three things in Box 22.j that children can do to protect themselves from porn, and practise these using role play.

Box 22.j Ways of protecting children from porn

Caregivers can:

- talk about porn with their children and other caregivers, family members, neighbours, housemaids, and friends, so that they understand and think critically about it; they can explain the negative effects of porn on children and adults, gender norms and practices, sexual safety, and legal and ethical issues;

- put password-protected blocks on porn to prevent children accessing it via computers and phones;

- in countries where all porn is illegal, campaign for enforcement of porn laws; for example, the closure of local video houses showing porn;

- campaign for cinema owners to refuse entry to porn films to children under 18 years;

- switch off the DVD player and lock up the plug;

- ensure that any porn in the house, such as DVDs and magazines, is locked up;

- if watching porn movies, ensure that no children can see or hear the film.

Children can:

- talk to peers about porn to share what they have learned, and help their peers become well informed;

- avoid watching porn, and be assertive when people try to persuade them to see it on DVDs, phones, or computers, in magazines, or at the cinema;

- tell an adult they trust if someone puts pressure on them to see porn.

Purpose: To enable participants to have better knowledge about, and skills for decision-making around, delaying, starting, and stopping sexual activity, and improved ability to keep to those decisions.

Contents	Materials required	Time required
Opening circle (see p.13)		15 mins
23.1 Why do children start having sex?		45 mins
23.2 Advantages and disadvantages of delaying, starting, and stopping having sex	Prepared flipcharts	60 mins
23.3 Sex and our life journey		30 mins
23.4 *For children aged 9–14 years and caregivers only* Should they have sex or not?	Drawings of characters from Exercise 23.1	45 mins
23.5 Sticking to our decisions		60 mins
Closing circle (see p.14)		15 mins

About 4.5 hrs

Box 23.a Information for facilitators

The majority of boys and girls between the ages of five and 14 years are not mature enough physically, mentally, socially, or emotionally to engage safely, healthily, and happily in sexual activity. When older people have sex with children of these age groups it is, in law, defined as sexual abuse. This session supports caregivers and children in thinking critically about whether children of this age are ready for sexual relationships, and in responding assertively to situations that may result in sex.

Most of the 5–8-year-old children will not have reached puberty and if they have sex it is likely only when forced, copying adults, or in need of material help or physical comfort. For these younger children, the focus of this session will be on the benefits of delaying their sexual debut, and thinking about why children might have sex either now or when they reach puberty.

By the age of around 12 years many children will reach puberty, and are more likely to be starting to engage in sexual activity. This is a crucial stage for supporting them in reinforcing their knowledge, virtues, confidence, and skills in delaying sex or stopping having sex until they are physically, mentally, emotionally, and socially mature.

Note: We will look further at the issue of forced sex and what we can do to protect children from sexual abuse in Session 26.

EXERCISE 23.1 WHY DO CHILDREN START HAVING SEX?

AIMS: To understand the different situations, relationships, and reasons why boys and girls of different ages might begin to engage in sexual activity, and then continue sexual activity.

DESCRIPTION: Identify different characters with whom people like them might have sex, and discuss the reasons why.

Directions

1. Divide the peer group into males and females. You may also wish to divide the children's peer groups into older and younger boys and girls. Explain that we are going to talk about why people of the same age and sex as them might start to have sex now, or when they are a bit older, and why they might continue to have sex.

2. Give participants several pieces of paper each and invite them to:
• (*children*) draw different types of people with whom people like them, or a bit older, might have sex for the first time (one person on each piece of paper);
• (*caregivers*) draw or write the types of people whom their boys and girls might have sex with for the first time (one person on each piece of paper).

For example: girls might draw a schoolmate, a teacher, an uncle, or a boy from their school choir.

3. Ask participants to explain the characters they have drawn or written down, as they place the pieces of paper in the centre of the group. Then invite participants to point out the characters with whom children of their age and sex, or a bit older, most commonly have sex for the first time.

4. Divide into smaller groups, and invite each group to choose one character drawing to work on further. Ask them to add a drawing of a child like them, or a bit older, to their chosen drawing. Ask them to discuss why the child started to have sex, why the other person had sex with the child, and to add the reasons to the drawing.

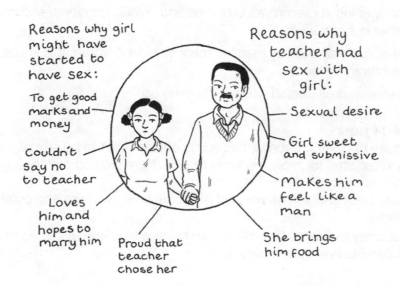

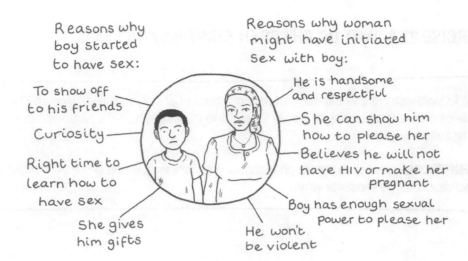

Reasons why boy started to have sex:

To show off to his friends

Curiosity

Right time to learn how to have sex

She gives him gifts

Reasons why woman might have initiated sex with boy:

He is handsome and respectful

She can show him how to please her

Believes he will not have HIV or make her pregnant

Boy has enough sexual power to please her

He won't be violent

5. Ask the groups to consider whether, and why, the child and other person might continue to have sex together, and to add these ideas to their drawing.

6. Ask the groups to present their ideas back to the rest of the groups.

Then ask: 'Is there a pattern regarding who has control? Is it the child like you, or the other person?'

7. Summarize what has been learned, adding information from Box 23.b if needed.

Box 23.b Why children might start having sex

Many children are forced into having sex for the first time, either by adults who abuse them or by other children who force them. They have not chosen to start having sex.

Children aged 5–8 years
Most children of this age will not feel sexual desire linked to another person because they have not yet reached puberty. They may start to have sex because:
- they see it happening in overcrowded homes and neighbourhoods, and may experiment with each other out of curiosity;
- they may be sexually abused by men, women, or older children; this abuse might involve gifts such as money or food;
- they may seek status as people who are growing up.

Children aged 9–14 years
These children are beginning puberty, and some of them start to be sexually active at this time. They often start for more than one reason. Here are some of those reasons, in addition to those above:
Boys or girls may seek and sometimes find affection, love, pleasure and comfort in their sexual relationships.
- It may be culturally expected that they begin to have sex, even if it is illegal and religious leaders and parents are against early sex.

- They may not know the disadvantages of having early sex, or have had the opportunity to discuss it with anyone who is well informed.
- Girls may not be able to resist the persistent advances of older boys and men. They may have been taught the gender norm of submitting to the needs of males.
- Boys or girls may have same-sex relationships, either voluntarily or forced.
- Boys or girls may start and continue sexual relationships to get gifts to meet their needs.
- Boys might start to have sex because they want to see themselves as men. Boys of this age may be treated as adults, expected to fend for themselves, separated from their families and homes, and working with adults. They may gain in self-esteem and respect from others if they have girlfriends.

EXERCISE 23.2 ADVANTAGES AND DISADVANTAGES OF DELAYING, STARTING, AND STOPPING SEX

AIM: To explore the advantages and disadvantages of delaying early sex, starting sexual activity at a young age, and stopping having sex after having started.

DESCRIPTION: Participants sing a song, then consider advantages and disadvantages of delaying having sex. *Children aged 9–14 years* and *caregivers* in their separate peer groups go on to consider advantages and disadvantages of starting having sex and stopping having sex.

Box 23.c Information for facilitators

It is important that boys and girls have an opportunity to think and talk about their understanding of the advantages and disadvantages of having sex, and that we listen with respect. At the same time, we need to support them in thinking more deeply about the reality of their reasons, their ability to manage the possible consequences of having sex, and the safety and health aspects of having sex at their age. The discussion in peer groups may raise these issues but, if not, the facilitator needs to bring new perspectives into the discussion. We need to do this without painting a negative or judgemental picture of sexual feelings, friendships, and intimacy. It is a matter of enjoying these benefits later in life, to provide the best chance of being happy, healthy, and safe.

 Some boys and girls in the group may already have had sexual experiences, and feel worried when talking about the advantages and disadvantages of having sex because they started early. Reassure participants that we can always decide to stop having sex until the right time, even if we have already had sex. This will help protect us. Remind people about the session on having an HIV test. If boys or girls have had sex and do not know whether they have HIV, a test can reduce anxiety, and support them in making good decisions and staying well.

Box 23.d Information for facilitators: Factors to consider about early sex

Physical maturity

Girls. The vagina and cervix are not fully grown until the end of puberty (around 16–18 years of age) when they develop protective skin and lubrication to protect women from bruising and sores during sexual intercourse. Girls having sex before they are mature are more likely to get bruising and sores, which make it easier for HIV and STIs to enter the body.

Childbirth is safer when the birth canal and organs are fully developed, at around 20 years of age. Younger girls who become pregnant have a higher risk of obstructed labour, fistulas, stillbirth, a small baby, and damage to their reproductive organs.

Boys. The penis grows in length and width during puberty, becoming fully grown by about 16 years of age. Condoms are designed for mature males, so they are too big for many boys during puberty (see Session 24 'All about condoms').

Myths. There is no truth in beliefs that girls and boys need to start having sex during puberty. Delaying having sex will not cause testicles to burst, nor penises to grow crooked. Neither does it affect when girls' periods start, nor cause vaginas to close up, nor increase the chance of the first child having abnormalities.

Mental and social maturity

The upper brain is not fully developed until sometime after puberty, usually in a person's early twenties. It is important for making good decisions, predicting consequences, controlling feelings, taking responsibility, and communicating and empathizing with others. For this reason, young people are more easily overwhelmed by sexual feelings than adults, and may make decisions that harm them and others.

In general, the younger the child, the less sexually competent they are. This relates to their capacity to, for example, be assertive about what they want and act on it; use contraception and condoms; and have an HIV test.

Maturity is also needed to assess a range of other factors, such as:
- whether the person we are attracted to is likely to be a good partner, or someone who may harm us (What virtues do they show? Do we have equal power? Do we agree things together? What is our relationship like?);
- whether we may regret having sex after we have done it;
- how having sex may affect achieving our vision of a good future.

The law

Regardless of whether the sex is forced or consensual (agreed to), sex with a child who is under the age of consent is illegal. The age of consent varies from country to country: for heterosexual sex it is 12 years in Angola, 16 in South Africa, and 18 in Tanzania. It can also vary by sex: in Botswana, for example, it is 14 for boys but 16 for girls. In many countries there is no age of consent for homosexual sex, as it is illegal for all ages. Laws about the age of consent are often not enforced, but most cultures treat forced sex with a child by an adult more seriously than sex between consenting children.

Culture

Many cultures expect children to have sex before they are physically, mentally, and socially mature. Such norms carry a high price for these societies and the children in them. But norms can and do change. This workshop process can contribute to change.

Directions

1. Keep the peer group split into males and females as in Exercise 23.1. Ideally, split the children's peer groups further, into older and younger boys and girls. Explain that we are now going to look at the advantages and disadvantages of delaying sexual activity.

2. Sing a pop or traditional song about delaying sex until the right time.

3. Draw two columns on a flipchart, marking one side 'advantages of delaying sex' and the other 'disadvantages of delaying sex'. With *caregivers*, explain that they should think about this in relation to their children's sexual activities, though the advantages and disadvantages may concern themselves and the wider family too.

4. Invite participants to think freely about the advantages of delaying sex at their age or a bit older, and to call them out one at a time, as you or a participant writes them in the 'advantages' column. Encourage everyone to call out whatever thoughts or feelings are in their heads, without judging or discussing them.

Repeat this process with the disadvantages of delaying sex at their age or a bit older.

5. When everyone has run out of ideas, discuss what they have written. As needed, add information from Box 23.d.

Box 23.d Some advantages of delaying or stopping sex

If we wait to start sex, or stop having sex until we are older:
- we can take time to find a loving relationship with someone we know and trust;
- our first sex may be better, because we will be more mature and prepared, and can enjoy it without worrying;
- by the end of puberty, our body will be mature enough to have sex safely;
- condoms will fit properly and our organs will not be injured by sexual intercourse, so we will have a lower risk of getting HIV and other STIs;
- when we do have a baby (ideally after we are 20 years old), we are more likely to deliver a healthy baby without harm to us or the baby;
- we will be more likely to have a more equal relationship and be able to say and do what we want assertively – it will be our choice;
- we will be less likely to be forced into having sex;
- we will be less likely to regret having sex;
- we will be better able to access and use contraceptives and condoms successfully to protect ourselves from unplanned pregnancy, HIV, and STIs (condoms greatly reduce the risk of these things happening, but they do not give 100% protection);
- we will be more likely to achieve our dreams, for example, by going to school, getting a job, and developing a harmonious, long-term relationship with faithfulness and trust;
- if we value sex as something to do only in a long-term relationship, we will feel happy with ourselves for upholding our values;
- if our friends and parents value sex as something to do only in a long-term relationship, our reputation will be better;
- we may have more time and energy to dedicate to our education and skills training;
- we will stay within the law.

---

6. Invite participants to:

- *(children aged 5–8 years)* talk or draw pictures about how delaying having sex until they are older can enable them to be safe, healthy, and happy.

- *(children aged 9–14 years and caregivers in separate peer groups)* repeat steps 4 and 5 to create a flipchart about the advantages and disadvantages of starting having sex. Ask the group to discuss the reality of the advantages they list, to check if their perceptions are accurate.

- Then ask them to repeat steps 4 and 5 for a third flipchart, about the advantages and disadvantages of stopping having sex. Emphasize that girls and boys who start having sex early do not necessarily need to continue to have sex.

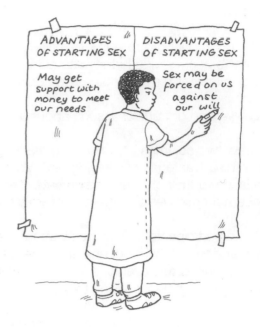

7. *All peer groups*. If girls and boys in the same age group feel comfortable sharing their work with each other, invite them to compare their charts.

Ask: 'What is similar and what is different for boys and girls in each case?'

Children aged 9–14 years and caregivers only in separate peer groups. Ask: 'What about the advantages and disadvantages of children having sex with more than one person? For example, imagine a boy has a girlfriend, breaks up with her, then has another girlfriend. Or that a girl has a boyfriend of her own age, and sometimes has sex with an older man.'

Contribute information from Box 23.e to the discussion as needed.

Box 23.e STI and HIV risk in relation to number of sexual partners

In general, the more partners a person has sex with without using a condom, the higher the chance that they will get HIV, or share it. Having unprotected sex with more than one sexual partner in the same time period, or with a sexual partner who is also having unprotected sex with someone else, increases the likelihood of getting HIV. This is because when someone first gets HIV there is a lot of HIV in their body fluids, making it easier to share HIV between people in the sexual network.

Some people believe that it is safe to have unprotected sex with one partner, then break up and have a new sexual partner, because they have only had one partner at a time. This is not true, although it is a bit safer than having more than one partner in the same time period. This belief would only be true if all three people had taken HIV tests, none of them had HIV, and all three were faithful to each other while in the relationship.

---

8. *All peer groups*. Ask: 'What have we learned from this exercise? How can we use this learning to keep safe, healthy, and happy as we grow up?'

EXERCISE 23.3 SEX AND OUR LIFE JOURNEY

> **AIMS:** To look at how having sex now might influence our life journey, now and in the future.
>
> **DESCRIPTION:** Participants dream of their vision for the future and draw it, then think about how to avoid challenges that might arise from sexual relations, which could prevent them from realizing their vision.

Directions

1. Remind participants of how they dreamed of a good future, drew a vision of it, and then worked out the steps needed to realize it, as they did for example during Exercise 1.5 'Our dreams'.

2. Invite participants to dream again about their vision of the future and to draw it, thinking about whether it features any sexual relationships. With *caregivers*, invite them to dream of their vision for their children, or for themselves.

Ask: 'If your dream includes a sexual partner or partners, how do they support you in reaching your vision?'

'Could the sexual partner or partners in your vision create challenges for you, and take you off your path?'

3. Bring participants back to the present, and ask: 'What virtues will you use to avoid any challenges that might result from sexual activity? How will we use our virtues to support each other in reaching our visions?'

4. Invite participants to share their ideas with the group, telling them:
- one virtue they will use;
- one thing they will do this year to avoid challenges to their vision that might result from sexual activity.

Discuss and agree on ways we will all use our virtues, as friends, to realize our visions.

EXERCISE 23.4 SHOULD THEY HAVE SEX OR NOT?

We suggest that children aged 5–8 years do not do this exercise.

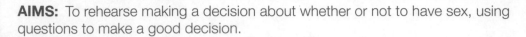

AIMS: To rehearse making a decision about whether or not to have sex, using questions to make a good decision.

DESCRIPTION: A boy and girl role play a couple making a decision about whether to have sex or not. The audience help them by asking questions. The actors make their decisions and the audience vote on their preference.

GROUPS: With children aged 9–14 years, you could either do the exercise with the whole group, or start with girls and boys separately and then bring them together to share their ideas.

Box 23.f Information for facilitators

This exercise builds skill in asking questions and listening. Encourage participants to think carefully about their questions and answers.

Remember that people may know that the negative consequences of unprotected sex can be devastating, but be overwhelmed by feelings at the time. Sexual feelings can be very powerful and can overcome people's plans and common sense.

Young people can be skilled negotiators about sex; for example, girls may negotiate for maximum material support before having sex, and boys may use deception to persuade a girl that they can give them long-term support. They can use these same skills to negotiate for delayed sex or safer sex.

Directions[58]

1. Explain that we are now going to practise making a decision about whether or not to have sex, using a role play about a couple. We are doing this to improve our ability to make safe and healthy decisions. We are definitely not saying that we should have sex with any of the characters in this exercise!

2. Show the drawings that the group made in Exercise 23.1, and decide which character you will all work on. Invite one person to play that character, and another to play the child who is thinking about having sex with the character.

3. Invite the pair to give themselves names which do not belong to any participants in the group. Ask them to leave the group and get into their roles. The 'child' and 'character' need to know why each is thinking of having sex with the other, and to agree on how long they have known each other, how and where they are together, and how they feel about each other.

4. Ask the rest of the group to pair up. Say: 'What questions will you ask the characters to help them make a good decision?' Ask them to:
• think of questions for both actors, to find out if they feel differently;

- think of open questions rather than closed ones, so the answer will make clear what the questioner thinks (for example, instead of asking: 'Don't you feel that it is wrong to have sex before marriage?', ask: 'What do you feel about having sex before marriage?');

- note down their questions if they want to;

- listen to what the characters say, and try to ask questions that build on the previous question and answer (for example, if the question is: 'Do you want to have a child with this person?', and the answer is no, the next question could be: 'What are you going to do to prevent pregnancy if you have sex?').

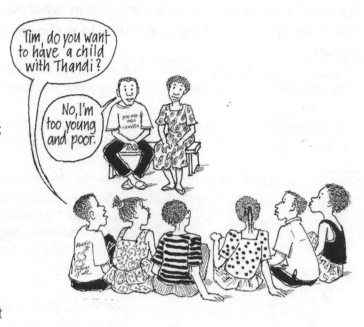

5. Invite the pair of characters to rejoin the group. Explain that the group members are going to help them decide whether or not to have sex by asking them some questions.

6. Ask the couple to introduce themselves, giving only their role-play names. Facilitate a role play, with the group asking the characters questions, and the characters answering in their roles.

7. If necessary, when people have asked all the questions they can think of, add in any key questions that have been missed, such as:

- If you do have sex, what will be your reasons for doing it? What virtues do these reasons express?

- Does this person show care and love for you? What are your feelings for them?

- Are you able to refuse this sex if you want to?

- Have you talked with this person about having sex?

- Are you physically mature enough to have sex safely?

- Are you old enough to have sex legally?

- How might having sex with this person affect reaching your vision for the future?

- How would your life change if you became pregnant or created a pregnancy?

- Could either of you have HIV or another STI? How do you know?

- What will you do to protect yourself and your partner from STIs and HIV?

- Would you be able to refuse sex without a condom with this person?

- Why might you regret having sex with this person?

8. When the two actors have answered all the questions, ask them to go away and decide, each of them privately, whether or not to have sex with the other.

9. While they are away, ask the group to vote on whether they think the pair should have sex or not.

10. Invite the two actors back in and ask each of them to reveal their decision and the reasons for it. Then tell them how the group voted. Encourage participants to consider the consequences of their decisions according to their responses, as indicated in Table 23.1.

Table 23.1 Responses to decision over whether or not to have sex

Decision made by actors and group	How to respond to the decision
The couple disagree with each other over whether or not to have sex.	Ask each of them what they will do now, and ask them to say something to each other in character.
The couple agree to have sex, but group thinks they shouldn't.	Invite the group to ask more questions to help the couple think clearly about the possible consequences of having sex.
The couple agree not to have sex but the group thinks they should.	Invite the group to explain to the couple why the group thinks they should have sex. Then invite the couple to explain to the group why they have decided not to have sex. If necessary, explain your concerns about the group's decision. See the next box for more suggestions.
Both the couple and the group think the couple should have sex.	As facilitator, ask more questions to help them think more deeply about the possible negative consequences. If needed, explain your concerns about the decision and ask the group to advise the couple on what would make their sexual activity safer (e.g. showing love in other ways, using outercourse, using condoms).
Both the couple and the group think that the couple should not have sex.	Go around the group asking each person to say one different reason why it is best if the couple do not have sex.

11. Ask people what they have learned from the activity, and summarize.

12. Thank the pair of actors for their role play and welcome their true selves back into the room, using their real names again.

13. Say: 'We will now look at what we can do to avoid sex until we are ready.'

 ## EXERCISE 23.5 STICKING TO OUR DECISIONS

AIMS: To look critically at what words may mean. To look at ways of keeping to our decision to say 'no' to sex. To practise saying assertively that we do not want to have sex.

DESCRIPTION: Participants practise saying 'no' to sex in different situations through role play.

Directions

1. Direct the relevant peer groups as follows:

Children aged 5–8 years. Ask them to imagine they have made a firm decision not to do something, which someone might pressure them to do. For example: not to go and play with friends by the river because it is dangerous, even though it is also fun; or not to cross a busy road without an adult, even though their friend lives on the other side of the road.

Ask them to pair up and role play the situation: one child tries to persuade the other, who must respond assertively.

Children aged 9–14 years. Ask the group to imagine that they have decided that they want to say 'no' to either starting to have sex, or continuing to have sex. Remind participants about Session 6 on assertiveness.

Explain that you want them to pair up and invent a role play where one person pressures the other to have sex; the second person must respond assertively. If they choose to pair up with someone of the same sex, then one of the pair may want to act as a character of the other sex.

You can give the pairs sentences from Table 23.2 to use to start their role play, or ask them to make up their own.

Table 23.2 Starter sentences for practising saying 'no' assertively

Child to child	Adult to child
I have to have sex with you now; I can't stop it, the urge is too strong.	You are so mature, not like others. Let me make you a man/woman.
I'm going to become ill if we don't make love. Don't deny me what I need.	You've kept me waiting too long. I can find another friend if don't love me enough to show it.
Please make love to me so I know I'm your girl/boy.	You're not a child anymore; you need to behave like a grown-up and satisfy me.
You've had sex before, so there's no point in saying 'no' now.	If you don't have sex with me again, I'll make trouble for you.
Let's play mummies and daddies. I've seen how they do it and it looks funny.	Be a good child, and I'll buy you something nice.

Caregivers. Explain that you want them to pair up and invent a role play demonstrating one of these situations:

• Someone like them is being pressured to have sex; they respond assertively to say 'no'.

• A caregiver is talking to their child about the pressure the child is facing from another child to have sex; they discuss how the child, and perhaps the caregiver, might respond assertively.

• A caregiver is talking to their child about the pressure the child is facing from an adult to have sex; they discuss how the caregiver and child might respond assertively.

2. *All peer groups*. After 10 minutes, clap your hands and ask the pairs to swap roles, so that each person has a chance to practise the other role. They can use the same situation, or a different one.

3. Ask some pairs to show their role play to the rest of the group. Invite discussion and add ideas, if needed, from Box 23.g and Box 23.h.

With *children aged 5–8 years*, explain that they can also use the skills they have practised in non-sexual situations to say 'no' to having sex.

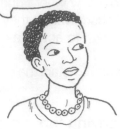

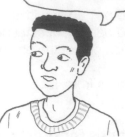

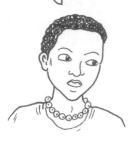

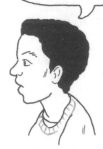

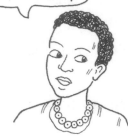

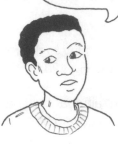

Box 23.g Ways of saying 'no' to starting or continuing to have sex

- I have made a decision to delay sex until I am older and ready.

- I'd like you to respect my views.

- Not having sex is the only 100% effective way to avoid pregnancy, getting an STI or sexually transmitted HIV. Right now I want to avoid all those things.

- I want to protect my fertility and life until I am ready to have a baby.

- I don't want to upset my parents, or keep secrets from them.

- I think sex before we are living together or married is wrong. I would feel bad if I went against my beliefs.

- Let me tell you what I want in my life and what I want to be doing in five years' time. Having a baby, paying fines, or getting sick would stop me from getting to where I want to be, and realizing my vision of a good future.

- I'm determined to get through primary school and try for secondary school. If I had sex with you, my mind would be distracted by you, and I wouldn't be able to concentrate.

- Let me tell you about what my caregivers hope for me, and how they would feel if I had a child or got sick.

- We don't have to have sex to love each other. Let's stay safe and focus on our visions for our future life. They are more important than a bit of fun today.

Box 23.h Ways of supporting a child in saying 'no' to starting or continuing to have sex

- Be a good role model in terms of your own virtues and behaviour. Share your values with your child; for example, tell them that you think it is best for children to delay having sex until they are mature. Explain why.

- Show empathy by sharing that you know it is difficult to say 'no' to sex.

- Discuss non-judgementally situations of people like them, such as children who have had to drop out of school owing to pregnancy, as a way of exploring the consequences of early sex. Talk together about why it may have happened, and what the relevant people could have done differently.

- Communicate that children who have had early sex don't have to keep having it. They can benefit by stopping.

- Encourage the child to have a vision of their future, and support them in working towards their vision.

- Try to meet children's basic needs, so it is easier for them to refuse having sex in exchange for gifts. Encourage them to consider the difference between needs and wants. Ask whether what we want now is always in line with our future visions for ourselves. Explore the possible high personal costs, in the longer term, of receiving gifts in exchange for sex.

- If the child is willing to talk to you, listen to their thoughts and feelings about the situation without being judgemental or angry. Support them in thinking about different actions they could take, and what they could say. Help them find ways of being assertive and staying safe.

- If the child is being pressured or forced to have sex, particularly if by an adult or older child who has power over them, you need to help them stop the abuse (see Session 26 on sexual abuse).

4. Ask: 'What virtues are the actors showing when they respond assertively?'

5. Explain that sometimes people may say one thing, but mean something else. For example, 'I love you' may mean exactly that, or it may just mean 'I want to have sex with you'. We are now going to practise being assertive, to try and find out what someone actually means when they say nice things to us.

6. Direct relevant peer groups as follows:

Children aged 5–8 years. Split into separate groups of boys and girls, each with a facilitator. Ask each group to think about what someone might say to them if they want to do something sexual with them. For example, a child might say: 'I love you. Let's play mummies and daddies, it looks fun.' An adult might say: 'I love you best. Let's do nice things to each other and I will give you a present.'

Ask: 'What do you think the person really means?' Discuss the groups' ideas or, if the children are comfortable using role play, invite them to act out questioning the person about what they really mean. Ask them to form small groups and take it in turns to practise saying 'no' to sex.

Children aged 9–14 years. Ask participants to pair up and to think of a situation in which someone like them hears a 'chat-up line' from someone who probably wants to become sexually intimate with them. Ask them to use role play to practise being assertive, by trying to find out what the person really means. If what they really mean is that they want to have sex, practise sticking to the decision to say 'no'. For example:

Person A: 'You're so pretty. Let's go for a walk together.'

Person B: 'Thanks for the compliment. Why do you want to go for a walk?'

Person A: 'There are too many people here. I want to be with just you, because you're special.'

Person B: 'Let's sit just over there, where it's not so noisy.'

Person A: 'But it would be much nicer to go for a walk.'

Person B: 'I feel perhaps you'd like to go for a walk so that we could get sexy together?'

Person A: 'Well, I do love you. Wouldn't it be good to get closer?'

Person B: 'Not for me. I feel safe and happy staying here with my friends, which include you. I'm not having sex until I'm older.'

Ask the pairs to think of a new situation and to swap roles, so that both people practise being assertive.

Invite participants to tell the whole group what their opening line was, and what they really meant by it. Remind them that sometimes people *do* mean what they say: it is fine to ask questions and look critically at how a person behaves, to check whether what they say is what they actually mean.

Ask: 'Would this way of being assertive work in real life?'

Caregivers. Ask them to either:

- practise for themselves ways of finding out what someone really means when they try to get close (following the same instructions as for the children aged 9–14 years); or
- role play a caregiver supporting their child in being assertive, in order to find out what someone who is trying to get close to the child really means.

7. Then ask the relevant peer groups:

Children of all ages. 'What else can you do to stick to your decision not to start having sex, or to stop having sex?'

'What can we do to support each other?'

Caregivers. 'What else can you do to support your children in delaying starting having sex, or in stopping having sex?'

If needed, remind participants what they learned in Session 21, about managing sexual feelings, safe ways of showing sexual love, and setting boundaries. Ask them to restate what they agreed then about setting boundaries, and about supporting each other in sticking to them.

8. *All peer groups*. Ask what participants have learned from this exercise. Summarize, and remind them that the decision to have sex needs to be agreed properly by individuals whose brains and bodies are mature, who care about each other, and who will take care to protect themselves from HIV, STIs, and unwanted pregnancy.

Closing circle

It is essential that this session is followed by Session 24 'All about condoms'.

Note: If using option 1 in Exercise 24.2 'Condoms are our friends', explain that in the next session, we will meet some visitors who feel comfortable using condoms and sharing their experience with us. Invite participants to write down any questions they have about condoms and to put them in the question box, or tell the facilitator.

Cluster key themes and share with the visitors before the workshop so they can prepare and select questions that they are comfortable to answer. Use the questions yourself in planning your session.

SESSION 24 ALL ABOUT CONDOMS

Do not do this session unless you have already done Sessions 12 (All about HIV), 21 (Our sexual feelings and sexual safety), and 23 (Delaying, starting, and stopping having sex).

Purpose: To gain correct and age-appropriate information about condoms; develop positive attitudes towards adults using condoms; learn to support each other in delaying starting sex until we are mature; and to reduce the likelihood of sharing STIs, including HIV, and unwanted pregnancy, if having sex.

Contents	Materials required	Time required
Opening circle (see p.13)		15 mins
24.1 What are condoms?	A plastic bag, plus outside and inside condoms	30 mins
24.2 Condoms are our friends	If using option 1, two visitors to talk about using condoms	40 mins
24.3 *For children aged 9–14 and caregivers only* How are outside condoms used?	Outside condoms, and bananas or other penis-shaped objects	40 mins
24.4 *For children aged 9–14 and caregivers only* How are inside condoms used?	Inside condoms	40 mins
24.5 Do condoms fit everyone?	*For children aged 5–8*: a bag of adults' clothes	30 mins
24.6 What are we doing now to stay safe?		30 mins
Closing circle (see p.14)		15 mins

About 4 hrs

Preparation

Exercise 24.2. If using option 1, invite a young man and woman who are willing to talk about how they use condoms successfully to join this session. Ideally, one of them might also be willing to share that they have HIV. Before the session, share with the visitors the questions that participants put into the question box at the end of Session 23, so they can select those they are comfortable answering and prepare their answers.

Exercise 24.4. This exercise could be useful to create demand for female 'inside' condoms, if they are available or could be. However, if female 'inside' condoms are not available to participants, and are not likely to become available in the near future, focus on male 'outside' condoms, and skip Exercise 24.4.

Box 24.a Information for facilitators

Some people believe that young people should not learn about condoms because it will encourage them to have sex. There is no evidence for this. Make it clear that this session is aimed at preparing young people for the future, when they have a sexual partner. Condoms are the only device we have to protect each other from STIs (including HIV), and which enable people with STIs (including HIV) to enjoy a sexual life safely. (It is only safe to have sex without a condom if the viral load of the person with HIV is undetectable, and no other STIs are present. But this can be difficult to monitor.)

Participants may have negative attitudes towards condoms due to religious influences, stigmatization of condoms, false information, and a preference for unprotected sex. It is important to enable them to explore the issue of condoms in more depth, and get correct information on the benefits of using them.

Children may know little about condoms, and those who do may not want to share their knowledge. Emphasize that what they learn in this session will help them stay safe when they are grown up enough to have sex.

Caregivers may not agree to their children learning about condoms. They may prefer to give strong guidance on abstinence only. Help them see the importance of children knowing how to stay safe when they do have sex. Research by a Christian organization in South Africa has shown that teaching abstinence only to children is more dangerous to the children's lives than giving them full information.[59]

Tailoring the session

Inside (female) and outside (male) condoms give users protection during vaginal, anal, and oral sex. However, in the text for this session we have focussed on their use for vaginal sex. Anal sex is illegal and stigmatized in many countries, although it certainly happens between males, and between females and males. People may engage in anal intercourse because they believe it is safe from the risk of HIV, STI, and pregnancy. However, HIV and other STIs can be transmitted through anal sex. Please handle this according to local laws and participants' best interests.

 ## EXERCISE 24.1 WHAT ARE CONDOMS?

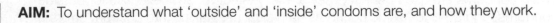

AIM: To understand what 'outside' and 'inside' condoms are, and how they work.

DESCRIPTION: Participants engage in a question and answer session and examine outside and inside condoms (or outside condoms only, if inside condoms are not available – see note above). Information is provided as appropriate for the relevant peer group.

Directions

1. Put a plastic bag on your hand and shake hands with some participants in your peer group. Ask the group what you are doing. They should remember the game from Exercise 12.4, when some people used plastic bags (representing condoms) to stop HIV spreading. Explain that today we are going to talk and learn all about condoms.

2. Say: 'Some religious leaders advise us that we should not use condoms; others say it is better to use condoms than to risk our health if, for example, in a marriage, one person has HIV and the other does not. If you feel that your faith prevents you from using condoms now or when you are grown-up, please still join in and learn about them; you may be able to help others with your knowledge.'

3. Ask: 'What is a condom?' As needed, add information from Box 24.b.

Show some condoms. As you open them, explain that you are checking for a damaged packet and that the use-by date is correct. Show how you are opening them carefully so they do not tear. Tell the group whether they are lubricated or not. Pass them around, so that people can feel and smell them.

Box 24.b What is a condom?

- Condoms are barrier devices used during sexual intercourse to prevent exchange of body fluids between sexual partners.

- 'Outside', or male, condoms are tubes which are closed at one end. They fit tightly over the penis when it is hard – so they are worn on the outside of men's bodies.

- 'Inside', or female, condoms vary in design, but all of them are tubes that are closed at one end. They fit inside the vagina, with the open end staying on the labia – so they are worn on the inside of women's bodies.

---

5. Ask: 'Why do people use condoms and how do they work?' As needed, add information from Box 24.c.

Box 24.c Why use condoms and how do they work?

- Condoms stop semen, vaginal fluids, and blood going from one partner into another during vaginal, anal, or oral sexual intercourse.

- People use them to protect themselves and their sexual partner from passing on or getting STIs (including HIV), and from creating a pregnancy. Some STIs, such as chlamydia, can cause infertility in males and females.

- When condoms are used perfectly they are very effective: 98% effective for outside condoms, and 95% for inside condoms. In typical use, taking into account errors often made by users, they are about 80–90% effective. That is a lot better than having no protection at all!

- When condoms are used perfectly for anal sex, they are about 70% effective.

---

6. Ask: 'Can children use condoms?'

Box 24.d Can children use condoms?

- Condoms are not designed for use by children. Outside condoms are too large for younger boys and fall off. Inside condoms may be too big and uncomfortable for younger girls.

- Most children need to mature physically for condoms to fit them properly, and so give them and their partners a high level of protection.

- It is always better for children to delay or stop having sex until they are mature in mind and body, and competent enough to have sex safely, healthily, and happily.

---

7. Ask: 'Do condoms cause any physical problems?'

Box 24.e Do condoms cause any physical problems?

- Around one in a hundred people is allergic to latex, the rubber material that outside condoms are made of. The allergy is more common among health workers who have a lot of exposure to latex (for example, through wearing latex gloves). Most inside condoms are not made of latex, and it is also possible to get outside condoms which are not made of latex.

- Condoms cannot get lost within the vagina or travel further into the female body: the hole from the vagina into the uterus is far too small for them to pass through.

- Condoms can come off in the rectum but will get pushed out during defecation.

- Condoms come in different sizes. If an outside condom is very tight at the top, it can cause discomfort. Try different sizes and brands, or inside condoms.

---

8. Ask: 'What are the main similarities and differences between outside and inside condoms?'

Box 24.f Outside and inside condoms: similarities and differences

Similarities
- Both types protect users during vaginal sex, anal sex, and oral sex.
- People can get and use them without a prescription.
- Both types may be available for free from health workers.
- Both types may be purchased in shops.
- Both types come in different brands and different sizes.
- Both types can reduce sensitivity a little, because they form a thin barrier between one partner's skin and the other partner's skin.
- Both types can reduce anxiety about HIV, STIs, or pregnancy from sex.
- Both types should be wrapped and thrown into a pit latrine or rubbish bin or buried, or burned, safely away from children or animals.

Differences
- Outside condoms are much more widely available, and cost less to buy, than inside condoms.
- Outside condoms have been used for many years, so people are used to them, whereas inside condoms are relatively new and unfamiliar.
- Inside condoms are still being developed and vary in design, whereas all outside condoms are essentially the same design.
- Outside condoms may feel tight for the man, whereas inside condoms do not.
- Outside condoms help some men have intercourse for longer before they ejaculate, but inside condoms do not have this effect.
- Inside condoms can be put in the vagina hours before having sex, whereas outside condoms can only be put on when the penis is hard, just before having sex.
- Inside condoms stay in place if the man loses his erection, or if the couple want to pause intercourse. Outside condoms should be removed if a man loses his erection and a new one put on when he regains his erection.

- When using inside condoms, the man can keep his penis inside the vagina after he has ejaculated, whereas when using outside condoms he needs to take his penis out before it goes soft.

 EXERCISE 24.2 CONDOMS ARE OUR FRIENDS

AIM: To develop positive attitudes towards condoms, now and in the future.

DESCRIPTION: *Option 1 (for caregivers and children aged 9–14 years).* A male and female, who are comfortable talking about their positive experiences of using condoms, join the session to discuss these with participants in their peer groups. *Option 2 (for all peer groups, or children aged 5–8 years).* Participants draw or make up stories, plays, or songs to express the benefits of using condoms.

Directions

Option 1 (caregivers and children aged 9–14 years)

1. Welcome the visitors, and invite them to answer participants' questions from the question box. They can either sit at the front, facing the participants, or, if the visitors prefer, you could use the 'fishbowl' method, where the participants sit in a circle facing inwards, and the visitors sit in the middle of the circle. The participants sit silently, listening to the visitors' conversation.

2. You can also invite people to ask questions during the session, but let the visitors know that if they don't wish to answer a particular question, they can say so and explain why.

3. If any important questions have been left out, ask them yourself.

Option 2 (for all peer groups)

1. Invite participants to think of creative ways of showing how condoms are our friends, because they can help us at certain points in our lives. The participants could work individually, in pairs, or in small groups. For example, they might:
- draw a picture of a friendly condom, writing down what it would say if it could speak;
- think about what a condom is like (for example, like an umbrella or a shield), and explain why;
- imagine that they are a condom character, which sits on people's shoulders and whispers in their ears to help them; what does it whisper?
- make up a story or song, where Mr or Ms Condom is a hero and rescues people from danger.

2. Ask participants to share what they have created, and affirm each others' work.

EXERCISE 24.3 HOW ARE OUTSIDE CONDOMS USED?

Children aged 5–8 years do not do this exercise, unless caregivers request it.

> **AIM:** To gain knowledge and skills in how to use outside condoms correctly.
>
> **DESCRIPTION:** Participants engage in a question and answer session and are given a demonstration; caregivers and, if appropriate, children aged 9–14 years, practise putting condoms on and taking them off.

Directions

1. Explain that in this session we are going to share our knowledge about how to use outside (male) condoms correctly. Even if we don't intend to use condoms, or are too young to use them now, it's good to learn, so we can teach others and know how to use them for the future.

2. Use the information in Box 24.g to lead a question and answer session.

Box 24.g Using outside condoms correctly

How can users be sure a condom is good?

- Obtain condoms from a place where they are covered and stored out of the sun.
- Check the package to make sure it is not open or torn. Check there is air pressure in the packet before opening.
- Check the date on the condom. If this is the date of expiry, and that date has passed, the condom is no longer safe. Throw it away and get a new one. If the date is the date of manufacture, add five years to it. If that date has passed, the condom is no longer safe. Throw it away and get a new one.
- If when you open the packet the condom is discoloured, or sticks to your fingers like glue, it is not safe. Throw it away and get a new one.

How can users protect condoms from damage?

- Direct light and heat can damage condoms, and so can sharp objects (for example, pens, fingernails) or friction (for example, if carried in a wallet for a long time). So we need to store them in a cool place (not carry them for a long time in our pocket), and keep them either in the box they came in, or in a small tin or other container.
- When using a condom, open the package carefully, taking care not to break the condom with your nails.
- If you want or need to use lubricant, make sure it is safe to use with condoms. It must not be oil-based (for example, Vaseline), as oils damage condoms.

How can users use outside condoms correctly?

1. Wait until the penis is hard and the woman is feeling sexy and wet inside before opening the condom package. Some people find playful, exciting ways to put on a condom as part of safe lovemaking.
2. Use water-based lubricant if the vagina is dry. Always use plenty of lubricant for anal sex, because the rectum does not make its own lubricant.

---

3. Make sure that the condom is the right way up, with the tip upwards and the roll on the outside, so that it can be unrolled on the penis properly. (If you put it in the palm of your hand, it should look like a little hat.)

4. If the man is not circumcised, pull the foreskin back before putting on the condom.

5. Hold the tip of the condom between finger and thumb, to squeeze out the air and so make room for the semen. This is very important, to stop the condom from bursting.

6. Place the condom on the head of the penis (with the condom tip squeezed) and unroll the condom all the way down to the base of the penis.

7. You can now enjoy intercourse safely!

8. After sex, while the penis is still hard, remove the penis from the vagina while holding the rim of the condom around the base of the penis, so that the semen doesn't spill.

9. Take the condom off, wrap it up, and throw it away safely so that children or animals can't find it and play with it. Bury it, burn it, or put it into a pit latrine. Do not try to flush it down a flush lavatory – it will float, or block the drain.

What are the main mistakes that people make (reducing effectiveness)?

• They use a condom which is too old, has been stored in heat or light, or is damaged.

• They damage the condom when opening it, for example, with teeth, a knife, or scissors, or with fingernails or jewellery.

• Before putting on the condom, they unroll it or blow it up to check for holes. This means they can't put it on correctly, and it doesn't fit properly.

• They start to put the condom on upside down. When they find that it is not unrolling, they turn it inside out and unroll it. In fact, they should throw it away and get a new one. A condom turned inside-out will have body fluid on its outside.

• They don't squeeze air out of the tip of the condom. The condom is then more likely to burst, because the tip is full of air when the man ejaculates, so there isn't space for his semen.

• They have intercourse when the woman's vagina is dry. They need to add safe lubrication (for example, saliva) and to do things to make the woman aroused and wetter. The friction of dry sex can make a condom burst.

• They use an oil-based lubricant, such as Vaseline or hand lotion, which can make the condom burst.

• They put the condom on too late, after the penis and vagina have been in contact and body fluids have been shared.

• They take the condom off too soon, before finishing intercourse.

• They use two condoms at the same time. This does not create double protection; it just increases the risk of breakage.

• They use a condom which has been used before. Condoms are only designed to be used once.

• They fail to use a condom at all!

What should we do if an outside condom breaks or comes off the penis?

• The man should take his penis out of the vagina, bringing the condom out too, if possible.

• If necessary, use fingers to take the condom out of the vagina, trying not to spill any of the fluid inside the condom.

• Go and see the family planning nurse. If there is a risk of pregnancy, she can give you emergency contraception. If one of you has HIV, get post-exposure prophylaxis. She can also check for other STIs.

3. Demonstrate putting a condom onto a banana or other acceptable object, and ask a question at each step to check that participants understand. Explain how to take the condom off.

4. If appropriate, invite participants to practise putting a condom on a suitable object by showing each other how to do it in small groups. Ask the person practising to describe what they are doing at each step, and ask others in their group to check that they are doing it well.

5. Point out that participants have just learned an important skill. Even if they never use a male condom themselves, they are now able to show others, such as their peers and children, how to do it correctly.

 EXERCISE 24.4 HOW ARE INSIDE CONDOMS USED?

Only use this exercise if inside condoms are available, or can be made available, to participants. Children aged 5–8 years do not do this exercise, unless caregivers request it.

AIM: To gain knowledge and skills in how to use inside condoms correctly.

DESCRIPTION: Participants engage in a question and answer session and are given a demonstration; caregivers and, if appropriate, children aged 9–14 years, practise putting condoms on and taking them off.

1. Lead a question and answer session in which participants can share their knowledge about using inside condoms. As needed, add information from Box 24.h.

Box 24.h Using inside condoms correctly

How can users be sure an inside condom is good?
See answers in Box 24.g.

How can users protect inside condoms from damage?
See answers in Box 24.g.

How can we use inside condoms correctly?
The design of inside condoms varies, but each kind comes with full instructions. The male general steps, which apply to all inside condoms, are:

1. Remove the condom from the package.

2. Find the ring at the closed end of the condom. Squeeze it together between a finger and thumb and then feed it gently into the vaginal opening. Push it into the vagina, as far as you can. The condom is slippery, so do this carefully and without twisting it inside the vagina. The open end of the condom and the ring at this open end should lie outside the vagina and cover the surrounding surface skin.

3. Once in place you can carry on with normal life with the condom in place. It won't fall out.

4. When ready to have intercourse, guide the penis into the condom, making sure it does not slip outside the condom and so come in contact with the vagina.

5. Enjoy sex! If the man takes his penis out for any reason, make sure it goes back into the condom correctly when you resume intercourse.

---

6. You can stay together after the man has ejaculated, if you wish. When you do pull apart, take the condom out of the vagina carefully, keeping the semen inside.

7. Wrap up the condom in paper and either bury it, burn it, or put the rubbish in a pit latrine, so that no children or animals will find and play with it. Do not put it down a flush lavatory, because it will float or block the drains.

What are the main mistakes that people make (reducing effectiveness)?

- They use a condom which is too old, has been stored in heat or light, or is damaged.
- They damage the condom when opening it, for example, with teeth, a knife, or scissors, or with fingernails or jewellery.
- They use an oil-based lubricant, such as Vaseline or hand lotion, which can damage some inside condoms. Users need to check which lubricants are safe to use, as this varies among female condoms.
- They put the condom on too late, after the penis and vagina have been in contact and body fluids have been shared.
- They allow the penis and vagina to come into contact by not guiding the penis into the condom correctly every time.
- They take the condom out too soon, before finishing intercourse.
- They fail to use a condom at all!

Are inside condoms difficult to use? What can help us use them?

Inside condoms are not difficult to use, but they are different – something new that we have to learn how to use. Many women do not like them much after their first try, but most do like them after four or five times of use. It takes a few tries to get used to them and skilled at putting them in.

What should we do if an inside condom breaks or slips out of place?

- Female condoms very rarely break. If this does happen, follow the same steps as set out for outside condoms in Box 24.g.
- Sometimes inside condoms get slightly attached to the penis, so that they don't stay in place properly. If this happens, add lubricant to the outside of the penis and to the inside of the condom.
- Sometimes inside condoms can slip completely inside the vagina during sex. If this happens, reposition the condom correctly, so that the labia are covered by the opening of the condom.

2. Demonstrate how to use an inside condom by making a small circle with your thumb and first finger, and using that to practise inserting it, as if the circle were a vagina. Alternatively you could make a clay model, or use a box with a hole in it.

3. If appropriate, get participants to practise inserting an inside condom by showing each other how to do it in small groups. Ask the person inserting it to describe what they are doing at each step, and ask others in the group to check that they are doing it well. Congratulate them on their new skill.

EXERCISE 24.5 DO CONDOMS FIT EVERYONE?

AIMS: To examine at what stage of development boys and girls can use condoms safely. To help participants make good decisions about using condoms. To support participants in their efforts to practise safer sex.

DESCRIPTION *Children aged 5–8 years.* Participants play a game and have a discussion. *Children aged 9–14 years.* Participants engage in discussion and pair work about condoms and the different ways they can respond to the fact that condoms are too big for them. *Caregivers.* Participants consider a scenario and discuss how best to support their children with regard to condoms.

Box 24.i Information for facilitators

Many people will not be comfortable with the idea of children using condoms. But the fact is that some children try to protect themselves by improvising a condom to meet their needs, for example, by tying clingfilm or plastic bags onto the penis, or putting rubber bands at the top of condoms to try and improve the fit. We need to respect children's efforts to have safer sex and discuss these ideas with them, so that they have the information they need to make good decisions. During the discussion we can also promote the benefits of delaying sex until their bodies and upper brains are fully developed.

Directions

Children aged 5–8 years

1. Ask the children to choose a game which involves movement, where each time someone is 'out'. Ask the children to close their eyes and pick out an item from a bag of adults' clothes. The clothes need to be far too big for the children. Have fun together seeing how the children look funny, and how the big clothes make it hard for them to play, for example when trying to run or catch a ball.

2. Ask why the clothes don't fit them. Ask whether they think that condoms would fit children of their age. Explain that condoms are designed to fit adults: they don't fit young children, and they don't fit many older children either.

3. Ask them to take off the big clothes, and to see if their own clothes fit better.

Ask: 'If companies make clothes for children, why don't they make condoms for children?'

Talk together about the issues you covered previously in Sessions 21 (Our sexual feelings and sexual safety) and 23 (Delaying, starting, and stopping having sex).

Children aged 9–14 years

1. Divide into males and females, or into older and younger children.

Ask the participants to pair up and to talk about a time when they tried on an adult's clothes, or tried to use something designed for use by an adult, such as a bike or a water pump.

2. Bring the pairs back into one group and ask a few people to share their funny stories.

Ask: 'Why do children like to try on grown-ups' things, or to use things designed for adults?'

Talk about how, as we grow and learn, we often mimic what adults do. It makes us feel grown up. If appropriate to the stories participants tell, ask questions to highlight the fact that the clothes didn't look good, or that it was difficult to use the items, because they were designed to fit adults, not children.

3. Ask: 'What about condoms? Do you think they fit boys and girls of your age? What have you heard?'

4. Ask: 'What do boys and girls do if condoms don't fit? What can happen?'

Invite participants, in pairs, to write or draw their answers on pieces of paper. Next, mix up the answers in a box or hat. Ask each person to take one idea from the hat, and read it out or show the picture.

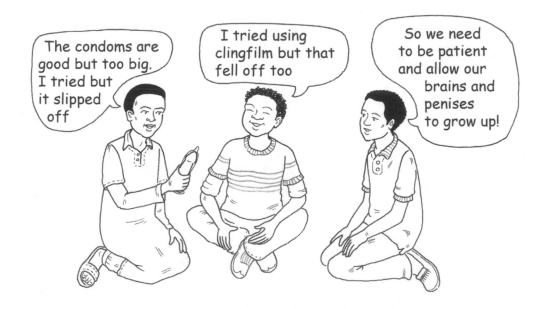

5. Discuss each idea one by one, as to whether it is safe and what challenges it involves.

6. Contribute to the discussion using ideas from Box 24.j, after allowing participants to give their ideas.

Box 24.j Information about condoms and children

Although outside condoms are available in different sizes, they are made to fit adults. The penis reaches its full length and girth by about age 16 years. For most younger boys, therefore, male condoms will be too big and may slip off the penis.

Inside condoms are made to fit adult women. They can be worn by girls, but may be too big and so feel uncomfortable to insert and wear.

Even if condoms do fit children's bodies, the act of intercourse does not fit with children's immature brains. Many young people, and especially women, regret their first sexual encounter, and this regret is greater the earlier in their life that encounter took place. It is safest to delay having sexual intercourse until both body and mind are mature.

Loving friends can enjoy being together without having sex, as we explored in Session 21 about sexual feelings and sexual safety.

Ideas for coping when condoms are too big

- Use an inside condom: practise getting used to inserting it until it is comfortable. Do not use it if it rubs or causes pain. Inside condoms are not affected by the size of the penis.
- Try to find smaller outside condoms, with a snug fit. Check that they grip the penis tightly and stay on before using with a partner.
- Try to find non-lubricated outside condoms. Don't put lubrication inside the condom; only use extra lubrication outside the condom if the vagina is dry and the friction is too great, or if having anal sex.
- Use a rubber band to help keep the outside condom on.
- Talk together about what's happening. For example, 'The condom is slipping off because my erection is coming and going!'
- Hold the rim of the outside condom to keep it on while having sex, and take it off as soon as the male ejaculates to avoid the semen escaping from the condom because the fit is not tight.

7. After the discussion, ask people to vote for the best option, including intercourse, outercourse, not having sex and masturbation; ask them to explain why the option they have chosen is best.

8. Summarize, and emphasize that delaying sex, especially intercourse, until we are physically and mentally mature is safer and more responsible, as we are then able to develop strong relationships and use condoms correctly.

Caregivers

1. Ask participants to form groups of four. Read out the following scenario:

'Imagine that you are looking for a pen among your 13-year-old son's/daughter's belongings. At the back of a box you find a packet of condoms with one missing. At that moment, you hear your child coming into the house.'

Ask participants, within their groups, to take turns to answer these questions:

- What do you feel?
- What do you think?
- What do you do?
- What do you think the outcome of your action will be?

2. Bring the groups together and invite them to share what they have learned from the exercise.

Ask: 'Do you feel that it is better to: i) teach children about condoms, but emphasize that they are intended for adults?; or ii) focus on the disadvantages of having sex when you are young, without suggesting how children could do it safely?'

3. Ask participants to discuss how we can:

- support our children as much as possible in delaying their sexual debut until they are able to fully consent to caring, wanted relationships; be in control of the situation; and be able to use condoms successfully.

- acknowledge that our children will have sexual relationships in the future, and often earlier than we did; and support them in keeping healthy and safe, including by using condoms.

 EXERCISE 24.6 WHAT ARE WE DOING NOW TO STAY SAFE?

AIM: To spot our abilities in staying safe around sex, and supporting others.

DESCRIPTION: Participants do ability-spotting and think about the future.

Directions

1. Say: 'Now that we have talked about the different ways that we can stay safe, let's tell each other about what we are already doing to keep ourselves healthy.'

2. With the relevant separate peer groups:

Children aged 9–14 years and caregivers. Ask participants to pair up and take it in turns to tell each other about a time when they felt good because they did something, or helped their friends to do something, that protected them and their friends from unwanted pregnancy, or from getting or passing on STIs (including HIV). For example, they might have said 'no' to a sexual relationship, or talked to a friend about safe ways of avoiding unwanted pregnancy.

Ask them to interview their partner in detail to spot the abilities that person showed, and to show appreciation of these and curiosity about the story.

Children aged 5–8 years. As for the older children, ask the children to pair up and tell each other a story about doing something that helped keep them or a friend safe, but in relation to general health and safety issues rather than sexual ones.

3. After 10 minutes, ask the pairs to switch roles.

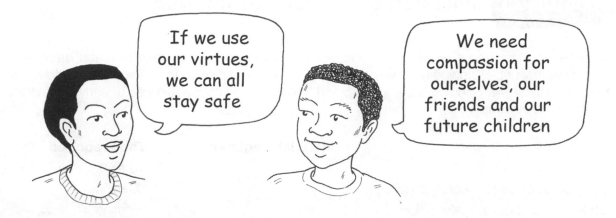

4. When both people have been interviewed, ask them to think together about what they imagine they might do in the future in this regard.

5. Bring the pairs back together into one large group. Ask participants to comment on anything that someone in their group is doing well to protect their health and that of others.

Closing circle

Ask people what they are happy to share with participants from other peer groups, and use their ideas about how to share it. For example, they may be willing to share their 'condoms are our friends' pictures or stories from Exercise 24.2.

Preparation for Session 25

Explain that in the next session 'Children by choice not chance', we have invited a visitor to tell us about having babies, and about having babies when we have HIV. Invite participants to write all their questions about babies and HIV and post them in the question box.

Sort out the questions into themes and share them with your visitor before running Session 25, so they can select the questions that they feel comfortable answering and prepare. Invite them to refer to HIV when answering the questions when that feels comfortable.

Purpose: To learn about fertility and conception; to think of steps to take to reach dreams of having healthy babies, including if we have HIV; to learn about how to take responsibility; to know safe and reliable ways to avoid pregnancy; and to explore the consequences of early pregnancy and how to cope with it.

Contents	Materials required	Time required
Opening circle (see p.13)		15 mins
25.1 Our dreams for healthy children		30 mins
25.2 How do people make babies?		45 mins
25.3 Meeting a woman with HIV and her baby	Flipchart of key themes, visitor and her baby	45 mins
25.4 Taking responsibility for our actions		45 mins
25.5 Managing our fertility	Contraceptives	60 mins
25.6 Consequences of early pregnancy		30 mins
25.7 Coping with an early pregnancy	Know abortion laws and availability of legal abortion	45 mins
Closing circle (see p.14)		15 mins

About 5.5 hrs

Preparation

Exercise 25.3. Invite a woman with HIV, who has had a positive experience of childbirth, and her baby to come to the group and talk about her experiences of having a baby and caring for it. You could invite the father of the baby to come too if the woman agrees. She (and the father of the baby) could be from among the participants. The woman will need to feel comfortable about being open about living with HIV, and the support she receives in keeping her baby well. At the end of Session 24 you asked participants to put any questions on this topic into the question box. So now, before this session, sort the questions into themes. Write out the themes and key questions on flipchart paper.

Exercise 25.5. Read Tables 25.1 and 25.2, so that you are well informed about what methods do and don't work to prevent pregnancy.

If caregivers request it, invite a family planning provider to visit at a convenient time to show them different contraceptives and explain how they work. If caregivers and providers agree, invite children aged 9–14 years to join the lesson if they are interested.

Exercise 25.6. Stick together four pieces of flipchart paper to make a big sheet for each of the male and female groups, marking each quarter as follows:

Advantages of having a baby when aged under 17 years	Disadvantages of having a baby when aged under 17 years
Disadvantages of waiting until older	Advantages of waiting until older

Exercise 25.7. Find out about the abortion laws in your country, and what services are legally available to community members.

EXERCISE 25.1 OUR DREAMS FOR HEALTHY CHILDREN

AIMS: *For children*. To dream about having children, and think about what we can do to have healthy children when the time is right for us.
For caregivers. To dream about what we wish for our children and grandchildren, and think of what steps to take to reach that dream.

DESCRIPTION: Participants dream about the future and then think about what steps they can take to reach that dream.

Directions

1. Direct the relevant peer groups as follows:

Children. Explain that we are going to dream about our future, and the place of having children in our future.

Caregivers. Explain that we are going to dream about our children's future, and how their having children fits into our future.

Invite participants to shut their eyes, relax, and take some deep breaths. If appropriate, remind them of Exercise 20.6, when they dreamed about a good long-term loving relationship (for themselves or for their children).

Ask them to focus on any dreams that they have had, or have now, about having children or grandchildren. Ask: 'Do your dreams involve having children, or your children having children?'

2. Now ask participants to imagine they are in the good future they have imagined for themselves, and that they have had a child or grandchild. Ask them to picture the situation as if they are really there, in their home with their baby or grandchild, and the people around them.

3. After five minutes, ask participants to open their eyes and interview each other in turn about their dream, as if they are still in the future.

For example, they might ask:
- What age and sex is the child? What does he or she look like?
- How are the child's health, growth, and wellbeing?
- How old are you and where are you living?
- Who are you living with?
- Who is the father/mother of the child?
- How does the family earn a living?
- Who looks after the child?

Ask each person to draw a picture, or make up a song, to remind them of how their future looks.

4. Ask them to think about, or add to their picture, what would need to happen in their life for them to reach their dream about having healthy children. For example, they might need to earn money, find a supportive partner, and use health services.

EXERCISE 25.2 HOW DO PEOPLE MAKE BABIES?

AIMS: To understand how people make babies and know the signs of pregnancy.

DESCRIPTION: Participants engage in question and answer sessions, are given explanations, and use role play to learn about pregnancy.

Directions

1. Explain that now we are going to talk about having babies. Ask: 'Who can tell us what we mean by pregnancy?'

If necessary, explain that pregnancy is the period between conception (when sperm from a man fertilizes a woman's egg) and the birth of the baby. Pregnancy usually lasts for about nine months.

2. Ask: 'How do women and men make babies?'

Remind participants about Exercise 19.2 in the session about growing up, when we learned about our sexual and reproductive organs. If necessary, explain how when a man ejaculates during intercourse with a woman, sperm in his semen swim into the uterus and fallopian tubes. If a sperm finds an egg that is ready, it will fertilize it and start to make a baby. This is called the foetus. The foetus will attach itself to the lining of the womb and then the woman will be pregnant.

Caregivers. Encourage caregivers to share and role play how they have talked, or might talk, to their children of various ages about how babies are made.

Children aged 9–14 years. Ask what explanation they would give if a younger child were to ask them: 'Where do babies come from? How do they get in their mummy's tummy?'

3. *All peer groups.* Ask: 'What are the *signs of pregnancy*?' As needed, add information from Box 25.a.

Box 25.a Signs of pregnancy

The first sign is that a woman or girl does not have a period for six weeks after she has had sexual intercourse.

Other signs can include any of the following:
- the need to urinate frequently;
- feeling more tired than usual;
- the desire to vomit, and actually being sick;
- feeling tenderness of the breasts;
- the belly and breasts getting bigger, with dark areas around the nipples, belly, and face;
- being choosy about food.

Explain that if a girl shows any of these signs and has had sexual intercourse, she should tell a trusted person, especially if she did not plan to have a baby. She can go to a health centre for a pregnancy test. It is best to know for sure whether she is pregnant as soon as possible, so that she can plan and make good decisions in her context. See Exercise 25.7.

---

4. Read the story of Sara and Vincent (see Box 25.b) to the group.

Box 25.b The story of Sara and Vincent[60]

Sara was a girl aged 11 years, and she had a friend called Vincent who was 12 years old. They liked each other very much, and their families knew that Sara and Vincent were good friends because they travelled to the same school together from the same neighbourhood.

One day, as Sara and Vincent were studying in Sara's bedroom, they felt attracted to each other and started kissing and touching each other. Eventually they had sexual intercourse because it came so naturally to them.

After a few weeks, Sara started feeling weak and wanted to vomit all the time. She told her mother, who suspected that she might have malaria and rushed her to the clinic. The doctors tested her and found that she was pregnant. This was shocking news to everyone, including Sara and Vincent. Sara didn't know about pregnancy and had not had her first period. Vincent had thought that he was too young to make Sara pregnant.

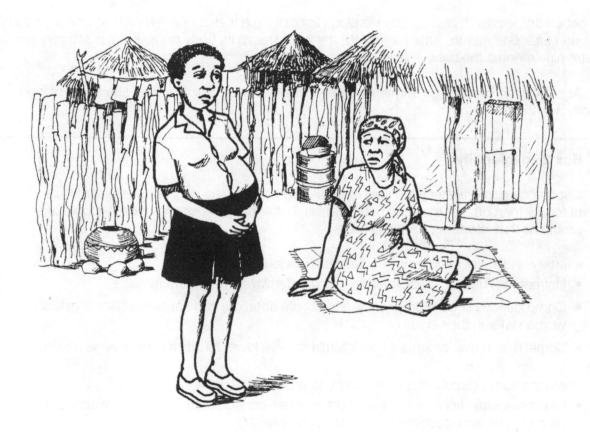

Ask: 'Can children make a baby before the girl starts her period?' Encourage participants to debate this, and ensure they have accurate information.

Ask: 'Can girls get pregnant the first time they have sexual intercourse?'

Box 25.c Can children make a baby before a girl's first period?

Girls can get pregnant before they experience any menstrual bleeding, because the first egg is released from an ovary two weeks *before* their first period. So in every girl's life, there are two weeks when she doesn't know that her body has matured enough to make a baby. There is no way of knowing when these two weeks are happening.

Boys usually start making sperm, which can create a pregnancy, around the age of 12–14 years, but it can happen earlier.

Pregnancy can happen the first time a boy and girl have sexual intercourse. It can also happen on the fourth time, or twenty third time, or any other time! Children who have sex and do not create a pregnancy may think they are 'safe' because they are too young. But at some point their bodies will mature, and pregnancy is then likely unless they use a condom correctly. However, it is better to wait until our minds and bodies are mature before having sex.

5. Ask: 'How does a baby develop in the uterus?'

If necessary, explain that the baby develops from being a foetus of a few cells to one the size of a bean after one month. After six months the baby has all its body parts, but it is still very small. After nine months the baby is ready to be born.

6. Ask: 'Why do people sometimes struggle to make a baby?' As needed, share information from Box 25.d.

Box 25.d Infertility

If someone is *infertile* they are unable to make a baby. Some people have lower levels of fertility than others; they can make babies, but it may take longer, because there are problems that interfere with the process.

Infertility and lower fertility may be caused in various ways:
- Untreated STIs can cause infertility or lower fertility in males and females.
- Complications in early pregnancy, and unsafe abortion, can cause infertility in girls and women later in their lives.
- Sometimes males or females are infertile or have lower fertility for no obvious reason.

There are some steps we can take to try to protect our fertility:
- We can abstain from sexual intercourse, or use condoms, to avoid STIs, which can damage the reproductive organs and cause infertility.
- If we have any signs of an STI, we should go at once to a clinic for treatment.
- We can abstain from sexual intercourse, or use condoms, to avoid early pregnancy and unsafe abortion. These can damage a girl's reproductive organs.

Signs of STIs

Signs of STIs include:

- pain on urination;
- unusual or smelly discharge from the genitals;
- any rash or spots on the genitals;
- pain in the lower belly.

However, some STIs have no physical signs, yet can cause infertility. This is why it is important for us all to try to protect ourselves from getting an STI as best we can.

 ## EXERCISE 25.3 MEETING A WOMAN WITH HIV AND HER BABY

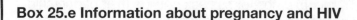

AIMS: The specific aims will depend on the questions asked by participants, but may be:

- to reassure participants that people with HIV can have healthy babies;
- to understand what having a baby, and meeting its needs, involves;
- to develop empathy with mothers and babies.

DESCRIPTION: Participants engage in a question and answer session with a woman living with HIV and her baby and partner if she agrees. If it is not possible to arrange a suitable visitor, the facilitator can run a question and answer session instead, using information from Box 25.e.

Box 25.e Information about pregnancy and HIV

People who have HIV can have healthy babies who do not have HIV. With the right support and medication, nearly all babies born to women with HIV can be free of HIV.

Babies who do have HIV can be given ARV treatment when they need it; with good care and correct medication they can grow up in good health and, when they are adults, have their own babies free of HIV.

Pregnancy, HIV, and rights
Pregnant girls and women are often tested for HIV, but not always in ways that respect their rights. A human rights approach to pregnancy and HIV testing includes:

- voluntary and confidential pre- and post-test counselling and testing;
- only testing with the woman or girl's informed consent (i.e. she understands enough about the test to make an informed choice whether to have it or not);
- not telling partners or others the test result without the woman or girl's express permission;
- if she has HIV, support in starting ARVs during her pregnancy (if not already on them) to protect herself and her baby;
- support in having normal vaginal delivery if viral load is undetectable and no other STIs are present;

- not pressuring the woman or girl to continue ARVs after delivery until she herself needs them (rather than for the sake of the child or her partner);
- not blaming the woman if her baby gets HIV.

Support to pregnant women

In addition to having their human rights respected, pregnant girls and women need support from those around them. Without support they may face rejection and violence if they have HIV, and be blamed if their baby gets HIV. This is bad for both the woman and her baby.

Planning for a healthy baby

Before conception. Ideally, both parents-to-be should have an HIV test. If one or both of them have HIV, they should use condoms to protect one another, except on days in the woman's menstrual cycle when they are most likely to make a baby. These days are about halfway between the start of one menstrual period and the start of the next period. There may be physical signs that the woman is fertile: vaginal discharge which is clear, stretchy and slippery; breast tenderness; bloating; mild tummy pain; and increased interest in sex.

If either partner has HIV, they may want to consider starting ARVs to minimize transmission risk and for the health of the woman.

Some women with HIV who haven't yet started treatment are advised to start treatment before conceiving in order to protect the baby during pregnancy, delivery, and breastfeeding. Yet they may also feel anxious about the effects of the treatment on the baby and on themselves. It is best for them to consult their doctor about this.

During pregnancy and delivery. The girl or woman attends the antenatal clinic as soon as she suspects pregnancy. She can bring her partner, or attend alone if she prefers. She tells the health provider if she knows that she, her partner, or both have HIV. If they have not had an HIV test, both partners are invited to have one. The woman may have another test later, as women can get HIV – for example, through unprotected sex – during pregnancy.

If either partner has HIV or another STI, injects drugs, or has sex outside their partnership, they should use condoms throughout pregnancy and breastfeeding, or decide not to have sexual intercourse.

The mother takes ARVs when her health provider advises her that her body needs them. She takes care to prevent illnesses, and has any illnesses treated quickly.

She delivers the baby at a health unit in a way that reduces the chance of HIV being shared with the baby. If she has an undetectable viral load and no other STIs, this can often be by normal vaginal delivery.

The baby is given ARVs during the pregnancy via the mother, during delivery, and while breastfeeding, to minimize its chances of getting HIV.

After delivery. The parents learn how to feed the baby in a way that reduces its chance of getting HIV from breast milk. (Explain how to do this based on local health ministry guidelines.)

Directions

1. Before the visitor(s) arrive(s), bring together all the participants, and ask them to rank the themes you have written down (see Preparation) so you can focus on the ones which are most important to them.

2. Welcome the visitors and their baby, and invite them to sit in the circle with the caregivers and children. Explain that if there are any questions they don't want to answer, they don't need to.

3. Invite participants to take it in turns to ask the visitors the questions under the theme(s) they ranked as most important.

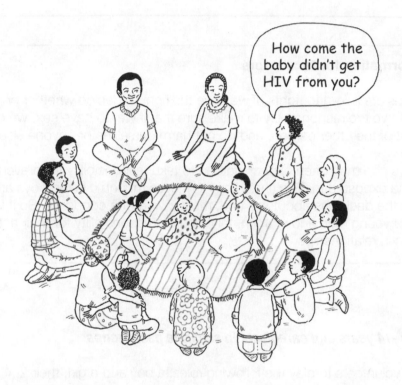

How come the baby didn't get HIV from you?

4. Invite participants to sing a song, and to play with the baby if the parents agree.

5. Continue working through the questions, theme by theme. Possible questions include:
- How was it having a baby when you have HIV? What did you and the health workers do to look after you and your baby?
- What is it like having a baby? What makes you feel happy? What is challenging?
- What is it like to be pregnant? What is delivery like?
- What did you need before the baby was born? What did you need after the baby was born? How did you get what you needed? How did others support you?
- What did the baby need before it was born? What did the baby need after it was born? How did/do you meet its needs?
- What did you have to think about and what preparations did you make for being a parent?
- How did your life change after having your baby?

6. Ask participants and the visitors to think to themselves: 'What do you think the baby is feeling – how do you know this?'

Invite a few participants to answer the questions, and then the parents. Are their answers the same or different? What might be the reasons for this?

EXERCISE 25.4 TAKING RESPONSIBILITY FOR OUR ACTIONS

AIMS: To understand the virtue of *responsibility*, and to use the Five Point Plan to support ourselves in taking responsibility for our actions.

DESCRIPTION: *Children aged 9–14 years and caregivers in separate peer groups.* Participants act out a story and analyse it to learn about shared responsibility. *All peer groups.* Participants learn about and practise using the Five Point Plan.

Box 25.f Information for facilitators

Responsibilities are linked to rights. If we have the right to decide whether or not to have sex, we also have the responsibility to make sure that if we do have sex, we do it with the full agreement of the other person, and do not harm ourselves or anyone else.

However, boys and men often expect women to take responsibility for preventing pregnancy and exposure to STIs (including HIV), even though it is the boys and men who tend to make the decisions about sex and, mostly, wear the condoms. So it is best if girls and boys, and young men and women, take shared responsibility for their actions and what happens in relationships.

Directions

Children aged 9–14 years and caregivers in separate peer groups

1. Ask for 8–10 volunteers to play the following roles: a boy and a girl, their 2–4 caregivers, 2 nurses, and 2–4 friends of the young people. Ask one of the volunteers to read out the story in Box 25.g.

Box 25.g The story of Kalimi and Kaguti

My name is Kalimi. I am a 14-year-old girl. I fell in love with Kaguti, a boy in the class above mine. We kissed and cuddled, but I refused to have sex with him because I was afraid of getting pregnant.

My caregiver saw me with him one day and told me that it was time that I got a friend who would pay for my needs, because she couldn't afford to anymore.

Our sexual feelings for each other were getting very strong, and Kaguti promised that he would not get me pregnant. He tried to get condoms, but the nurse said that he was too young. But he said that if we had sex a week after my period, and he pulled out, then I couldn't get pregnant. I didn't know anything about sex – no one had talked to me about it – but Kaguti seemed to know what he was doing. He said he would bring me a present too, so I knew that he loved me, and I knew my caregiver would be pleased. We had a nice time.

Next month I did not get my period and I felt like vomiting all the time. I was pregnant.

Kaguti said that it could not be his baby because he pulled out in time and I was in the 'safe' period. His friend said that he had seen me with another boy, so it must have been that boy who made me pregnant. My caregiver was very angry and slapped me. What am I going to do?

2. Ask the volunteers to take 10 minutes to create a short drama of Kalimi's story.

While they are preparing their role play, ask the rest of the group to divide into pairs and to discuss whether this type of situation happens in their community. If so, what are the positive things about it? What are the challenges?

3. Ask the actors to perform the drama to the rest of the group.

4. At the end of the play, ask the actors to stay where they are and remain in character. For each character in turn, ask the audience: 'What responsibility did this person have for the pregnancy?'

5. Explain the Five Point Plan for taking responsibility:
    1. *Acknowledge* what we have done.
    2. *Accept* our part of the responsibility for it.
    3. *Apologize* for this.
    4. *Act* to make things turn out as well as possible for everyone.
    5. *Think* about how we can avoid doing it again.

Write the five steps of *acknowledge*, *accept*, *apologize*, *act*, and *think* on a flipchart.

6. Ask each of the characters in the play to stand up and use the Five Point Plan. What does their character need to acknowledge and accept, what should they apologize for, what action will they take now, and what do they think they can do to avoid doing it again?

7. Ask for comments from the audience.

8. Ask people what they have learned from the activity. Summarize.

Children aged 5–8 years

1. Ask children to share things that have happened recently in their lives where everything went right. For example: 'I helped cooked a meal; it was delicious and everybody liked the food.'

2. Now ask them to share things when something went a little bit wrong. For example: 'I helped cook a meal and I burned my finger. I cried because it really hurt. My sister laughed at me and I punched her.'

3. Explain that whether things go right or wrong, there are usually several people who share some responsibility for what has happened. Talk about one of the children's examples and ask: 'Who had some responsibility?' For example:
- The person supervising the child's cooking didn't protect them from getting burned.
- The sister who laughed did not show compassion and provoked the child's anger.

- The child who punched did not manage to stay on their hub and cope with their feelings of upset and anger.

4. Explain the Five Point Plan for taking responsibility:
    1. *Acknowledge* what we have done.
    2. *Accept* our part of the responsibility for it.
    3. *Apologize* for this.
    4. *Act* to make things turn out as well as possible for everyone.
    5. *Think* about how we can avoid doing it again.

Using the example you just discussed, ask for volunteers to act out the situation. Then ask each character to use the Five Point Plan. For example, the sister might say:

'I *acknowledge* that it was mean of me to laugh.

I *accept* that he hit me because I provoked him.

I *apologize* for provoking him.

I can *act* by helping him next time.

I *think* I will show more empathy when my brother cries in the future.'

5. Practise using the Five Point Plan by repeating step 4 for another situation.

6. Ask: 'Are there times when it is good to share responsibility with others?' Possible examples are making shared decisions in a friendship, or (when we are older) in a relationship.

7. Emphasize that sometimes things happen that are not our responsibility at all. When children are sexually abused they often blame themselves, but this is *not their responsibility*. It is the responsibility of the abuser, and of the adults who are supposed to protect the child.

 ## EXERCISE 25.5 MANAGING OUR FERTILITY

AIMS: To gain accurate knowledge about different ways of preventing pregnancy. To feel positive about using a safe way of preventing pregnancy. To know how to give, and ask for, help in avoiding pregnancy.

DESCRIPTION: Participants list all the ways they know of avoiding pregnancy, and discuss them to learn which are safe and which are not. The facilitator shows different contraceptives and explains how they work.

Directions

1. Explain that we are going to talk about how people who have decided to have sex can avoid pregnancy.

2. Say: 'The safest way to avoid pregnancy is not to have sex. But if people are going to have sex, how can they try to avoid pregnancy?'

Ask participants to call out all the ways that people use to try to avoid pregnancy, and note them down. If necessary, remind them that our focus now is on ways of preventing pregnancy if people are having sex; we talked about delaying starting, or stopping, having sex in Session 23.

3. Ask participants to shut their eyes. Read out one of the ways they identified. Ask them to raise their hands if they think that it is true, drop their hands if they think it is false, and cross their hands over their chest if they don't know. Count the vote, and ask them to open their eyes. Tell them the vote, and discuss:

- Why is it true or not true?
- Is it a good method for avoiding pregnancy for young people?

Help people share ideas, and give them correct information from Tables 25.1 and 25.2 if needed.

Table 25.1 Methods used to prevent pregnancy: true

You can prevent pregnancy if:	Reasons
You engage in mutual masturbation or outercourse (*reliability depends on what this involves*)	If a male and female touch each other without allowing the penis to touch the clitoris or vulva, and do not transfer any body fluids from the male to female genitals (for example, on their hands), then pregnancy will not happen.
You have oral intercourse (*100% reliable*)	Even if semen goes into the mouth, there is no way that sperm can get into the fallopian tubes and fertilize an egg.
You use the fertility cycle to calculate when the woman is most likely to be fertile, and have sex when she is less likely to get pregnant. (*50% reliable*)	This can work if periods are *very regular*, with the same number of days each month, and if the woman is very aware of her cycle. It also needs cooperation between partners, and discipline. Counselling by an experienced person is best. It is *not* safe for young people, since periods may not be regular.
The female takes emergency contraception within 72 hours of having sex without using a contraceptive (*55–95% reliable*)	If a female doesn't want to get pregnant, but has had intercourse (by choice or by force) without using a contraceptive, or has used a condom and it has burst, she should seek help from a health centre within 72 hours (ideally within 24 hours) to get emergency contraception. She takes a pill which prevents or delays the release of an egg. The earlier the pill is taken, the more effective it is in preventing pregnancy. She can also take a short course of ARVs to reduce the chance of her getting HIV, and get tests to see if she has got any other STIs. If she has had forced sex, other support should also be available, such as a full medical exam and counselling.
You use male and/or female condoms (*80–90% reliable*)	Condoms protect against pregnancy and sharing HIV, or more HIV, and other STIs. They are the best method for young people. They need to fit and be used correctly every time.
The female uses the cap (diaphragm) (*80% reliable*)	The cap is a latex barrier, which the female inserts in her vagina before having sex. It covers the cervix and stops sperm swimming into the uterus. Women need to get a cap that fits correctly from a health centre, and use it every time they have sex.

You can prevent pregnancy if:	Reasons
The female takes a contraceptive pill every day (*99% reliable*)	These methods use hormones to stop eggs from being released. They are best used when a girl has had periods for some time and they have become regular. However, contraceptive *injections* may increase the risk for females of getting HIV through sex, and contraceptive *implants* may be less effective if used at the same time as certain ARVs, so we are advised to use alternative methods to these two if possible.
The female gets a contraceptive injection every 2 months (*99% reliable*)	
The female gets a contraceptive implant every 3–5 years (*99% reliable*)	
The female has an intra-uterine device (IUD) fitted (*99% reliable*)	IUDs are small devices that are fitted by a health worker into the womb, and which stay there for five or more years. They prevent pregnancy by disturbing the process of fertilization and growth.
You get sterilized (*100% reliable*)	For males, sterilization is a simple operation to cut tubes and prevent sperm going into semen; for females, it is an operation to prevent eggs travelling to the womb. This permanent method is only used when a man or woman clearly decides, with no force, that he or she no longer wants to be able to have children. It cannot be reversed.

Table 25.2 Methods used to prevent pregnancy: false

You can get pregnant if:	Reasons
The female is having sex for the first time	If the girl has ovulated, she can get pregnant the first time she has sex.
You have sex before the female starts her periods	Girls ovulate before starting their periods (see Box 25.c).
You have sex during your period (when bleeding)	It is possible to be fertile when bleeding, if the female's menstrual cycle is a short one of 21 days. Blood, including menstrual blood, is also one of the body fluids that can contain enough HIV to pass HIV on.
You have sex before the age of 15	On average, boys start making sperm between the ages of 12 and 14 years; girls may start their periods from nine years onwards.
You have sex standing up You wash after sex You urinate after sex You jump up and down after sex You have sex in water	Millions of sperm are produced and quickly swim into the womb; none of these actions stop them.
You drink water after sex	This has no effect on sperm or egg.
|One or other partner, or both, has been circumcised (males) or had genital cutting (females)	This has no effect on sperm or egg.
the male takes out his penis before ejaculating	Sperm can leak out of the penis before the male ejaculates, and he may not pull out in time. Boys may have less control than men over when they ejaculate.
You have anal intercourse	If semen comes out of the anus after ejaculation, the sperm can swim into the vagina and uterus and fertilize an egg.

You can get pregnant if:	Reasons
You engage in mutual masturbation or outercourse (*reliability depends on what this involves*)	If outercourse involves playing with the penis around the vulva or clitoris, it can result in pregnancy because fluid from the penis may get onto the vulva, and sperm may swim into the vagina even if the male does not ejaculate. This is because the fluid that comes from the penis before ejaculation can contain sperm, and they are good swimmers.

4. Repeat Step 3 for each of the ways that participants have identified. Add any key ways from Table 25.1 which have not been mentioned.

Children aged 5–8 years. The younger children do not need much detail. Select methods to discuss according to what they say helps people to avoid pregnancy, and which methods are most common among young people.

5. Summarize by saying that condoms are the best device for young people, because they protect against pregnancy and prevent sharing and getting (more) STIs, including HIV. However, for many people condoms are 80–90% effective, because they make mistakes when using them. Young women can best be supported by using condoms as well as another more reliable contraceptive, such as the pill.

6. Explain that older teenagers who have decided to have a sexual relationship may be able to get counselling on their lives and safe methods of contraception from family planning/ contraceptive service providers. Ask: 'Where can young people and adults get such supportive services locally?'

7. Remind participants that not starting sex, or stopping having sex, are the safest ways for children to avoid pregnancy and STIs, including HIV.

 ## EXERCISE 25.6 CONSEQUENCES OF EARLY PREGNANCY

AIMS: To understand the advantages and disadvantages of early pregnancy.

DESCRIPTION: Peer groups divide into males and females, brainstorm the advantages and disadvantages of early and later pregnancy, and come together to share similarities and differences between advantages and disadvantages for males and females.

Directions

1. Divide your peer group into males and females.

2. Explain and give out the prepared flipcharts to the groups (see Preparation). Invite them to brainstorm all their ideas, without discussion, and fill in the four pieces of flipchart paper. Use different colours to highlight any advantages and disadvantages that only apply to either boys or girls.

3. Bring the peer groups together and invite them to share their flipcharts. Add information as needed from Box 25.i.

Box 25.i Information about early pregnancy

Early pregnancy is dangerous for girls

The girl's body is not developed enough, and she may have problems delivering the baby because her hips are too narrow. The baby may get stuck and may tear the vagina when it comes out. This can leave a hole between the vagina and bladder or rectum, which causes urine and faeces to leak out.

- Girls are more likely to die in childbirth than grown women.
- Babies born to girls are more likely to die in the uterus or within a month of birth, or to be very small.

Pregnancy is safer if girls and women:

- wait until they are at least 18 years old before becoming pregnant;
- have a gap of at least three years between having children;
- have no more than four children;
- have their babies before they are 35 years old.

Early pregnancy can:

- spoil boys' and girls' chances of getting a good education;
- lead to gender-based violence against girls;
- negatively affect the future of the child.

Taking responsibility

Avoiding pregnancy is the responsibility of both partners; it is not the responsibility of the female alone. Equally, when a pregnancy occurs, it is the responsibility of both partners.

4. Invite them to comment on any differences in advantages and disadvantages between males and females.

5. Ask: 'What have we learned from this activity?'

 EXERCISE 25.7 COPING WITH AN EARLY PREGNANCY

AIMS: To think about who has responsibility for deciding how to cope with early pregnancy, and consider different options for coping.

DESCRIPTION: Participants use the story of Kalimi and Kaguti to consider the options available to them. *Children* discuss who Kalimi can turn to for help; *caregivers* discuss how they can help a child such as Kalimi.

Directions

1. Divide participants into groups of five. In these groups, read out Kalimi and Kaguti's story (see Box 25.g) again. Remind each other which people in the story have some responsibility for Kalimi being pregnant, and why.

2. Say: 'Kalimi asks "What am I going to do?" Who do you think has responsibility for supporting Kalimi in her decision? Why them?'

3. Ask the groups to create role plays showing Kalimi talking about the pregnancy with Kaguti, her caregiver, and the nurse.

4. Ask: 'What options does Kalimi have concerning this pregnancy?' If necessary, probe for key options that the participants do not mention. For example, they may not like to mention abortion.

5. Divide into the same number of pairs or groups as there are options. For example:
- Kalimi and Kaguti take responsibility together for caring for the baby with support from friends and family;
- Kalimi raises the baby with help from her caregiver;
- Kalimi raises the baby by herself;
- Kalimi and her family ask another person to bring up her baby;
- Kalimi has a legal abortion;
- Kalimi has an illegal abortion;
- Kaguti's caregiver looks after the baby with support from Kaguti.

Give each group one option and ask: 'What are the good and less good points of this choice for everyone concerned?'

6. Ask each group to report back briefly. As needed, add information from Box 25.j.

Box 25.j Information about abortion

Abortion is the ending of a pregnancy before the baby has grown enough to live outside the uterus. There are two types of abortion:
- *Natural abortion*. The pregnancy stops on its own before the baby can survive outside. This is also called miscarriage. We cannot make a natural abortion happen, it just happens.
- *Medical abortion*. People do something to end the pregnancy.

Countries have different laws about medical abortion. In most countries in Africa, it is allowed to save a woman or girl's life. In many, it is also permitted to preserve her physical or mental health. In some, it is allowed if the pregnancy is due to rape or incest, and if the foetus is severely damaged.

Medical abortion is *safe* for girls and women if:
- they tell a trusted person, who helps them have a safe abortion as soon as possible after missing a period, and not more than three months after;
- the abortion is carried out by a qualified medical practitioner in a very clean place;
- they go to a health worker at once if they develop complications after the abortion, such as continuous bleeding, smelly fluid coming from the vagina, pain in the lower belly, or fever and chills.

Abortion is *unsafe* when it is carried out in a dirty environment by an unqualified person, who uses methods such as an overdose of drugs, or using a sharp object, to get the foetus out. These methods are very dangerous for girls and women and can cause infertility or death.

Things to remember

It is always better to avoid unwanted pregnancy than have an abortion.
- It is best to delay sexual intercourse until we are mature enough to avoid unwanted pregnancy and the dangers of unsafe abortion.
- People who are having sexual intercourse can avoid pregnancy by using a condom and other 'true' methods listed in Table 25.1.
- Emergency contraception can prevent a pregnancy if taken within 72 hours of having unprotected sex.

7. Direct the relevant peer groups as follows:

Children. Discuss who Kalimi can go to for help, thinking about who you would go to in this situation.

Caregivers. Identify ways in which you could support a child in Kalimi's situation.

Closing circle

Ask participants to bring their ability necklaces to the next meeting, Session 26, which is about protecting each other from sexual abuse.

Purpose: To support caregivers and children in: understanding the difference between caring touches and abusive sexual touches; talking more openly about sexual abuse and recognizing its consequences; identifying and describing characteristics of unsafe situations; and practising ways that caregivers, children, families, and communities can protect children from sexual abuse.

Contents	Materials required	Time required
Opening circle (see p.13)		15 mins
26.1 Unsafe situations		30 mins
26.2 Points of contact		20 mins
26.3 Caring, sexual, and confusing touches	Prepared slips of paper	40 mins
26.4 Protecting ourselves and our children		60 mins
26.5 Practising responses to sexual approaches		45 mins
26.6 *Homework*: Awareness of ourselves in our environment		10 mins
Closing circle (see p.14)		15 mins

About 4 hrs

Preparation

Exercise 26.1. For this you may want to make up locally relevant stories about children being in unsafe situations.

Exercise 26.3. For this you need to prepare slips of paper, half of which describe situations in which touches are caring, and half of which describe touches which are sexual and harmful. Use examples from Table 26.1, or make up situations appropriate to the age of the participants. Each group of three in your peer group will need one slip describing a caring touch, and one slip describing a sexual or confusing touch.

Box 26.a Information for facilitators

Child sexual abuse happens in all countries and communities and involves people from all backgrounds. The person abusing the child may be male or female; they may abuse a child of the same or different sex as themselves; and they may be a peer of the child, an older child, or an adult.

Most sexual abuse of children aged between five and eight years is carried out by people they know and trust, such as a family member or older friends. Sexual abuse of children aged from nine to 14 years is also carried out by 'boyfriends' or 'girlfriends' who force them to engage in sexual activity.

Remember, some caregivers may have been sexually abused when they were children, or may be being abused now. Equally, some children may have been abused or continue to be abused now. Before you start the workshop, ensure that your organization has a Child Protection Policy, and that you are familiar with your role and the official procedures for handling suspected or reported child sexual abuse. (See Introduction, p.10) Be ready to follow up with

---

caregivers or children if you suspect or know that a child is being abused. *Before you start the session, make sure that support is available during the meeting and afterwards from someone whom participants trust.*

Never pressurize a child to talk about abuse unless they are ready. If a child wants to tell someone about abuse, wait until after the session and introduce them and their caregiver, if appropriate, to the counsellor or support person.

Take care not to create unnecessary anxiety in children. Remind them that the majority of people they meet are kind and responsible towards children. Finish Sessions 26 and 27 on a positive note, focussing on using our virtues and abilities to protect each other.

Watch out for participants trying to put some responsibility for sexual abuse onto the child who has been abused, for example, for being out alone in the dark, or for wearing certain clothes: explain that it is never their fault. Although there are things that children can do to try to protect themselves, they may not always succeed. It is always the responsibility of adults, of whatever age, to behave in a moral way and protect children from abuse. Older children and peers also have a responsibility to use their virtues and not persuade or force children to engage in any sexual activity.

Note: In this and the next session we are focussing on harmful *sexual* touching, rather than the violent punishments that we talked about in Session 9.

Introduction

1. Explain that in this session we are going to talk about *sexual abuse*: what it is, how it can affect children, and how we can work together to protect our children and each other. In our next session (Session 27) we will talk about what we can do if a child is being, or has been, sexually abused.

2. Explain that, as this is a sensitive topic, we need to be extra careful to treat each other with respect and kindness during these two sessions.

3. Reassure children, by reminding them that most people we meet are kind and responsible. Also, there is a lot that we can do to keep ourselves and each other safe.

4. Say that it is best to talk about suspected or known instances of sexual abuse privately, after the meeting, rather than in the group. It is safer to talk about such things with a counsellor or trusted adult quietly first, and to think carefully about whom else to tell. This helps protect children from further harm. Remind participants that they can talk privately to the trusted person during the session or afterwards.

EXERCISE 26.1 UNSAFE SITUATIONS

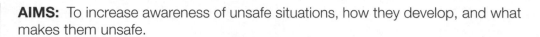

AIMS: To increase awareness of unsafe situations, how they develop, and what makes them unsafe.

DESCRIPTION: Participants listen to a story, answer questions, and consider what tends to make situations unsafe with regard to sexual abuse.

 Be very aware of the body language and behaviour of participants; someone might have been abused in one of the situations described. Make sure that your supportive adult is around in case anyone becomes upset or withdrawn.

Directions

1. If you wish, split the group into males and females.

2. Explain that we are going to start by reading a story of a situation where sexual approaches and abuse happened. We will then discuss some questions about the story. In the rest of the session we will use what we learn from this exercise to look at how we can protect ourselves, our children, and our friends and families, from sexual abuse.

3. Read out the story of Layla or the story of Kali (see Box 26.b), or make up your own story to suit your context and peer group, such as a story about a boy being sexually abused. Ask the questions following the story, and discuss them.

Box 26.b Stories about sexual abuse

Option 1: The story of Layla
Layla was nine years old. She was walking along the road on her way to school, feeling sad and tired. A youngish man came and walked with her. She was a bit worried, but he said in a very kind way, 'You are looking sad and tired, let me get you a Coke and you can tell me what is wrong.' He said his name was Anza and he was a lay preacher. She then recognized him as the uncle of a girl at school. Her auntie had told her not to talk to strangers, but as she knew who he was, she thought this would be OK.

As she drank her Coke, she told him that she was an orphan and lived in a faraway village with her auntie. She missed her mum, and her big sister had gone to the city. She was struggling to go to school. Her auntie could not afford to give her a uniform that fitted, or buy her books. Anza gently put his arm round her and said: 'I can see you are a brave and clever girl and want to do well in school. I would like to help you.' He had a motorbike and drove her to school. After school he was waiting for her, and drove her back to her village. He stopped outside the village. Layla wanted him to meet her auntie but he said, 'It's best if we keep our meeting a secret, because your auntie might not understand that we are friends.'

Layla continued to meet Anza, and he was very kind. He gave her nice cuddles and helped by giving her soap, pomade, a new school dress, and her books and pens for school. She

---

felt much better, and her schoolmates were friendlier to her. She enjoyed her cuddles with Anza, but he was touching her in new ways that made her feel uncomfortable. He said: 'I love you, and we should show our love for each other completely.' She didn't really know what he meant, but he had helped her so much that she wanted to please him. She felt that she could not say 'no' when he took her into his room.

Questions:
- What happened in the story?
- Do things like this happen to children like us (ours) in our community?
- What did Layla like about Anza and her meetings with him?
- What did she not like about her meetings with Anza?
- How did Anza touch her? Were the touches caring or sexual?
- Who had the power in this relationship?
- Why did Anza ask Layla to keep their meetings secret?
- What were the things in the situation that put Layla at risk of sexual abuse?
- What could Layla have done differently?
- What could Layla's relatives and friends have done differently?
- What could Anza's relatives and friends have done differently?

Option 2: The story of Kali
Sarah and Kali were eight years old and travelled to school together on the bus. It was often very crowded. One day a man told Kali to sit on his lap, so that more people could enter the bus. As the journey continued, the man started to rub his body against her and she could feel his hard penis against her private parts. He put his jacket over her lap and touched her private parts. Kali did not know what to do; she felt embarrassed and ashamed, and afraid that if she said anything people would not believe her and that the man would be angry.

Questions:
- What happened in the story?
- Do things like this happen to children like us (ours) in our community?
- How did the man touch Kali? Were the touches caring or sexual? What were the things that put Kali at risk of sexual abuse in this situation?
- Did she know the person who abused her?
- Who had the power in this relationship?
- What could Kali have done differently?
- What could the other passengers on the bus have done differently?

4. After the discussion, ask: 'In general, what things tend to make situations unsafe with regard to sexual abuse?' As needed, add points from Box 26.c to help participants understand the characteristics of unsafe situations.

Box 26.c Characteristics of unsafe situations

The situations in which children are abused vary, but they share common characteristics:

- Any situation where the abuse can happen *unseen by others*. This mainly involves the abuser being alone with the child, for example: in a room with the door closed, in a home when everyone else is out, or in the bush. If other people are around, then the abuse needs to be done in a way that is not visible to them.

- Any situation where children are alone with someone who has some kind of *power over them* increases risk. The person might be: older or bigger; trusted to protect the child; have influence over their future; give money or gifts; be loved and trusted by the child; be able to help others whom the child cares about; have total control over the child's survival. Power over the child links to getting the *child's silence*: abusers do not want the child to tell anyone about the abuse. The child may keep quiet willingly (a special secret), or out of obedience or fear.

- Any situation where the abuse is known about by one or more other people but they *will not intervene* to prevent it, for example: where the abuser has power over the other people too; where the other people do not believe the child; and where the other people find it easier to take no action.

- *Vulnerable children*, such as orphans, children with disabilities, homeless children, and very poor children, are more vulnerable to sexual abuse. They may: not have a person who cares for them deeply and protects them; have low self-esteem; lack safe shelter; or be desperate for love, kindness, attention, promises of support, and resources to meet their basic needs.

 EXERCISE 26.2 POINTS OF CONTACT

 AIM: To encourage teamwork, laughter, trust, and shared problem-solving.

DESCRIPTION: Option 1: A fun game that involves participants working together in different-sized groups. Option 2: A game encouraging participants to be aware of how they feel when different parts of their body are touched, and to build confidence in refusing uncomfortable contact.

GROUPS: Caregivers and children could play this game together or in their peer groups. They may want to divide into males and females for option 1, and they should be divided for option 2.

Directions

Option 1

1. Explain to participants that there are seven points of the body that can make contact with the floor in this game: two hands, two feet, two elbows, and one forehead.

2. Call out a number between one and seven, and ask each participant to touch the floor with that number of points of the body. Do this again.

3. Now ask people to play the game together in pairs. Instruct them: 'You cannot call out a number higher than 14 (two people each using all seven contact points), but you can call out lower numbers.'

4. Ask participants to play again in groups of three, then of four. Have fun calling numbers lower than the size of the group: for example, a group of four people can go as low as two points of contact if two people carry the other two, hold hands to balance each other, and stand on one leg each!

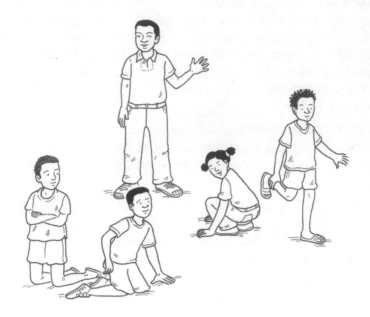

Option 2

1. Ask everyone to skip or run around. Tell them that when you call out a body part, they have to touch that part of their body with that part of another person's body. Ask them to say 'no' firmly if they don't feel comfortable doing so. Start with easier parts such as hands, elbows, and knees, then mix in more intimate parts such as noses, bottoms, lips, or stomachs.

2. Invite participants to tell everyone, if they would like, how they felt and what they learned from this activity.

 EXERCISE 26.3 CARING, SEXUAL, AND CONFUSING TOUCHES

AIMS: To recognize the difference between caring touches, sexual touches, and confusing touches, between children and older people. To know that sexual touching between adults and children can cause serious emotional and physical harm to children, and is against children's rights and the law.

DESCRIPTION: Participants engage in a question and answer session, practise telling the difference between caring touching and sexual touching, and discuss the influence of different touches on children's development and wellbeing.

Box 26.d Information for facilitators

Caring touches. These are essential for bonding between children and adults and each other. They support a child's emotional and social development. Caring touches promote the development of compassion to the self and others, security and confidence, and the ability to form close and lasting relationships with others.

Sexual touching. This is a special type of touch which ideally gives pleasure, soothes and comforts, and can lead to intercourse and conception. If it happens with mutual consent between mature people who care for each other, sexual touch increases wellbeing, and strengthens bonding and lasting relationships between sexual partners.

Child sexual abuse. This is when an adult touches a child in a sexual, harmful, and unwanted way, or has sex or sexual activities with them. It includes: exposing the genitals to a child or looking at a child's genitals; touching a child's genitals; making a child touch the adult's genitals or someone else's genitals; fondling the breasts and sexual kissing; having oral, vaginal, or anal sex with a child; showing sexual magazines, pictures, or audio tracks or films, or telling sexy stories or jokes to a child.

Any type of sexual touching between an adult and a child is wrong. This is true even if the person says 'I love you' or the child loves them too, or they give the child presents. Sexual abuse is never the fault of the child, even if a part of them enjoys the attention and touching from a loved person. It is always the older person's responsibility to behave in a moral way.

Note: Sexual abuse also happens to adults, and includes rape and any kind of sexual activity without consent. All sexual activity with children before the age of consent is considered abuse. This applies even if the abuser is also a child of similar age. This can result in situations where both children wish to engage in sexual activity but the older child, and often the boy, is treated as a criminal. This is likely to be very damaging to both children who would be better served by counselling and education.

Table 26.1 summarizes the differences between caring and sexual touches between adults and children. Use this information in the discussions as appropriate.

Table 26.1 Differences between caring and sexual touches

Questions	Caring touch	Sexual touch
'How might the child feel about the touching?'	The child might feel happy and supported, as if something is being given or shared with them.	The child may feel uncomfortable, ashamed, dirty, guilty, angry, or scared; as if someone is taking something away from them. If the abuser is acting in a loving and kind way, the child might enjoy the touching.
'How might the adult feel about the child?'	The adult might feel compassionate, caring, loving, wanting to give and receive love and comfort; they might wish to help, or get the child's attention.	The adult may not be concerned about the effect of their action on the child. They may not believe it is harmful. They may think it is a normal part of childhood. They may believe that the child wants to have sex.
'Does what the adult says match what they do?'	The words match the touches. The words are caring and match the reasons for the touch.	Words may not match acts. The adult may say they love the child, but take no notice when the child says 'no', or shows distress. The adult is concerned with getting pleasure for themselves.
'Which part of the child's body do adults touch and/or ask children to touch?'	This is usually any part except sexual parts.	This is mainly sexual organs: penis, vagina, vulva, breasts, buttocks, mouth.
'In what ways might the adult touch the child?'	They may touch gently, without force, on non-sexual parts. Touches include hugging, holding hands, stroking the hair or face, and non-sexual kissing.	They may use force or they may be gentle. The touches are sexual and arouse the abuser. They include sexual kissing, stroking sexual organs, sucking or licking sexual organs, and anal or vaginal intercourse.
'What might be the reasons that the adult touches the child and/ or asks the child to touch them?'	Reasons might be: • to show love and care for the child; • to support the child; • to keep the child healthy; • to get the child's attention; • for health reasons, if touching the penis or vulva, e.g. dressing circumcision wound, washing a sick child, changing a nappy.	Reasons might be: • to get sexual pleasure; • they are sexually attracted to children; • to have sex without paying for it or having any arguments; • they believe that men/women cannot control their sexual urges and have a right to use children (and women) to satisfy them; • to groom the child so they can provide sex to friends or for money; • to frighten the child so they are obedient; • to exert power over the child.
'Does the adult tell the child to keep the touch secret or threaten them in some way?'	No: the touch is caring so there is nothing to hide.	Yes: the adult does not want others to know about their sexually or physically abusive touching.

Directions

1. Divide the peer groups into males and females. Explain that we are now going to talk more about different kinds of touching and how they make us feel. It is very important that we learn to recognize the difference between caring touches, which are motivated by care and make us feel good, and sexual touches, which make us feel uncomfortable. When we are children, we may not know whether what is happening to us is acceptable or unacceptable.

2. Invite participants to mention the touches we talked about in the stories of Layla or Kali, or their own story, in Exercise 26.1.

3. Say: 'First we will talk about *caring touching*.'

Remind participants about Session 8 'The power of love', when we talked about how we can show love to our children, caregivers, friends, or family.

Ask: 'Who can remember some of the physical ways that we show love to our family and friends?' Invite participants to think of and show as many physical ways of showing caring love as they can.

Ask: 'How does caring touching feel? Most people find that kind and caring touching feels like something is being given or shared with you.'

Ask: 'Which parts of our bodies are involved in caring touches?' You can explain that caring touches do not usually involve our sexual organs, except sometimes when an adult is caring for a child, for example, washing a baby.

Ask: 'What are the reasons that the person is touching you, or asking you to touch them?' If necessary, explain that caring touches are usually done to help us, to show non-sexual love (or professional care), or to get pleasure and comfort from being close to a loved person.

Explain: 'Some adults use caring touches at first to encourage a child to love and trust them, and then start to use sexual touches that lead to sexual activity.'

4. Say: 'Now let's talk about *sexual touching*.'

Remind participants about Session 21, when we talked about our sexual feelings and sexual safety, and safe and unsafe ways in which adults show sexual love to each other.

Explain: 'When mature people who care about each other agree to touch each other in a sexual way, it gives them pleasure and comfort, strengthens their relationship, and can lead to pregnancy. This type of sexual touching increases physical and emotional wellbeing. Masturbation – privately touching our own genitals – can also give pleasure and help us manage our sexual feelings safely.

'But some sexual touching is *not* good. One type of harmful sexual touching is when older people touch children's sexual organs, or ask a child to touch theirs or do other sexual activities with them to satisfy their own sexual feelings. Then the adult is not managing their sexual feelings safely, and is not thinking about the effect of their actions on the child. This type of sexual touching is sexual abuse. It usually makes children feel uncomfortable or scared, as if someone is taking something away from them and they are doing something wrong. This can be when someone touches their buttocks, breasts, or private parts, or holds them too tightly against their will. Our societies see these touches as wrong: *any* sexual activity with a child before the age of consent, not only sexual intercourse, is against the law.'

Ask: 'Can you think of other examples of sexual touching between older people and children? How do children feel when they are touched this way?'

Use information from Table 26.2 to talk about all the forms of harmful sexual touching that an adult might try to do with a child.

Table 26.2 Examples of caring, sexual, and confusing touches

Situation	Place and type of touching	How does child feel?	Reason for the adult's/peer's touching
Caring touches			
Mother washes 8-year-old girl who is sick all over	Washes girl gently all over, including between legs	Happy, being loved	To keep daughter clean, healthy, and comfortable
Female nurse dresses penis of 14-year-old boy after circumcision	Puts antiseptic on boy's penis and wraps it with a bandage	Embarrassed but happy that the nurse is helping him heal	To protect wound from infection and help penis heal
Caregiver kisses 5-year-old child's tummy	Pulls up top to show tummy and gives noisy kisses	Happy because laughing, and close to caregiver	It's fun to make child laugh and show love
Uncle sits child on their lap and hugs child	Strokes child's hair and puts arm around the child's shoulders	Happy, loved, and comforted	To show love and get comfort from touching
Boyfriend hugs girlfriend who is upset about an argument with her friend	Puts arms around girl's shoulder and waist loosely, and rocks her gently	Comforted and supported	To show love and compassion, and to give comfort
Confusing touches			
Caregiver kisses 5-year-old child's tummy and continues kissing to pubic area	Pulls up top to give noisy kisses, continues down abdomen to pubic area	Not sure what to feel: game felt nice but now feels different; wants it to stop	To use game as an excuse for sexual touching
Boyfriend hugs upset girlfriend tightly	Hugs her so her breasts are touching his chest and moves his body against her	Feels happy that he wants to comfort her, but uncomfortable with the closeness	To try and arouse her sexual feelings and have sex with her
Sexual touches			
Stepfather says he must check 8-year-old girl before she goes to school	Touches girl's breasts and vagina	Uncomfortable, scared, ashamed	To get sexual pleasure, and feeling of power over girl
Woman takes 11-year-old boy into empty house and says she will make him a man	Holds boy's penis and puts it inside her vagina	Ashamed, uncomfortable, embarrassed, aroused	To get sexual pleasure
Caregiver kisses 7-year-old child	Deep open-mouth kissing, using tongue	Uncomfortable and scared	To enjoy sexual feelings and satisfaction

Situation	Place and type of touching	How does child feel?	Reason for the adult's/peer's touching
uncle sits child on their lap and hugs child	rubs his penis against child	embarrassed and scared, powerless, wants to get away	to enjoy sexual feelings
boyfriend hugs upset girlfriend	puts his hand up her blouse and touches her nipples	feels very sexy but doesn't want to have sex, confused about how to say no	to make her feel sexy and persuade her to have sex

5. Say: 'Now let's talk about *confusing touching*.'

Explain: 'Sometimes a touch is not clearly caring or sexual. Hugs, kissing, and tickling can be confusing when we don't know what a person means by their actions, or when the person says something that does not fit with the touch.'

Ask: 'Can you think of examples of confusing touching? How do children feel when a touch is confusing? What do children do when a touch is confusing?'

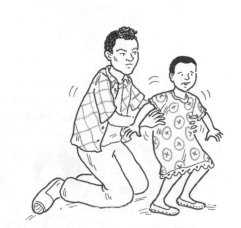

6. Ask: 'Can anyone suggest a way that we can tell whether a touch is caring or not? Can you give us an example?' Explain that we are going to practise deciding whether a touch is caring or sexual using some questions (see Box 26.e).

Box 26.e Is a touch caring or sexual? Questions to ask

- How does the child feel about the touching?
- How does the older person feel about the child?
- What does the older person say to the child? Do the words match the touching?
- Which part of the child's body do older people touch and/or ask children to touch?
- In what ways does the older person touch the child?
- What are the reasons that the older person touches the child and/or asks the child to touch them?
- Does the older person tell the child to keep the touching a secret?
- Does the older person threaten the child that if they tell someone, the older person will accuse them of starting it, or of doing something the child doesn't want known?

---

7. Choose two situations, one caring and one sexual or confusing, from Table 26.2, which are appropriate for the age group; alternatively, make up your own. Read one situation out (just the words in the first column), then ask participants the first question from Box 26.e. Continue though the questions, writing each one on a flipchart so participants can refer back to them at step 8. At the end, ask whether the situation showed caring touches, sexual touches, or confusing touches. Repeat with the other situation.

8. Explain that we will now practise in groups of three. Give each group two slips of paper that you prepared in advance (see 'Preparation'): one describing a situation where a touch is caring, and the other a situation where a touch is sexual.

Remember: don't add which kind of touch it is – they need to work this out for themselves. Ask them to use the questions you wrote down at step 7 to agree on which one is caring and which one is sexual.

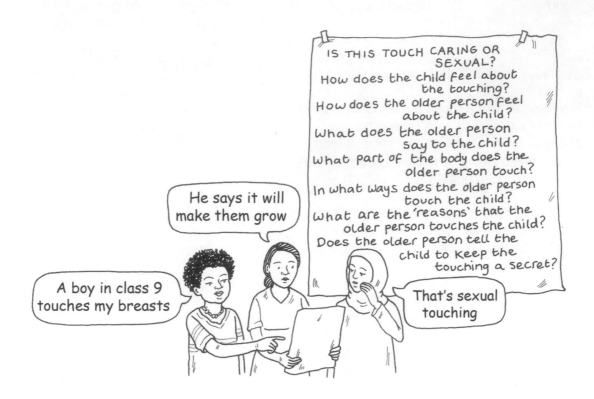

9. Bring the groups together and ask them to put the slips for the caring touches on one side of the floor, and the sexual touches on the other. If anyone disagrees with where a slip is put, discuss the questions until agreement is reached.

10. Ask: 'What effect do you think caring touches have on children as they develop, and later in their lives?'

If necessary, clarify that caring touches make children feel valued, loved, and secure. They grow up having compassion for themselves and others. They have higher self-esteem and are more able to form trusting, loving relationships in their lives.

11. Ask: 'What effect do you think sexual touches have on children as they develop, and later in their lives?'

As needed, add information from Box 26.f.

12. Explain that there are lots of things that we can do to protect each other from sexual abuse, and that is what we are going to talk about in the next exercise.

Box 26.f Effects of sexual abuse on children

Sexual abuse of children can be very harmful to them. It can cause them to:
- feel sad and low, angry or withdrawn, dirty, guilty, and confused;
- have lower self-esteem;
- engage in risky sexual behaviour;
- have problems developing relationships for the rest of their lives;
- abuse others, or fail to prevent abuse as it may be normal to them.

However, if families, communities, and services believe children who report abuse, and love and support them as they grow up, they can survive the abuse and recover from these effects. This is the topic of our next session.

Note that children may be concerned about different consequences of abuse from those that adults are concerned by. For example, a caregiver might be concerned about an abused girl's loss of virginity. But the girl may have thought that the abuse was a way of feeling loved and valued; and she may then feel loss and jealousy if the abuser leaves her alone and starts to abuse her younger sister instead. It is important to allow abused children to talk about the things that are worrying them, such as this. But never put pressure on them to talk until they are ready. Children who are sexually abused are often afraid to talk about it. We will talk more about this in the next session.

Often, people who abuse children sexually have themselves been abused as children. So there can be a lifelong effect of this behaviour across generations. This is not to excuse these adults – but it can help us understand that they too have somehow been damaged by these experiences. Fortunately these long-term legacies can be broken if we know how to intervene.

Note: We must never blame a child for being abused – it is never their fault. It is always the responsibility of adults to protect children. Blaming the children makes the consequences of sexual abuse even worse.

 EXERCISE 26.4 PROTECTING OURSELVES AND OUR CHILDREN

AIMS: To identify times and places in our community where sexual abuse might take place. To spot strategies and abilities that participants use to protect themselves and others from harmful touches. To build on these strategies and abilities to protect ourselves and others.

DESCRIPTION: Participants brainstorm places and times where sexual abuse may happen; do ability-spotting; and identify actions that could be taken to protect children from sexual abuse and make a mind map of them.

Box 26.g Information for facilitators

Changes are needed in (potential) perpetrators, community gender norms and values, and in service providers, to make it safe for children to assert their rights and for caregivers to protect their children. In this exercise we are looking at things that children and caregivers can do. Participants may want to join up with community groups to address the other issues.[62]

Directions

1. Divide your peer group into males and females.

2. Ask the group to think of and draw two maps, one for day and one for night; or to write times and places in which sexual abuse might happen to children like them, or to the children in their care, by day and by night. Don't forget to include spaces inside houses as well as places in the neighbourhood, such as the bus station or on the way to school. Select the five most common places and times.

Remind them that most people are kind and responsible: we are thinking about situations where it would be easier for someone to sexually abuse a child, but that does not mean that sexual abuse does happen or will happen in these places.

3. Divide participants into groups of four and ask each group to take one of the situations in which a child of their age is approached by an older person for sexual touching.

4. Ask them to answer these questions:
- What is the relationship between the child and older person? (for example, boyfriend, relative, stranger, acquaintance, teacher)
- What is the older person doing? What is the child doing?
- How does the child feel? How does the adult feel?
- What characteristics make this situation unsafe? (Refer back to Box 26.c if needed.)
- How could we all use our virtues together to support both these people in this situation?

5. Next invite participants to pair up and spot abilities and virtues that they have used to protect themselves or others from child sexual abuse.

Ask them to ask each other: 'Tell me about a time when you did something to protect yourself or someone else from child sexual abuse.' Suggest that they use their 'where, what, when, who, and how' questions to learn more about the story, and add the abilities and virtues to each other's necklaces.

Then ask them to ask each other: 'What other strategies have you used? How might you use these abilities in the future?'

6. Come together in the peer group. Write 'safety' in the middle of a flipchart sheet. Ask participants to share their ideas about how to make situations safer, and all the ways they have used to protect themselves or their children, and others. Add the ideas to the sheet as they say them. As needed, add information from Box 26.h for children, and from Box 26.i for caregivers.

7. Explain that you will keep the mind map for the next Exercise (26.5), and for Session 27, when we will share it with the other peer groups.

Box 26.h What can children do to protect themselves and each other from sexual abuse?

- Know that it is wrong for older people to touch your sexual organs and body to give themselves sexual pleasure. Tell your friends about this, and let adults know that you know your rights.

- Be assertive.

- Know that you always have the right to say 'no' to any behaviour which you do not like. This includes someone touching you, talking to you, looking at you, showing you something, or giving you something unusual to eat or smoke. It also includes touches that you do not like or want from your peers.

- Be alert to whether touches are caring, confusing, or sexual. If you are not sure, or are not sure what to do, talk to a trusted friend or adult.

- Watch out for danger signs, for example: if someone asks you to keep any touching or any sexual activity secret, or threatens you with a consequence if you do not keep the secret.

- Be careful about offers of favours, gifts or money, or help with schoolwork or promise of success in exams: all of these may be linked to an expectation of sex in return. If you would like to take up the offer, involve a trusted adult and tell your friends, so there is no secrecy, and do not be alone with the person making the offer.

- Say 'no' clearly and strongly to anyone doing something that makes you feel bad. Say that you will tell someone what they are doing.

- Run away, or shout for help, so that others will hear you and come. Be prepared to make a big noise in order to protect yourself or someone else.

- Try to move in pairs or groups with friends, especially in places that you think are less safe because there are few people around or because it is dark.

- Some girls decide to wear clothes such as undershorts and trousers, which make it more difficult for boys and men to touch their genitals. This is not to suggest that abuse is ever girls' fault because of what they are wearing. It is a way of dressing that gives girls in some places more confidence to be assertive with males who attempt to harass or abuse them.

- Trust your feelings about people: if you feel uneasy with someone, even if they haven't done anything, get away from them.

- Tell an adult you trust if you don't like the behaviour of someone, even if it is a relative or family friend. Tell a trusted adult if anyone touches you in a way you don't like, touches your private parts, asks you to take off your clothes, or talks to you about sexy things or having sex.

- If the first person you tell doesn't believe you, or tries to tell you it isn't a problem, tell another person, until someone takes it seriously.

Box 26.i What can caregivers and family members do to prevent sexual abuse of children?

- Be aware that children are at risk, whatever class and environment, and close family members need to be protective and above suspicion.

- Teach your children that males and females can control their sexual feelings, that sexual abuse is violence and that violence is wrong; and that everyone has a right to say 'no' to sexual touching at any time.

- Give your children lots of love and attention. If they feel sad and alone it is easy for someone to seduce them with kind words, cuddles, promises, and sympathy. This is psychological violence, because it lulls children into a false sense of security.

- Talk to your children about the difference between caring and sexual touch and how they can protect themselves.

- With your children, make a list of five people that they can speak to if they ever feel scared or abused.

- Give your children permission to say 'no' loudly if anyone tries to hurt them. Tell them they should run away and tell someone they can trust.

- Communicate with your children at home. Find opportunities to speak to them about their day, for example, at meal times and weekends, and ask them to tell you about one good thing that happened and one thing that they didn't like.

- Know the signs of sexual abuse (see Session 27) and always listen to a child who reports abusive behaviour. Take it seriously and find out more about the situation, even if it is difficult for you.

- Be aware and keep your eyes and ears wide open so you can recognize unsafe situations and abuse. Sexual abuse is often more common from family members and friends than from strangers. Children may hide the abuse if they are worried that the abuser may go to prison, or that the family would split up.

- Understand that care and love can sometimes slide into exploitation and abuse.

- Be aware of your children's safety when they sleep in the same room as others, particularly older children and adults.

- Look at the things that protect your children and those that might be unsafe in your household and neighbourhood. Make a plan with the whole family to keep the children safe.

- Talk with other family members, including males, about their roles as loving and protective family members. Talk about how you can work together to ensure that the children are safe so that no one can suspect them of child sexual abuse.

8. Invite each group to write or draw a manifesto to say what they will do to keep children safe. Perhaps they can write it as a song that they can sing and remember. Box 26.j gives an example of a children's manifesto.

Box 26.j Example of a children's manifesto

If someone touches me sexually:

I will tell them to stop.

I will say that I will tell someone.

I will run away if I can.

I will shout for help very loudly.

I will tell someone I trust what happened.

This way I can stay safe and happy.

 EXERCISE 26.5 PRACTISING RESPONSES TO SEXUAL APPROACHES

AIMS: To understand our options for responding to sexual approaches (threats) and when to use them. To develop confidence and skills in using these options.

DESCRIPTION: Participants are given information on ways of responding to threats, and rehearse and assess different ways of responding in threatening situations.

GROUPS: This exercise could be done in groups of caregivers with other people's children, or in separate peer groups.

Box 26.k Information for facilitators

When we feel threatened, our lower brains immediately become active and tell our bodies to prepare for *flight, fight, freeze* or *appease*.

This is a survival situation in which we may have to act before we bring in our upper brains to make a decision. Children's upper brains are still developing, and they are taught from an early age to show respect to older people by doing what they ask. We need to teach them that it's OK to say 'no', and practise how to do this in the safest way. In many situations, the safest response for children is to be respectful and nice to the older person (to appease them), and try to leave the place safely.

It is very difficult for any of us to know the best way of dealing with a sexual approach or threat, because the response of the other person is unpredictable. Assertiveness, fighting, or shouting might lead to violence, or the person might leave the scene; running away may increase the excitement of the chase, or allow the child to reach a safe place; freezing or appeasing might lead to the perpetrator doing whatever they wish, or having compassion for the child, or acting morally because they were shown respect. Box 26.l contains some ideas.

Directions

1. Explain that in this exercise we are going to practise what to do if an older person approaches a child for sexual activity. This will support children in feeling more confident and able to resist sexual advances.

2. Invite participants to show their mind maps from Exercise 26.4 on how to protect themselves and each other from sexual abuse. Explain that in this exercise we will practise these skills and add others.

3. Remind participants of what they learned in Session 2 'Using our brains' about how we react to threats.

Ask: 'What do we do when we are threatened?'

If necessary, remind them that when we feel threatened, for example, by someone who wants to touch us sexually without our consent, our lower brains immediately become active and tell our bodies to prepare for *flight, fight, freeze* or *appease*. If we have time to connect with our upper brains, we can think of options and decide what action to take, helped by our body's readiness.

4. Ask some volunteers to role play the story of Layla or Kali from Exercise 26.1, or another story, in front of the whole group, up to the point where the older person is asking the child to do something that he or she is uncomfortable with. This might be getting close physically, suggesting going somewhere quiet, or asking for sexual touching.

5. Invite participants to suggest ways that the child could respond in that situation. These can either be acted out by the role players, or the person making the suggestion can step into the role of the child and demonstrate their suggested method.

For each new method ask everyone: 'What are the good points about this response?'

'What are the difficulties with this response?'

6. Encourage people, in turn, to try out all the possibilities, including flight, fight, freeze, and appease. Continue until people run out of ideas.

7. If there are any approaches in Box 26.l that participants have not thought of, demonstrate them yourself.

Ask: 'Which way do you think works best in this situation? What are your reasons for thinking this?'

8. Then ask: 'How can we all use our virtues together to support this adult and child in staying on their hubs, so that the adult acts responsibly and the child stays safe?'

Box 26.I Ways of responding to sexual approaches

Flight: Run away to other people or to a place to hide, if these are nearby and you can run faster than the abuser. Or jump up and shout, 'Ouch, I've got cramp!', to escape from the abuser's lap or arm without shaming or confronting them. Then move away fast.

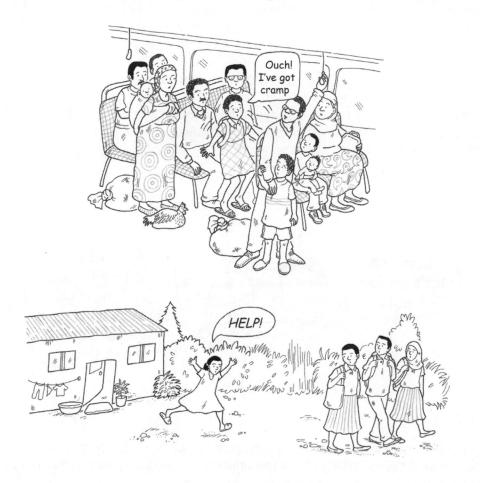

Fight: Be assertive: tell the abuser that what they are doing is wrong, it is your body, and they have no right to touch you. For example:

'Stop that! It is a sin and a crime.'

'If you touch me like that, I'll tell my mother/father/brother/teacher/the police.'

'My body belongs to me; it is not yours to touch.'

Shout and yell, and use your strength to hurt and surprise the person, and then run away. For example, poke or gouge their eyes, kick their knee, kick between a male's legs, or push the heel of your hand forcefully up and under their nose. This may work if you are big and strong, there are people within hearing distance, you are determined to hurt them, and you have learned some fighting skills. If not, it is likely to be safer to appease the adult.

Freeze: Hide and keep absolutely still. Act as if you are dead or very sick. This may make the abuser give up. Or it can make an abuser believe that you have given up, or that you have 'agreed' to what they want to do. While seemingly unaware, watch out for an opportunity to get away.

Appease: Try to please the abuser, calm them down, give them respect, or make them feel compassion.

You might try to calm them down by using 'I' statements, acknowledging their strengths, or giving them respect and dignity, for example: 'When you touch me in that way, I feel very unhappy. I would be glad if you behaved in your usual wise and respectful way.'

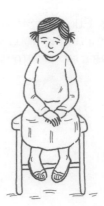

You might say things that are not true, in order to appease the person and get away from them. For example, say that you would like to please them, but not now because you feel unwell. Or you might say you will meet them another time. This is likely to result in the person approaching you again, so you must get support quickly to stop them.

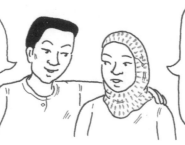

Come on, let's go for a walk

My mother is waiting for me so I must go now. Perhaps we'll see each other next time

You might call forth their virtues of compassion or responsibility by crying, urinating, telling them about your dreams, talking about the virtues promoted by your religion, or asking them to imagine that you are their own daughter or son.

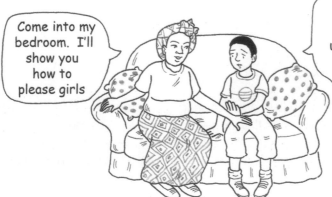

Come into my bedroom. I'll show you how to please girls

I trust you to care for me. I feel so unhappy when you do things that my caregiver, teacher and priest have told me are wrong

9. Now repeat steps 5 to 8 for another role play story.

10. If there is time, divide participants into groups of three and give each small group a situation from the mind maps they drew in Exercise 26.4. Ask them to take it in turns to role play the child, adult, and observer, and show what they would say and do in this situation. Ask the group members to give feedback to each other on the good and risky points of their responses, and agree on which ways they think will work best.

11. Invite the small groups to show their best role play to the whole group, and explain their reasons for choosing that one.

12. Choose one of the role plays, and ask participants to imagine that in this situation, the person does not stop trying to touch them in spite of their resistance. What would they do then?

13. Ask participants to summarize what they have learned from the exercise and how they will use it and/or share it with others.

14. Explain that we will keep the mind maps to use in Session 27.

Box 26.m Alternative activity for children aged 5–8 years

Younger children may enjoy drawing on their fingers to make puppets, which they can use to practise saying 'no' to sexual touch. Ask them to imagine that one finger is a child, and the other a person who wants to touch the child in a sexual way. Invite them to practise what the child could say or do, and to show their ideas to a friend.

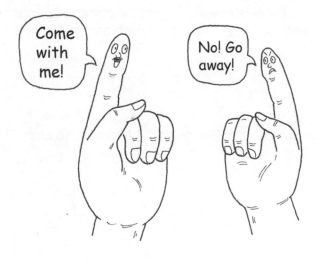

EXERCISE 26.6 HOMEWORK: AWARENESS OF OURSELVES IN OUR ENVIRONMENT

AIMS: To help caregivers and children pay attention to what is going on around them.

DESCRIPTION: A mindfulness exercise which can help participants become more aware of their environment.

Directions

1. Explain that sometimes we are deep in our own thoughts and do not pay attention to what is going on around us, or our own behaviour. Being more aware of ourselves in the environment may help us make good decisions and stay safe.

2. Ask participants to do one of these activities outside the workshop:

I am a camera: Invite participants to imagine that they are video cameras. Their lens is focussing on all the details about their own experience, and playing it back as it is happening.

I am a newspaper reporter. Invite participants to write or draw their step-by-step experience of one hour in their day.

I am a TV reporter. Invite participants to walk around the community together in pairs (this could be a caregiver and child); each says aloud what they can see and what is happening around them as they walk along.

Closing circle

Remember to keep the mind map from Exercise 26.4 to use in Session 27.

SESSION 27 SUPPORTING SURVIVORS OF SEXUAL ABUSE

Note: It is essential that participants have done Session 26 before doing this session.

Purpose: To recognize signs and symptoms of possible sexual abuse; to support caregivers and children in communicating about it; to support children who are being, or have been, abused, and their caregivers; and to put in place protective measures in the home and community.

Contents	Materials required	Time required
Opening circle (see p.13)		25–30 mins
27.1 Telling trusted people about child sexual abuse	Prepare three stories	45 mins
27.2 Signs of sexual abuse and supporting children in talking about it		60 mins
27.3 *For children aged 9–14 years and caregivers only* Supporting survivors of abuse		60 mins
27.4 Protecting children from further abuse		30–60 mins
27.5 Imagining a safe haven		20 mins
Closing circle (see p.14)		15 mins

About 4.5–5 hrs

Preparation

Exercise 27.1. We have provided a story for each peer group, but you may want to prepare other stories so that each sex is featured in the stories of abuse, or use stories that emerged in Session 26. You will find a picture of the characters in the story of Miriam in the Annex, so that you can point to places on the body where the abuser touched the child.

Exercise 27.4. Prepare case studies relevant to girls and boys aged 5–8 years, and 9–14 years, perhaps using one of the unsafe situations or stories already discussed. Give enough information in the case studies for groups to make a detailed protection plan.

Box 27.a Information for facilitators

Never force or pressure children to talk about possible sexual abuse, or invite them to do so in a group. This breaks confidentiality, and can result in gossip, punishment, and rejection by the family. Encourage them to talk about sexual abuse which might happen to 'people like them' in the group, and encourage them to talk to you afterwards about their concerns.

Ask privately about possible abuse in a gentle and general way, and observe body language and facial expression carefully. Support families in starting to put protective measures in place without having full evidence of abuse. This protects the child and helps them communicate more about any abuse. Refer families and children who may have been abused to skilled counsellors, who can work with them on a detailed strategy to protect the child.

It is essential that support is in place at the session and in the community for children and caregivers who need it following this session (see: Introduction, p.11).

Opening circle

In addition to following the usual Opening circle process, ask participants how they got on with their homework (Exercise 26.6), about being aware in our environment. Invite people who tried this to share what they learned and any observations on how we can support each other in staying safe. Invite participants to perform an energetic and uplifting local song and dance, related to today's virtue.

 EXERCISE 27.1 TELLING TRUSTED PEOPLE ABOUT CHILD SEXUAL ABUSE

AIMS: To understand the importance of telling a trusted person about sexual abuse, even if the abuser tells us to keep it a secret. To think about how we can use our virtues to support a friend who is being abused.

DESCRIPTION: The caregivers' and children's peer groups divide into males and females, as appropriate, and read and discuss stories relevant to them. The abusers in this exercise are the types of people who would be known to participants, such as family members and teachers.

Directions[63]

1. Divide the peer groups into males and females.

2. Remind participants about Exercise 26.2 in the last session, and invite them to mention some caring, confusing, and sexual touches. Then invite them to explain what we mean by child sexual abuse.

3. Explain: 'Children and caregivers often cannot talk easily or openly if they are being abused, or their child is being abused. In this exercise we are going to read a story about sexual abuse

and answer questions about it. This will support us in seeing how important it is to recognize child sexual abuse, and protect children even if they are not able to speak about it.'

Say that we will discuss these questions further in the next exercise – this is an introduction to the topic. Write yourself brief notes to remind you of the important points that arise in discussion.

Caregivers

> **Box 27.b For caregivers: The story of David**
>
> I am a 26-year-old man. From when I was four years old until I was eight, my auntie, who lived with us, would touch my private parts and make me touch hers.
>
> I was scared. She would give me sweets to make me feel a little better.
>
> Now I am married to a good woman, but every day I become angry and I ask myself:
>
> 'Why couldn't someone stop what happened to me?'

4. Read out the story of David (see Box 27.b), then ask the following questions:
- Does this happen to boys in our community? Does this happen to girls?
- How do children behave when an adult or older child touches their private parts or has sexual activity with them?
- Do boys and girls show their feelings differently?
- How do children behave when the person who touches their private parts tells them to keep it a secret?
- How can we talk to a child if we think they have been sexually abused?

5. Ask: 'How can we all use our virtues together to help each other if we are scared or have a secret that makes us sad or angry?'

Children aged 5–8 years

4. Read out Part A of the story of Miriam (see Box 27.c).

Use the picture of Miriam and her cousin in the Annex to illustrate what is happening in the story as you tell it. Point to the various body parts on each picture, as the story requires.

5. At the end of Part A, ask: 'Do you know what a secret is?' (The children answer.)

'Do you think Miriam told anybody that her cousin was touching her here and here?' (point to Miriam's breast and pubic area on her picture)

**Box 27.c For children aged 5–8 years:
The story of Miriam**

Part A. This is a story about a six-year-old girl called Miriam. Miriam is very unhappy.

She has a cousin who lives in her house. He is 17 years old. This cousin touches her here (point to breasts on the picture of Miriam), and here (point to pubic area), and she has to touch him here (point to pubic area on the picture of her cousin) almost every day. He tells her that if she doesn't agree, he will do things that scare her, and she cries.

Her cousin gives her sweets to make her feel a little better. He tells her: 'This is our special secret. Don't tell anybody.'

Part B. Miriam thinks: 'Am I doing something bad?' But she doesn't want to keep this secret. Sometimes she cries at night because she doesn't know what to do. She wants her cousin to stop. But she is too scared to tell anybody.

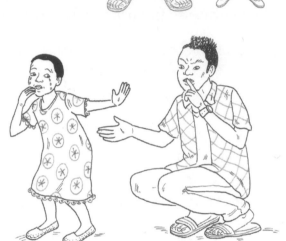

6. Now read out Part B. At the end, ask the following questions:

• What could Miriam do?

• Why does her cousin want to her to keep what he does a secret?

• Why does Miriam not tell anyone?

• What could help her to talk?

• How could we all use our virtues together to help her and her cousin get back on their hubs?

• Who can children like us talk to if we have a secret that is scaring us or making us sad?

7. Give each child a piece of paper and ask them to draw a picture of themselves in the middle, and then to draw people they could talk to around them in a circle. Remind them of the people they named as their supporters to help them across the river in Exercise 1.8, those they included on the bracelet of helpers they made in Exercise 10.5, and those they named as supporters during Exercise 19.4 about puberty.

Say: 'If you are scared or sad about a secret, you can also come to me after the meeting today, or go to any of your helpers and tell them.'

8. Ask: 'What would help you talk to your helpers if something were happening to you that made you scared or sad?'

9. Ask: 'How can we all use our virtues together to help each other if we are scared or have a secret that makes us sad?'

Children aged 9–14 years

Box 27.d For children aged 9–14 years: The story of Mary

Mary is an 12-year-old girl. She is starting to show signs of becoming a woman. Her teacher tried to touch her breasts whenever he found her alone. One day he asked her to go to his house to talk about her maths results. Mary had always been eager to participate in class and played basketball after school. But now her friends noticed that she was very quiet in class, and hurried home as soon as school was over. Whenever the teacher walked by she looked away and her hands shook. They asked her what was wrong, but she said she was fine and that they should leave her alone.

One day Mary's friends overheard the teacher telling Mary sternly to go to his house. They followed her and could see she was crying. They stopped her before she reached the house and led her to a quiet place. There she told them that the teacher was demanding sex from her. She was afraid to say anything in case he caused her to fail her exams. Her friends talked with her and praised her courage for telling them. She agreed to report the teacher to the school guidance counsellor and tell her caregiver. They then reported the teacher to the headteacher so that he could not harm other children. The teacher left the school, and learned to see the harm that his behaviour caused children. Mary's friends were very proud of her courage and compassion in protecting others from abuse.

---

4. Read out the story of Mary (Box 27.d), then ask the following questions:
- Why did Mary's friends suspect that she might have been abused?
- Why do you think that Mary didn't tell anybody at first?
- How did Mary's friends support her to talk about it with them and her mother and the guidance counsellor?
- How did Mary and her friends protect other children from abuse? What can we do in our community to protect children from abuse?

5. Ask: 'How can we all use our virtues together to help each other if we are scared or have a secret that makes us sad?'

 ## EXERCISE 27.2 SIGNS OF SEXUAL ABUSE AND SUPPORTING CHILDREN IN TALKING ABOUT IT

AIMS: To recognize signs and symptoms that a child might have been, or is being, sexually abused. To support caregivers and children in talking about sexual abuse.

DESCRIPTION: In small groups, participants discuss signs and symptoms of sexual abuse. They create a 'brick wall', showing reasons why children find it difficult to talk about sexual abuse, and use role plays to find solutions.

Box 27.e Information for facilitators

It is important that children are able to speak about sexual abuse, but we must remember that adults may respond in negative and harmful ways. For example, they may disregard what the child is saying, or accuse them of lying or engaging in sexual activity, and punish them. So we need to keep reinforcing the message to children that they are not to blame, and help them know who else they can talk to if their caregiver responds in an unhelpful way.

Directions

1. Explain that some children report sexual abuse to their caregiver or another person at the time of the abuse. Others do not feel able to talk about it. In this session we will talk about signs of possible sexual abuse, and how to help children talk about abuse. Explain that we should never force or pressure a child to talk about abuse until they are ready. We can learn a lot from the child's non-verbal communication, and take steps to protect the child without insisting on verbal information.

2. Ask: 'What signs might make us think about the possibility that someone is abusing a child sexually?'

Explain that some of the signs might also be caused by other problems, but we do need to consider the possibility of sexual abuse. As needed, add in possible signs of abuse from Box 27.f.

Note: Children aged 5–8 years do not need to know all the signs; they can just learn that a child's behaviour could be affected in all sorts of ways.

Box 27.f Possible signs that a child is being sexually abused

- Child shows sudden change in behaviour that can't be explained;
- Child bursts into tears easily;
- Child wants lots of attention;
- Child is overly affectionate, or knowledgeable in a sexual way inappropriate to their age;
- Child suddenly draws sexually explicit pictures;
- Child shows medical problems, such as chronic itching, pain in the genitals or when urinating, symptoms of STIs or pregnancy, having trouble walking or sitting;
- Child shows signs of physical abuse, such as bruises or cuts, with refusal to discuss or explain them;
- Child shows a change in possessions and the availability of money;
- Child's personality changes, becoming, for example, insecure, clingy, angry, or hostile to caregivers;
- Child shows fear of returning home or having caregiver contacted;
- Child's attitude to school and performance at school changes;
- Child regresses to younger behaviour patterns, such as thumb-sucking or bringing out discarded cuddly toys;
- Child shows sudden loss of appetite or compulsive eating;

- Child is anxious, isolated or withdrawn;
- Child shows inability to concentrate;
- Child shows lack of trust in, or fear of, someone they know well; for instance, not wanting to be alone with a relative or child minder for no obvious reason;
- Child starts to lie or steal;
- Child starts to wet the bed, has bad dreams in the day or night;
- Child becomes worried about clothing being removed, or physical activities;
- Child tries to be 'ultra-good' or perfect, or overreacts to criticism;
- Child shows non-verbal signs such as slamming doors, coming home late from school, being withdrawn or silent;
- Among more extreme reactions, child shows signs of depression, self-mutilation, suicide attempts, running away, taking drug overdoses, anorexia, using alcohol or other drugs, and obsessive washing of self or clothes.

3. Draw a wall made of bricks on the ground, board, or wall. Invite participants to pair up and think of reasons why children might not want to talk about being abused, and to put one reason on each brick in the wall. Ask them to think of as many reasons as possible. If necessary, use the ideas in Box 27.g as prompts.

Note: With children aged 5–8 years, we suggest that you only talk about the reasons that they come up with, and try to find ways to deal with these.

Box 27.g Reasons children might not talk about being sexually abused

- They don't know how to talk about it.
- They feel shame and guilt.
- They blame themselves.
- They don't know that child sexual abuse is wrong.
- They love the person who has abused them and rely on them for attention, love, and support.
- They get pleasure from being chosen, touching, and intimacy.
- They need or want the money and gifts they are offered.
- They fear that the abuser might go to prison or leave the house.
- They fear that the abuser will act on their threats, or punish or kill them.
- They fear that the abuser might hurt someone else the child loves.
- They fear that the family will break up, with uncertain consequences.
- They fear that the partner of the abuser will hate them.
- They fear rejection, by their family and wider community.
- They think that no one would believe them.
- They fear spoiling their own reputation, jeopardizing their own chances of a marriage later.
- They fear bringing shame on the family (even though the child has done nothing wrong).
- When they previously told someone, either they were not taken seriously, were told off or punished, or no action was taken, but their feeling of powerlessness and blame increased.

---

4. Explain that many of these reasons are to do with the way we respond to threats, particularly if we are children with little power. Our lower brain focusses on survival, and may rightly decide that it is safer to freeze, or do as the powerful person says (appease), than fight (in this case by telling others). Explain that some of the bricks in the wall we have drawn are difficult and unsafe to remove without protective and supportive action from the family, community, and services.

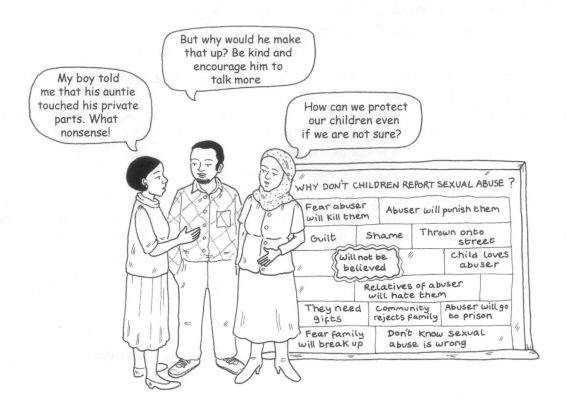

5. Invite participants to pair up and to choose a brick that they think they can help with; ask them to rehearse what they might say to their child or friend or other involved person, to help them to talk about the abuse or to help a child talk about the abuse.

6. Say: 'Share what you have learned about your brick and how to deal with this barrier to talking about abuse.' If everyone agrees, remove the brick from the wall.

7. Keep the bricks that are too difficult to remove to discuss during a follow-up session with family, services, and community members.

8. Next, direct relevant peer groups as follows:

Children. Explain that, unfortunately, adults may not react well when children tell them about abuse. Ask: 'What unhelpful reactions might a child get from an adult?'

For example, an adult might:
- not believe the child, or ignore what they have said;
- accuse the child of lying;
- say that what the child is describing is normal, and they are making a fuss about nothing;
- threaten the child with what they will do if the child ever mentions it again;
- accuse the child of seducing the adult, or of inviting the abuse;

- say they will do something, but then do nothing.

Explore each possibility in turn, ensuring that the children understand that the poor reaction is because the adult is wrong in some way, not because the child is wrong to speak up about sexual abuse.

Ask: 'How can a child try to reduce the chance of getting a negative reaction from the adult that they tell?'

Encourage them to think about whom else the abuser has power over, who loves the abuser, and who might want to protect the abuser. Ideally, they need to tell someone who shows virtues, and who will be willing and able to take action to protect them, even if this action involves challenging the abuser.

Ask: 'What if a child tells an adult about abuse, and the adult doesn't believe them, or doesn't take action? What should the child do then?'

If necessary, explain that they need to keep telling people until someone does take it seriously, and takes action to protect them.

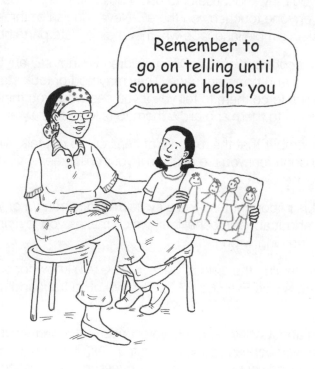

Caregivers. Explain that many children never talk about their experience of sexual abuse. However, there are ways in which we can support a child to talk.

Ask them to form small groups and to suggest 'opening lines' in response to the question: 'What could we say to try to start a conversation with a child whom we suspect is being sexually abused?'

Ask each small group to suggest one different 'opening line' in turn, until they run out of ideas. Then ask: 'What other techniques might we use?' and invite them to call out answers. As needed, add information from Box 27.h.

Box 27.h Ways of helping a child talk about sexual abuse

Time and place. Have this conversation somewhere that the child feels comfortable and private, when you are not in a hurry.

Opening question. Find a way of beginning a conversation in an open and caring way. For example:

- 'I love you and want to help you be happy. I wonder, is someone making you unhappy? Are you afraid of something? Whatever you say, I will not be angry with you. I just want to know what is troubling you, so I can protect and support you better.'
- 'Have you got a problem at home or at school?'
- 'I've noticed you have got some new things recently. I wonder who gave them to you? It's nice to have new things, but people who give gifts often expect something in return. Can we explore this together?'
- 'I sometimes wonder if things have been happening to you in a sexual way, which should not happen to any child. Has anyone been touching you in ways that make you feel uncomfortable or hurt you?' (Note that sexual abuse can feel good to the child, so asking about discomfort or pain may not get the information that you are looking for.)

Get more specific. You may find it useful to use a doll and point to between its legs or chest, asking: 'Has anyone touched you there?' Never punish or threaten the child, or show shock, but ask in simple language whether their private parts hurt.

Be alert to non-verbal communication. Often children will not say anything. Observe their facial expressions and body language. They may nod or look startled. Allow them to remain silent. Do not force them to tell you if you see what you think is positive body language. Go on talking to them and allow them to talk when they are ready.

Accept silence. Remember that the majority of children do not talk about the abuse they experience, so don't feel you are a failure if your child keeps silent. Feel proud for observing a potential problem.

Stay on your hub. It is important that you stay calm and in control of your emotions, even if the child tells you about abusive behaviour, which makes you feel angry. Reassure them that they have done nothing wrong.

Take action. Start protecting the child at once, before you know for sure the abuse has happened or the details (see Exercise 27.3). This will build trust and make it easier for them to talk.

Follow up. Ask again about whatever made you concerned. If there was something your child said or did that made you concerned, ask about that. Ask in a non-judgemental way, and take care to avoid shaming your child as you ask questions. 'I' questions can be very helpful, for example: 'I'm concerned because I heard you say that you are not allowed to lock the bathroom door.'

Talk. Discuss secrets and threats with your child, and how abusers use this to trap children. Talk about times that it's OK not to keep a secret, even if they made a promise.

Identify supporters. Show understanding that the child might prefer to talk to someone else: mention names of other possible supporters, or talk more generally about whom the child trusts and respects and who could help them with any problems they may face.

Build a trusting relationship with your child. Let them know it is OK to come to you if someone is making them uncomfortable. Be sure to keep any promises you make. If you tell your child that they can talk to you, be sure to make time for them when they do come to you.

EXERCISE 27.3 SUPPORTING SURVIVORS OF ABUSE

We recommend that children aged 5–8 years do not do this exercise.

AIMS: To support caregivers in understanding what to do if their child is sexually abused. To support children in knowing what to do if they or their friends are sexually abused. To support participants in providing continuing support to survivors of abuse.

DESCRIPTION: Participants draw a pathway and draw, on pieces of paper, the steps to helping someone who is abused.

Directions

1. Remind participants of the work they did in Session 26 about protecting each other from sexual abuse. Put up the mind map they made, which showed ways of keeping children safe. Explain we can use some of those strategies to protect children from further sexual abuse.

2. Explain that we are going to draw a pathway to show the steps to take if we suspect a child is being abused, but we don't know for certain and they haven't told us.

Ask: 'What would you do?'

Ask them to write or draw each action on a different piece of paper, and then lay them on the floor in some kind of order. As needed, add information from Box 27.i.

Box 27.i Steps to take if we suspect a child is being abused

For children

- Try to talk with our friend, but accept that they may not want to talk.

- Talk with an adult about our concerns. Ask them what they will do. Talk with another adult if the first adult does not take us seriously.

- Give our friend love and support.

- If possible, try to protect our friend, for example, by helping them avoid being alone with the suspected abuser. But we should not put ourselves at risk of abuse or violence.

- Keep watching for signs of abuse and repeat the same steps as needed.

For caregivers

- Try to talk with the child, but accept that they may not want to talk.

- Talk to other adults that we trust about our concern, and make a plan to protect the child. Think about all the ways in which they may be vulnerable to abuse during the day and night, and find ways to protect them.

- Give the child love and support, and help them know that we and other adults want to help and protect them.

- If appropriate, arrange for them to have a medical check-up for injuries, infections including HIV, and pregnancy.

---

3. Ask participants to add in additional steps to take if a child actually tells us that they are being, or have been, sexually abused. Write each idea on a separate piece of paper and add them to the appropriate places in the path. As needed, add information from Box 27.j.

Box 27.j Additional steps to take if a child tells us they are being abused

For children and caregivers

- Listen, but do not press for information.
- Stay calm and reassure them; don't panic or appear shocked.
- Believe what we are being told.
- Say that we are glad that they have told us; thank them for sharing with us.
- Stress that they are not to blame.
- If it will help the child cope, say that the person who has abused them has a problem and needs support from professionals to stop doing this in future.
- Say that we will do our best to help protect and support them.
- Discuss what we will do next.

For caregivers only

Consider the following to help protect the child from more abuse:

- Involve all family members and other relevant people (for example, police, social services, school staff) in making a plan to protect the child from more abuse.
- Involve the person who has done the abusing if they are a member of the family and are still present in the child's life. This requires a skilled child protection worker to ensure the child's safety, if the abuser does not feel he has done wrong or may/does continue the abuse. Usually it requires the abuser to move out of the family home for a time, and involves the police or community courts.
- In some communities, the abuser pays a fine for harming the child and the matter is closed. In some, a male who abuses a girl is obliged to marry her, even if she is below the age of consent. This further violates her rights and continues the abuse.
- Ask each family member to discuss what a person in their family role could do to protect the child from further abuse. For example: 'What would an auntie or uncle do to protect this child and others in the family from sexual abuse?' Also ask children to think of what they can do to try to protect themselves or their siblings. Get everyone to think of realistic things that they can do. (We look at this in detail in Exercise 27.4.)

Seek help from others, as appropriate:

- If necessary, contact the police and victim support unit, community support systems, and/or social services. If our child has told another adult, such as a teacher or school nurse, contact them. We may be able to work together to support our child.
- If the abuse may affect, or has affected, how our child behaves or performs at school, we may wish to liaise with school staff if we think they will treat the information sensitively and confidentially.

Find ways of expressing and dealing with feelings:

- Seek help from a counsellor for ourselves and our child.
- Acknowledge that the child may have angry, sad or even guilty feelings, including towards us, about what happened. Stress to the child that the abuse was not their fault.
- Acknowledge that we may need support to deal with our own feelings. We may feel anger at the person who has abused the child, and perhaps guilt for not managing to protect the child in our care.

4. When the path is finished, walk along it together, calling out some of the main points. When you reach the end of the path, remind everyone that many people who have experienced sexual abuse find it helpful to see themselves as survivors, not victims. They have survived the experience, and go on to live their lives. We can all support survivors by using our virtues to be good friends and caregivers.

 ## EXERCISE 27.4 PROTECTING CHILDREN FROM FURTHER ABUSE

AIM: To enable participants to take immediate action to protect a child who is being or may have been abused from further harm, and begin a process of finding more harmonious ways of relating if the abuse is in the family.

DESCRIPTION: Using a case study (see Preparation), participants talk through 24 hours in the life of a child who may have been, or is being, abused, in order to make a plan to protect them. They build on their work in Exercise 26.4 'Protecting ourselves and our children'.

GROUPS: Caregivers and children aged 9–14 years, as described in the directions.

Box 27.k Information for facilitators

This exercise is useful for all caregivers, whether abuse is happening in their home or not. It will support them in preventing abuse and make it easier for them to take action if they suspect, or are told about, abuse in the future. The exercise intends to introduce participants to the idea of protection with family support, and the experience of using one tool to support this. It is important to have a skilled person with some experience in dealing with sexual abuse to facilitate the process with a family in which abuse *has* happened. Try out the exercise, giving lots of support to groups, and paying attention to how children (and caregivers) are responding. Offer support to anyone who gets upset or wants to stop doing the exercise.

Directions[64]

1. Explain that we are going to talk about how to ensure that children are protected from further abuse if we know or suspect that they are being abused. We will discuss a case study and do an activity to look in detail about how a child might be protected from their abuser 24 hours a day.

2. Say: 'We have seen that many children – and often their caregivers – keep quiet about sexual abuse, because they fear that they will lose their practical and emotional support. They also fear violence.'

Explain that the approach we will explore now aims to protect the child even where there is no definite evidence of abuse, while working to transform and keep the family together.

The aims of the support are to:
- create a partnership between all who are involved in the family to provide care and protection for the child/children;

- immediately secure the safety of the child and support all family members in putting in place protective measures to ensure that abuse does not happen again.

3. Bring the caregivers and children aged 9–14 years together and divide into single-sex groups. Then ask them to form groups of six: three caregivers and three children, separating children from their own caregivers. Give each group a case study relating to the age and sex of their children.

4. Ask each group member to choose one of the following roles:
- caregiver;
- family member – male;
- family member – female;
- child – of the same age and sex as the peer group;
- older child, who is at risk of being abused;
- older child, who either is being abused or has been abused.

5. Ask each group to read the case study and draw a road to show the life of the child at risk of abuse over one day and night. Ask them to draw each main event, for example: getting up; bathing; getting dressed; travelling to school; school; travelling home from school; attending youth club; doing homework; fetching water; working in the garden; eating; bathing; going to bed.

Ask them, for each of these steps, to discuss whether the child is at risk of further abuse and the reasons for this. They should mark these times and places on the road. Draw the people who are around at that time.

6. Ask participants, at each point in the day, to discuss the question relating to their character from the options below:
- *Caregiver*. What would a caregiver do to protect his or her children from sexual abuse?
- *Male family member*. What would a father, uncle, grandfather, brother or cousin do to protect their children from sexual abuse?
- *Female family member*. What would a mother, auntie, grandmother, sister, cousin do to protect the children from sexual abuse?
- *Child*. What could children do to protect themselves and each other from sexual abuse?

7. Ask participants to write or draw beside each step their ideas for protection. Discuss how realistic they are and revise them if necessary.

8. Ask: 'What have we learned from this exercise? How might we use this knowledge in the future?'

9. Invite all the peer groups to come together and share their mind maps from Exercise 26.4, showing actions that children and caregivers can do to protect children from abuse. Join up the protective actions and things that make situations safer onto one big mind map. Explain that this shows the whole picture, and also that we all have some responsibility to work together to keep children safe.

10. If you have time ask if anyone would like to draw another road, this time about a day in the life of a child, for example, over the weekend, during the school holidays, during a visit to a relative, or going to a religious festival. If so, take the lead from the person who has suggested this, and repeat the exercise. Participants might like to do this at home.

11. Explain that in the next exercise we will do a meditation about safe places in our lives, to remind ourselves that we can be safe and happy if we work together.

EXERCISE 27.5 IMAGINING A SAFE HAVEN

AIMS: To help participants focus their attention, relax, and have a way of feeling safe in their daily lives.

DESCRIPTION: Participants in their three separate peer groups are led through a meditation exercise, building on earlier relaxation and meditation activities.

Directions

1. Read the following script in a calm voice:

Begin by sitting in a comfortable position, with your back straight and shoulders relaxed. Softly close your eyes. Breathe in and out a few times slowly, deeply and evenly, to calm yourself down, with your mouth slightly open and with a little smile on your face. Just focus on your breathing. Allow the picture in your mind to become blank.

Now imagine a place that feels comfortable, safe, and relaxing. It might be a garden, a lake, or your own bed. Imagine it slowly appearing before you, becoming clearer and clearer.

Look to your left. What do you see? Look to your right. What is over there? Look closer.

Breathe in. What do you smell? Walk around your place. Look closer at certain things. Stay focussed on your place.

Listen. What do you hear in your safe place?

Touch. What do you enjoy touching in your place? How does that thing feel?

How does the place make you feel?

What do you do to express your feelings? Perhaps you move in a certain way, or sing.

Going on breathing in gently … and breathing out gently … breathing in gently … and breathing out gently …

Would you like anyone to share your place, or do you prefer to be alone at this time? It's fine either way. If you want to, invite your person to join you in your mind. Welcome them with a hug or kiss.

What are you feelings now?

If you find your thoughts wandering, observe them, and then focus on bringing the image of your place back into focus in front of you.

2. Allow participants some time. Then say:

'When you are ready, put your hand in front of your eyes. Open your eyes. Slowly spread your fingers to allow light in. When you are ready, slowly remove your hand.'

3. Children may like to draw the scene they imagined. They can save this drawing to remind them of their safe, relaxing place.

Closing circle

Mix up caregivers and children and ask them to form circles of 10. One by one, ask each group of 10 to put their hands in the middle of their circle, on top of each other. Invite them to make a promise to work together to keep all children safe from harm. Invite them to raise their hands in the air and give their neighbours 'high fives'.

Note: Remind participants to bring their ability necklaces to the next session (Session 28), about learning and contributing.

Purpose: To help participants talk about the tasks they enjoy, and how their abilities contribute to the family and community; to find ways to make tasks easier and more enjoyable; to practise virtues related to work; to look at how children spend their day and how this influences their wellbeing.

Contents	Materials required	Time required
Opening circle (see p.13)		15 mins
28.1 Work we enjoy		45 mins
28.2 Ways of making tasks easier		45 mins
28.3 The virtue of diligence		30 mins
28.4 How do we spend our day?		60 mins
Closing circle (see p.14)		15 mins

About 3.5 hrs

Box 28.a Information for facilitators

In this session we are talking about children's and adults' work activities at home, at school, and in the community. These activities have a range of purposes, such as learning and developing skills (for example, reading), meeting household domestic needs (for example, cooking or caring for someone who is ill), or bringing in money or material resources (for example, growing food or trading).

Making a contribution to the world through activities is an important means of developing abilities and confidence, gaining a sense of belonging, feeling significant, and developing self-compassion from a young age. It's good if children are able to grow up seeing work as rewarding and enjoyable. Diligence and responsibility are important virtues for life and success. Team work makes tasks easier, and increased cooperation between boys and girls in sharing tasks nurtures equality. Being aware of how boys and girls spend their time can change gender attitudes and develops skills that are useful throughout life.

EXERCISE 28.1 WORK WE ENJOY

AIMS: To appreciate the different activities and tasks that we do, which contribute to our development, meeting our needs, and achieving our visions of a good future. To celebrate our skills and the activities we enjoy.

DESCRIPTION: Participants mime different activities that they do and enjoy, identify the abilities that they use, and compare tasks done by males and females.

Directions

1. Explain that we are going to talk about the different activities and tasks which contribute to our development, meeting our needs, and achieving our visions of a good future.

---

2. Ask each person in turn to say one thing about their family that they feel grateful for, to do with how their family meets their needs. Go round the group again, this time with participants saying one thing their family does to support them in growing up to reach their vision of a good future.

Explain that it helps us and others if we value what we have, and appreciate what our family is doing for us. Many of us are poor, but often our caregivers are doing their best. If we are grateful, respectful, and helpful, adults are more likely to support us.

3. Explain that in this exercise we will show with our bodies all the tasks we do that contribute to our learning, and to meeting our family needs and future hopes. We need food, water, shelter, clothes, health, and relationships to develop well, and as we get older we have to work to acquire these. If we think of our life journey, we see that we are able to do more and more to support our households and work towards our visions as we grow up. Many of us have responsibilities at home, and work at school, in addition to finding ways of bringing food into the house.

Let's give ourselves a big clap and cheer for all the important work we do!

We will start with a game to look at tasks that we enjoy and the abilities we use. Later in the session we will look at tasks that we find more difficult, and find ways of making them more manageable.

4. Ask participants to stand in two circles, one of males and one of females. For each circle, invite someone to go into the centre and mime a task that they enjoy doing, without saying anything. Invite the others to guess what they are doing. If necessary, ask the actor to say what they were doing, and to explain why they like that task.

5. Ask participants to call out the abilities the actor uses to do the task.

6. Invite the next person to go to the centre and mime a different task that they like doing. Continue until everyone has had a turn.

7. Bring everyone back together and ask each group to summarize the different types of tasks they mimed and the reasons why they enjoy these tasks.

Ask: 'Are some tasks only done by girls? Or only by boys?'

'Why are some tasks only done by boys or by girls?'

'Is this fair?'

'What would be the benefits if both boys and girls did these tasks?'

Explain that we will look at the importance of different jobs in the next session, 29, which is about livelihoods.

EXERCISE 28.2 WAYS OF MAKING TASKS EASIER

AIM: To support caregivers and children in communicating well about doing tasks, and in finding ways of making difficult tasks easier.

DESCRIPTION: Participants do role plays showing a task that most children find difficult and how to make it easier. The peer groups make a mind map of all the things that made the task easier.

Directions

1. Divide participants into males and females. Ask: 'What are some tasks that you/your children find difficult to do? Why are they difficult?'

Make a list of difficult tasks.

2. Divide into groups of three or four, and ask each group to choose one of the difficult tasks.

3. Ask each group to think of how the task could be made easier, and to develop a role play to show this.

4. Ask each group to perform their role play to the whole peer group, and invite others to suggest ways of making the task easier. Encourage children to think from their caregivers' perspective, to help them develop realistic ideas.

Draw all the ideas on a mind map as you go along, adding ideas from Box 28.b. Write or draw, for example, 'Ways of making it easier to fetch water' in the centre of the map. Then draw or write the different suggestions around it in bubbles, with lines connecting the bubbles where the ideas are linked.

Box 28.b Ways of making tasks easier for children to do

- Use good communication skills: i) show respect, kindness and appreciation; ii) understand and acknowledge how the child experiences the task; iii) give a clear explanation of the task to be done, one task at a time.

- Show appreciation and praise when the task is done, and perhaps give a reward of some sort – a hug or small treat.

- Share tasks with trusted others, for company and safety.

- Share tasks fairly within the family, for example, boys and girls can share tasks or take turns to do them using a rota.

- Find ways of making the task easier and more suitable for children.

- Have adults take over tasks that involve risks to children's health, for example, carrying heavy loads and going to insecure places.

EXERCISE 28.3 THE VIRTUE OF DILIGENCE

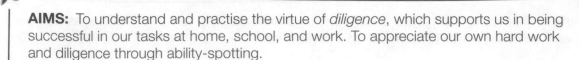

AIMS: To understand and practise the virtue of *diligence*, which supports us in being successful in our tasks at home, school, and work. To appreciate our own hard work and diligence through ability-spotting.

DESCRIPTION: Participants do ability-spotting in pairs, thinking of a time when they have been hard-working and diligent.

Directions[65]

1. Explain to the whole peer group that we are going to talk about a virtue called *diligence*.

Ask: 'Who can tell us the meaning of diligence?'

'Who can give us an example of people like us being diligent?'

Together, explain the meaning of 'diligence', adding information from Box 28.c if needed.

Box 28.c The virtue of diligence

Diligence is working hard, not giving up, and doing the best job we can. When we work diligently we can accomplish wonderful things.

When we practise diligence we develop ourselves and our families, and support each other in reaching the good life we wish for ourselves.

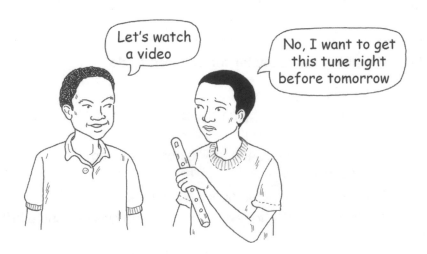

Consider these two sayings about diligence:
- 'Diligence is the mother of good fortune.'
- 'Life doesn't require that we be the best – only that we try our best.'

---

2. Ask participants to pair up and to interview each other, asking: 'Tell me about a time when you worked diligently and felt proud of yourself. What was the result?'

Encourage them to be curious and ask basic questions – where? when? how? who? what? – to expand the story, spot abilities, and add these to their necklaces.

Then invite each partner to ask the other: 'What other times have you been diligent?'

'How will you use this virtue to achieve your vision of an ideal future?'

3. Bring everyone back together and invite one or two participants to share their stories with the whole group.

4. Ask: 'Why is this virtue important in our lives?'

 ## EXERCISE 28.4 HOW DO WE SPEND OUR DAY?

AIM: To become more aware of how much time we spend on different activities through the day, and how that influences our lives.

DESCRIPTION: Participants draw timelines of their typical school and non-school days, and discuss the good things about them and what they might want to change.

Box 28.d Information for facilitators

Children need a balance of daily activities which meet their needs for learning in or out of school, playing, eating and drinking, resting, contributing to the household, interacting with peers and family, and exercising. They need support in balancing the virtue of diligence with other virtues, so that they stay in the middle of their river of wellbeing – not working too hard, nor doing less than the best they can.

Children benefit from time when caregivers focus purely on them. Even if it's only for 10 minutes a day, children will feel happy that this is their time, when they decide what to do together. This might be playing a game, reading a book together, or singing a song. Children may also enjoy doing tasks with their caretakers, such as shelling beans, if they can chat at the same time.

Caregivers have a responsibility to be aware of their child's daily activities, and to do their best to keep these in balance.

Some children are not able to attend school because they have too much domestic, care work, or economic work to do, or because they are ill. Strategies are needed to change this. Remind participants of Session 17 on going to school, and see Exercise 29.5 about protecting children from harmful work, in the next session about livelihoods.

Be alert to gender differences in this exercise: it is likely, for example, that girls do more tasks and have less time to do homework or play. Bringing caregivers and children together at the end of the exercise should enable caregivers to appreciate the contribution that children make, and provide a chance to change gender and generational norms.

Directions

1. Divide participants into males and females, and give each person two sheets of A4 paper and crayons. Ask them, on one of the sheets, to draw six columns, and give each pair of columns a heading (using words or symbols) for morning, afternoon, and evening. Start with a school day.

Children. Ask them to write or draw the time they get up and the time they go to bed at the beginning and end of the day. Then, in the first column of each pair of columns, ask them to add drawings or words about their activities in the morning, afternoon, and evening.

Caregivers. Ask them to do a timeline for their own activities, including those that involve their children.

Then ask participants to use the second column of each pair of columns to show how much time is spent on each activity. For example, draw one tick, two ticks, or three ticks, to show roughly how long it takes. See Table 28.1 for an example.

Table 28.1 Sample daily activities sheet

Morning (activity)	Morning (time spent)	Afternoon (activity)	Afternoon (time spent)	Evening (activity)	Evening (time spent)
06:30 Get up		Walk home from school	√√	Play with friend	√
Breakfast	√	Homework	√	Help caregiver cook dinner	√√
Walk to school	√√	Fetch wood	√√√	Have dinner	√
Maths	√	Fetch water	√√	Go to bed	
Biology	√				
Swahili	√				
Gardening	√				
Lunch	√				

Repeat this with a non-school day.

2. Ask participants to interview each other in pairs, asking: 'What do you like about your timeline? Why do you like that?'

'Would you like to change the pattern of activities: either the activities themselves or the time you spend on them? How and why would you like to change them?'

Invite them to use a different colour to mark on the sheet the changes they would like to make.

3. Bring the pairs together to make mind maps: one for the males' answers, and one for the females'. Write the words 'how we spend our days' in the middle. On the right put the things people like about their time-line. On the left put the things people would like to change. Use a different-coloured pen to show the change.

4. Ask the relevant peer groups:

Children. 'What would you like to say about your mind map to your caregiver?'

Caregiver. 'What would you like to say to your child about your mind map?'

5. Bring all peer groups together and ask them to lay out their timelines and mind maps. Together, talk about what they show, and similarities and differences between boys and girls of different ages in relation to:
- types of work done in school, at home, and to make money;
- leisure time;
- time spent with caregivers and other children.

6. Invite the children to pair up with their caregivers and share anything from their timelines that they wish.

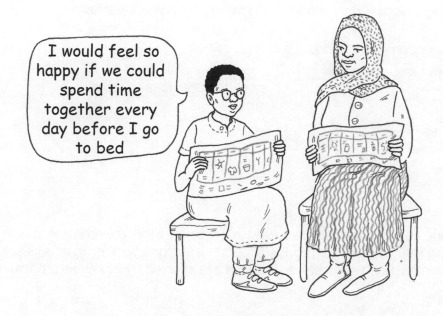

7. Invite participants to share their mind maps from Exercise 28.2 with the whole group, showing their ideas about changes they would like to see to make difficult tasks easier.

8. Explain that we will use the learning from this exercise again in the next session, which is about livelihoods.

Closing circle

Purpose: To gain a clearer sense of how we can find work we enjoy, and avoid harmful work; to evaluate ways of meeting our needs and wants now, and to think about ways of using resources wisely; and to plan economic activities as a step along our path to our vision of a good future.

Contents	Materials required	Time required
Opening circle (see p.13)		15 mins
29.1 The web of work	A ball of string, and an essential item such as clothing or food	30 mins
29.2 My dream occupation	Prepared flipchart of flower	30 mins
29.3 A tool to assess occupations		40 mins
29.4 Our path to an occupation that suits us		40 mins
29.5 Protecting children from harmful work	Knowledge of child labour laws	40 mins
29.6 Acquiring income and goods		40 mins
29.7 Using our resources wisely	Four sheets of flipchart paper stuck together for each small group	90 mins
29.8 Helping each other get started		40 mins
Closing circle (see p.14)		15 mins

About 6.5 hrs

Preparation

Find out if there are any organizations locally that support vulnerable children in going to school, help protect inheritance rights, or provide support for income-generating activities, and savings and credit schemes. Such services can help families affected by HIV avoid a downward spiral of poverty.

Exercise 29.1. Bring an essential item, or a picture of one, such as an item of food or a cotton shirt. Choose something that involves a chain of workers; not, for example, a vegetable grown in your own garden, which only involved you!

Exercise 29.2. Draw a big picture of a flower with questions on each petal, as illustrated in the picture on page 396. You may also want to prepare drawings of flowers with seven petals for children aged 5–8 years.

Exercise 29.7. Stick together four sheets of flip paper for each smaller group (total of 7) See picture on page 405.

Exercise 29.8. If you are in contact with people from any local organizations which offer economic support to vulnerable children and their families, you may wish to invite them to join this exercise.

EXERCISE 29.1 THE WEB OF WORK

AIM: To show how occupations link together in a web, and how all are valuable to our society.

DESCRIPTION: All participants come together to track the pathway and occupations that lead to an item being available for us to use.

Directions

1. Show the essential item you have brought and explain that we are going to identify all the workers who, together, make it available to us. This article is something that everyone, from a prime minister to the smallest child, needs to have.

Ask: 'What would happen to the prime minister if he/she did not eat food every day?'

'What would happen if he/she came to work without clothes?'

2. Ask everyone to stand in a circle, and ask someone to hold the item and the end of a ball of string. Explain that we are going to track backwards to the source of the item, and reveal the web of people who played their part in producing it. We will act as people with different occupations, and show the connections with the string. See the example in Box 29.a.

Box 29.a Example of a web of work

The item is some fried fish. Ask one person to hold the fish in one hand, and the end of the ball of string in the other.

Ask: 'What work was done before the fish was put on the plate?' The answer might be: 'It was cooked.'

Ask: 'Who cooked it?' Invite someone across the circle from you to act as the cook, and to take the ball of string, unwinding the string so that they are connected to the person holding the cooked fish.

Ask: 'What work was done before the fish was cooked?' The answer might be: 'Someone purchased it from the market.'

Ask: 'Who purchased it?' Invite someone else across the circle to act as the purchaser, and extend the string to them.

Ask: 'What work was done before the fish got to the market?' The answer might be: 'The fish seller purchased the fish from the lakeside and carried the fish on the bus.' Invite someone else across the circle to act as the fish seller in the web.

Ask: 'Who drove the bus?' Invite someone else to be the bus driver.

Ask: 'What work was done to bring the fish to the lakeside?' Invite someone to be the net puller who brought it to shore.

Ask: 'Who caught the fish?' Invite someone else to be the person who caught the fish.

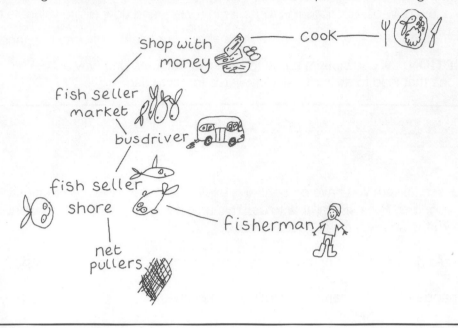

3. Invite participants to look at the web of workers you have created with the string pattern you are all now holding, and ask:

'Which work is done by males, females, or both?'

'What abilities and virtues are needed to do the various types of work?'

4. Invite participants to try removing various workers from the web and see what happens.

Ask: 'What happens if someone is struggling and drops out of the web?'

'What can we do to ensure that no one drops out?'

Explain that if someone is struggling, it makes the whole web weak. So it helps if we can all support them, rather than criticizing and blaming them. Then if at some stage we are struggling, we can count on their support.

5. Ask: 'What can we learn from this activity?'

If necessary, support participants in understanding that all work has its value to society: the work of a farmer or driver is as important in supporting the whole society as that of a doctor or lawyer. All occupations – and the people who do them – deserve respect.

Equally, everyone should be able to earn a decent living from their work in the web. In the household, income should be shared, so that children can be well nourished and go to school, women can get fair rewards for their work, and men and women can discuss how to use their resources together. The same is true of society.

Finally, the web shows us that when we all cooperate to work together, we can all strengthen our achievements, build our economy, and earn enough to live a good life.

EXERCISE 29.2 MY DREAM OCCUPATION

AIMS: To dream that we are working in an occupation that fits our preferences and talents in our vision of a good future. To think about our talents, preferences, and motivations for future work, and use this tool when we are older and considering occupations.

DESCRIPTION: Participants imagine that they are doing work in the future that suits them very well, and write answers to questions on the drawing of a flower.

Box 29.b Information for facilitator

In this exercise we help children think about their preferences for different aspects of work; this is more helpful than asking what they want to be when they grow up, without thinking about the reality of that work and their talents. They and their caregivers can use this same tool as they grow up and learn more about themselves and work opportunities. Being positive about work and knowing what we have to offer greatly strengthens our motivation and the interest of employers.

Directions[66]

1. Explain that the better we know ourselves and what we like in relation to work, the easier it can be to take up occupations that suit us. If we enjoy our work and feel positive about it, we will do our work better and feel happier.

2. Show and explain the picture of the flower that you have prepared. Ask everyone to draw their own flower, with seven empty petals. Explain that before we fill in the petals, we are going to dream.

3. Invite participants to sit together in pairs and shut their eyes.

Read out the following directions and questions. With *caregivers*, adapt the wording so that they are dreaming of the type of work they would like for their child; something they think would suit them and give them a good future.

Say: 'We are going to dream, and imagine that we are 20 years old and that we are working in an occupation that makes us happy. I am going to ask you the questions on the flower one by one, and ask you to imagine your answer to that question. You don't have to know what your occupation is; just imagine the different aspects of it that make you feel good.So now, imagine that you are 20 years old and you are in an occupation that suits you.'

Question 1. 'What is your purpose in life? What do you live for? What do you feel passionate about? How does your work fit with your passions?'

Question 2. 'What areas of knowledge are you using in your occupation? What subjects do you like at school and what you are good at? Now imagine you are using this very knowledge in your occupation. For example, is it about plants or animals, music, mechanics, health …?'

Question 3. 'What skills and abilities are you using? Think about your necklace. For example, are you communicating with people? Are you creating art or drama? Are you producing or selling something?'

Question 4. 'What are your working conditions like? Do you work inside or outside? Are you in a team or do you work alone? Are you moving about or sitting at a desk? Do you have to stick to time or can you be flexible? How many hours do you work every day? Do you have enough time for your partner and children?'

Question 5. 'What sort of people are you working with? Do you have a boss or do you work for yourself? How much responsibility do you have? What benefits does your work bring to the community? Who benefits from it?'

Question 6. 'Where are you living? Is it in the town or a rural area? Do you stay in one place or travel?'

Question 7. 'What rewards do you get for your work? What income do you get? What satisfaction do you get?'

4. Invite participants to open their eyes, but to continue to imagine they are in their future role. Ask them to write a few words, or draw a picture, on each petal of their flower, to remind themselves of their answers.

5. Ask participants to pair up and interview each other to find out more and add to their pictures.

Questions

Answers

6. Ask participants to see individually if they can think of one or two occupations that might fit with their flower.

7. Put all the flowers on the floor or wall, and invite participants to share one thing they have learned about themselves, and one thing they have learned about their partner, from this exercise.

8. Explain that we will now do an exercise to analyse different occupations.

 EXERCISE 29.3 A TOOL TO ASSESS OCCUPATIONS

AIMS: To use the learning from the flower exercise to rate occupations.

DESCRIPTION: Participants talk about all the occupations they can think of, then individually choose three occupations that might suit them (their children), and score it against each factor in their own flower.

Box 29.c Information for facilitators

Children may not know what occupation would suit them, but this tool will enable them to think critically about the characteristics of a job or business, and judge how well it would suit their talents and vision of the future. The tool also supports children in being realistic about the future. This is not to have low expectations, but to understand what is needed to reach preferred occupations.

Acknowledge that many people have to take whatever work opportunities are available, but they can keep their dreams in mind and use any work experience to build general skills and perhaps to save and invest in new skills.

Directions

1. Divide your peer group into males and females. Explain that we are going to use what we learned in the last exercise to see how different occupations might suit us (our children) in the future.

2. Invite each participant to say some occupations that might interest them (their children) when they are about 20 years old. After hearing lots of ideas, ask them each to focus on one of them.

3. Ask them to write, or draw a symbol for, this occupation in the corner of their flower picture, and then to score how well it fits each petal factor, for example:
- Low   1 point
- Medium   2 points
- High   3 points
- Don't know ?

For example, a girl may think she knows a lot about trading, so puts 3 points by that petal; but she thinks the rewards are likely to be low, so puts 1 point by that petal.

4. Ask participants to add up the scores and write the total by the word or symbol for the job.

5. Ask everyone to repeat the activity for two more occupations, using different-coloured pens, and compare the results.

6. Bring participants together to share their flowers.

Ask: 'What can we learn from this activity?'

7. Explain that some factors may be more important to us than others when we choose an occupation. For example, we may be willing to have a lower income and work longer hours, because we are passionate about the work.

8. Ask the relevant peer groups:

Children. 'How can this tool help us as we grow up?'

Caregivers. 'How might we use this tool, and the flower from Exercise 29.2, for ourselves?' Point out that our talents, skills, and ideas change as we grow. It's good to do this exercise again, for example every year.

 ## EXERCISE 29.4 OUR PATH TO AN OCCUPATION THAT SUITS US

AIM: To think about what we (our children) need to do to take up an occupation that suits us/them.

DESCRIPTION: Participants imagine that they are doing their chosen occupation and work backwards to imagine the steps they (their children) did to take it up. This is called 'backlighting'.

Box 29.d Information for facilitators

Participants may not have a single occupation in mind, which is fine. Ask them to think about the preferences they identified in Exercise 29.2, and the types of jobs that appeal to them. For example, they might feel that they want to run their own business, or become some kind of health worker. Ask them to choose one occupation that suits them which they can backlight in this exercise.

Encourage participants to be realistic about their chosen occupation and the amount of time they have to take it up. For example, if a participant wants to become president, ask them to think first about the steps needed to become a politician.

Directions

1. Explain that we will now think about the occupation which suits us (our children) to understand how we (they) would take up that profession. Ask participants to work individually, or in small groups if there are several people interested in the same occupation. Ask them to imagine they (their children) are in the future, doing their chosen occupation, while they work backwards to imagine the steps they took to get there (backlighting).

 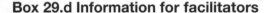

2. Give each person or group some paper and crayons or pencils. Ask them to start by drawing their occupation or idea at the top of the paper.

Ask: 'What happened just before you (your child) started this work?' For example, 'I passed my Teaching Certificate.'

Draw symbols or write a few words to show this event.

3. Thinking backwards, ask: 'What were you (they) doing before that?' For example, 'I studied at the Teacher Training College for two years.'

4. Continue going back in time until you reach the present day.

5. Go back up along the path and ask what resources you needed for each step and how you acquired those resources. Ask: 'Who helped you (them)? How did you afford the college fees?'

6. Explain that in the next but one exercise, we will look at the present time and see what resources we need, and how we can each use our resources wisely, to start along our path towards the occupations that suit us (our children). First, however, we will look at how we can protect children from harmful work.

 ## EXERCISE 29.5 PROTECTING CHILDREN FROM HARMFUL WORK

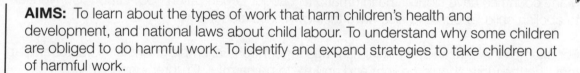

AIMS: To learn about the types of work that harm children's health and development, and national laws about child labour. To understand why some children are obliged to do harmful work. To identify and expand strategies to take children out of harmful work.

DESCRIPTION: Participants list harmful work that children might do, read and reflect on a story, and share positive methods that families have used to keep their children in school and protect them from harmful work.

Box 29.e Information for facilitators

This is an essential topic, because poverty is a major cause and consequence of HIV, and children affected by HIV are very vulnerable to being exploited by others and obliged to do harmful work.

Directions[67]

1. Explain that we are going to look at how we might protect children from harmful work.

2. Ask: 'What do we mean by harmful work? What makes work harmful?'

'Who can give some examples?'

As needed, add information from Box 29.f.

Box 29.f What work is harmful to children?

Work is harmful to children's health and development if:

- It deprives them of their rights to go to school, play, and enjoy leisure and rest.
- It goes on for too long with no rest. For example, girls doing domestic work often work for 14 hours a day, seven days a week.
- It is not appropriate to the child's age and development. For example, lifting heavy loads of water or firewood over long distances can cause permanent physical damage, especially when a child is young.
- It involves abusive punishment and little or no appreciation, payment, love, or care.
- The working environment is dangerous to children's health and safety. For example, in commercial agriculture, a building site, mining, or a busy road.
- It involves forced sexual activities and risk of violence. For example, sex work and forced sex in domestic service.

2. Ask: 'What does the law say about children working in our country?'

Explain the laws, and add information from Box 29.g as needed.

Box 29.g Child labour laws and rights

Many countries have signed the International Labour Organization (ILO) Labour Convention to abolish child labour, and also have their own child labour laws.

For example, in Tanzania, the minimum age for contractual employment is 14 years, and at that age the work should be light and unlikely to be harmful. Children under 18 years are not allowed to work in ships, mines, or on hazardous worksites.

However, in many countries child labour is common and the law is weakly enforced.

3. Tell one of the following three stories (see Box 29.h), or make up your own story, to feature the kind of harmful labour that is common in local communities.

After telling the story, ask the following questions:

- Does this happen in our community and school?
- Which rights are violated in this situation?
- What are the reasons that children do harmful work?
- What effect does this have on their lives?
- If it happened to us or our friends, what could we do to support each other?

Box 29.h Stories about harmful labour

Option 1: The young farmers

Huseina was eight years old when she and her younger brother Juma were orphaned and sent to live with relatives a long way away. Their new caregivers were poor, and didn't enrol them in school. Instead the children had to work long hours in the market and on the farm. One day a woman at the market asked them why they were not in school. They explained what had happened, and learned that the woman worked for a local non-governmental organization, and wanted to help them. She arranged to visit the caregivers, and they talked together about the children's needs and visions, and the benefits of going to school. She got a small grant to help them with school expenses, and the family found ways of sharing household tasks and prioritizing the use of family income so that Huseina and Juma could return to school. They still had to help with tasks after school, but were glad to be able to learn and play with other children once again.

Option 2: Meeting Chiku's needs

When Chiku's parents died she went to live with her auntie and uncle in the city. She was 13 years old. She had five cousins who were going to school, and her auntie and uncle struggled to make ends meet. They complained about the additional cost of keeping Chiku, and she was afraid to ask them for anything. One day her auntie said: 'Chiku, your dress is torn and too small, and your skin looks rough – you are a disgrace! You see how nice your friend Kisima next door looks, why don't you try to be like her?' Chiku talked to Kisima, who told her that a man called Idi gave her money for her things, and he could find Chiku a friend too.

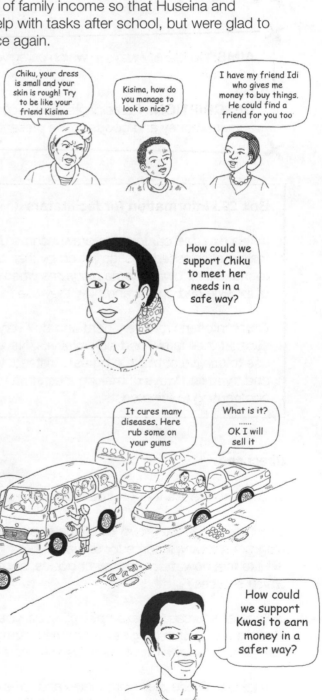

Chiku, your dress is small and your skin is rough! Try to be like your friend Kisima

Kisima, how do you manage to look so nice?

I have my friend Idi who gives me money to buy things. He could find a friend for you too

How could we support Chiku to meet her needs in a safe way?

It cures many diseases. Here rub some on your gums

What is it? ...... OK I will sell it

How could we support Kwasi to earn money in a safer way?

Option 3: Kwasi the 'medicine' seller

When his mother died, Kwasi was left to look after his two younger sisters. He was 11 years old and wanted to stay in school and keep his sisters in school too. How could he earn enough money for the family? He tried selling soft drinks to drivers, but the money was never enough and he hated moving amid the traffic; he had seen other children hit by cars. One day a man approached him and said, 'Would you like to sell this medicine for me? I will give you 1,000 shillings a bag.' The medicine was a white powder; the man said that it cured many diseases. He invited Kwasi to rub a little bit on his gums. It made him feel happy. He didn't know that it was an illegal drug: cocaine. He agreed to sell the medicine.

4. Ask participants to form small groups and to tell positive stories of how families they know (it could be their own) have managed to keep their children away from harmful work and send them to school. What abilities and strategies have people used to support themselves or their friends? Ask the groups to put all their ideas on a mind map, with 'ways to protect our children from harmful work' in the middle. Ask them to see how different parts of the mind map link up.

5. Bring the groups together and share the mind maps.

Ask: 'Is there anything that we can do locally, together, to address the issue of child labour?'

 ## EXERCISE 29.6 ACQUIRING INCOME AND GOODS

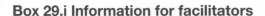

AIMS: To identify ways in which caregivers and children acquire money or goods at this time.

DESCRIPTION: Participants draw income diagrams to show how people like them acquire money and goods at the present time.

Box 29.i Information for facilitators

In this exercise participants draw income diagrams for people like them, so that no one feels embarrassed or stigmatized by their own economic situation. Encourage participants to make their own income diagrams when they go home, and to think about their sources of income and goods and how they use them.

Children often work very hard and do everything they can, including dangerous things, to support their family and sick relatives. Never be judgemental about strategies that children use to survive or make progress. Instead, talk about the good and challenging points, and try to find ways of making their strategies safer, or identify alternative strategies for contributing to living costs.

Directions

1. Direct the relevant peer groups as follows:

Children. Divide the group into females and males. Invite them to work together to draw a diagram showing income for someone like them. Invite them to ask themselves: 'For this boy/girl like me, how much money or goods, such as food or clothes, does he/she get roughly from which sources?'

Include all sources, for example: gifts; activities that may be disapproved of, such as begging, stealing and exchanging sex for money; farming; or getting money from the family or an NGO. Ask people to write numbers or use symbols to represent, for example, 1,000 shillings.

Caregivers. Divide them into males and females and divide these again into two groups of caregivers of 5-8 years and 9-14 years children. . Invite each group to draw a diagram showing income for someone like them; for a child like theirs; and any other income in the household.

All peer groups. Ask caregivers and children to write or draw the income sources down the left side of the flipchart paper, with their amounts, and leave the right side blank for Exercise 29.7. Tell them not to spend a lot of time working out the amounts, just to do it roughly.

2. Explain that we will now discuss the good and challenging points about ways that people like us acquire money and goods at present, and possible alternatives. Then in Exercise 29.7 we will look at how we use these resources, and how we might use them differently. In Exercise 29.8 we will look at safe local opportunities, currently available, to gain livelihood skills and earn resources.

3. Direct children and caregivers as follows:

Children. Ask children, in their peer groups, to form groups of three boys or three girls. Give each group one of the sources of income or goods drawn on their diagram made in step 1.

Caregivers. Ask caregivers to divide into groups of three. Give some groups one of their own sources of income; some groups one of their child's source of income; and some groups another source of income from their diagrams made in step 1.

4. *All peer groups*. Ask the groups to discuss: 'What are the good points about this way of getting money or goods to meet our needs at this time?'

'What are the challenging points about this way of getting money or goods to meet our needs at this time?'

Ask them to create a role play where: one person is thinking about using this way to meet their needs; one is in favour of it; and the other believes there are better ways of getting money and goods.

5. Ask each group of three, in turn, to show their role play to the rest of the peer group. After each one, ask the following questions:

- What are the positive things about this way of acquiring things?
- What are the negative things about this way of acquiring things?
- What would you do if you were making a decision about this option? What are your reasons?

If any participant feels that there are better ways of meeting the person's needs, ask: 'What alternative suggestions do you have? How would you show your friend love, and what would you say and do to support them in finding an alternative?'

 EXERCISE 29.7 USING OUR RESOURCES WISELY

AIMS: To think about how we use our resources, and ways of reducing and prioritizing expenditure.

DESCRIPTION: Participants add expenditure on different items, for a person like them, to their income diagram, and total up income and expenditure; they identify things that they would like to have, but do not divide them into needs and wants – instead they allocate each item to one of three categories (survival, feeling good, and making progress); they look at the immediate and future costs and benefits of an item; and they share ways of spending less, using resources wisely, avoiding waste, and saving for the future.

Box 29.j Information for facilitators

It is good to have opportunities to think about the things we need and want, and the benefits they bring. We may say in a judgemental way that people 'need' things to survive, such as food, shelter, and clothing, but they only 'want' mobile phones and nice clothes. However, we need to understand what the phone and clothes may mean for a person's self-compassion, connection with others, and success in achieving their vision of their future.

People usually define 'needs' as those things that people need to survive and have a reasonable quality of life. 'Wants' are things that people would like to have, but they are able to manage without them. However, it is not always easy to separate the two, because the 'wants' may be important for meeting the 'needs'. It is important to discuss this topic, and become aware about the difference between things that advertising is pushing us to buy, and things that will really support a good life.

Directions

1. Explain that in this exercise we will look at expenditure for a person like us and add it to our income diagram. We are going to look at our needs at this time; things that we have to buy, produce, or get. We will look at things we need to survive, to feel good about ourselves, to be part of our community, and to make progress towards the vision we have for our good future. We will see whether we want to change how we use our resources in a way that improves our lives.

2. Divide your peer group into males and females and make sure that they have their income diagrams from Exercise 29.6.

3. Ask: 'What does a girl or boy like you (your child) spend income on at this time?'

Ask them to draw or write each item on separate pieces of paper and keep them for later in the exercise. Then ask them to make a rough estimate of what they might spend on each item; and add these items and costs to their income diagram, using the columns on the right-hand side.

4. Ask them to add up the amount of income and expenditure, and put the totals at the bottom of the columns.

Ask: 'What do we learn from our income and expenditure diagram?'

'Which amount is greater, the income or the expenditure?'

'If the expenditure is greater, how can we manage?'

5. Explain that we will look in more detail about how we use our resources later in the exercise. In the meantime, direct the relevant peer groups as follows:

Children. Ask the boys to lay out the pieces of paper showing items of expenditure they prepared in step 3. Then ask them to work together to draw or write on separate small pieces of paper all the additional items that a boy like them might like to have. Ask girls to do the same for a girl of their age. Encourage them to think of as many items as they can.

Caregivers. Ask them to divide into three groups: one looking at their own needs/wants, one looking at their children's, and one looking at their households' needs/wants. Each group should then draw or write on separate small pieces of paper the relevant needs/wants. They do not have to decide whether they are needs or wants, or label them as such.

When they have finished, ask the group to give you their paper slips.

6. Ask participants in their groups to draw a picture of the person like them on the four sheets of flip paper stuck together you prepared, or on the ground. Ask them to draw three big circles around the person, one inside the other, leaving enough space to put the slips in each one. Ask them to write 'Survival' in the first circle (closest to the person).

This is for all the things needed to thrive and grow up into a person with a strong body, heart, and mind; for example, food, water, shelter, clothing and education, love and friendship, hugs, a gentle touch, and a sense of safety.

7. Now ask participants to write 'Feeling Good' in the second (middle) circle.

This is all the things we need to feel good, connect with others, make friends, be attractive, and be accepted as a member of the community. Examples might be: soap and moisturizer, decent clothes that fit us, a mobile phone, enough money to meet up with friends and attend events. It may also include things we use to relax and stay in our river of wellbeing, such as music or alcohol. Buying clothes or objects that are admired by our peer group can also make us feel good.

8. Ask participants to write 'Making Progress' in the third (widest) circle.

This is for all the items needed to move along the path to reach our vision of the future. For example, items which may help us: connect with sources of support; be accepted by a school, college, or training course; get a loan or a job; or attract a good potential spouse or partner.

Remind people of their backlit path to a good future; what did they need? Examples might be a mobile phone, money to travel, books, access to the internet, nice clothes.

9. Mix up all the slips of paper marked with items that participants would like to have, and give them out to participants. Ask them to take it in turns to place them in one of the circles, explaining why they feel it is a need for survival, for feeling good, or for making progress towards their vision of their future. If anyone disagrees, ask them to suggest a new place and to explain their reasons. Try to agree where to put the item, but if people can't agree, put that piece of paper to one side. Some items may

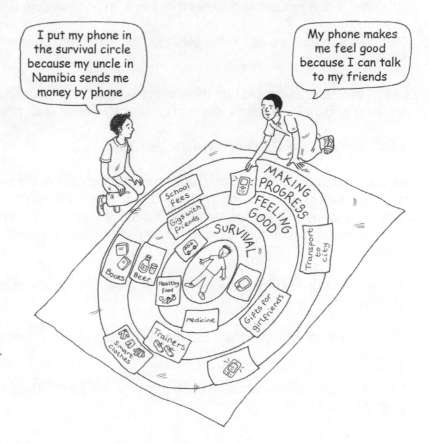

belong to more than one category. That's fine: place them across the lines, or make another slip for the same item.

10. When you've sorted all the pieces of paper, ask: 'What have we learned from this exercise?'

Ask: 'Are there any items which may make us feel good, but may be harmful for us? (for example: alcohol, cigarettes, unhealthy food).

'If we had to cut five items, which would we take out?'

'Which of the items in the Feeling Good circle also help us progress towards our vision of the future?'

11. As a group, estimate roughly what proportion of resources is spent on the three different circles.

Ask: 'Does anyone think we should spend more on a particular circle? What are your reasons?'

Then ask: 'If we spend more on this circle, which circle would we spend less on? What are your reasons?'

12. Select an item which participants think is important, and which is fairly costly, perhaps where there were differing views; for example, a mobile phone. Explain that we are going to look at the benefits and costs of having that item, now and in the future, to help us explore whether it is a good use of our resources.

13. Make two columns on a piece of flipchart paper, headed 'Benefits' and 'Costs'. Divide the columns into two. Label them so the top half of the columns is for benefits and costs 'now', and the bottom half for benefits and costs 'in the future'. Ask the relevant peer groups:

Children. 'What are all the benefits that this item gives people like us, now and in the future?'

Caregivers. 'What are all the benefits that this item gives children like ours, now and in the future?'

List all the benefits people can think of in the 'now' and 'future' benefits column. These can be any kind of benefit: practical, economic, social, or emotional; now or in the future.

14. Ask: 'What are all the costs of this item?'

Include the actual price and any running costs; the cost of the work needed to pay for it (hours of work, risks, time lost to studying); and the 'opportunity cost' (what else you might have done with that money). There may be other costs. For example, for a mobile phone there are risks, such as having it stolen, access to pornography, and the possibility of risky interactions with adults.

15. Say: 'Put up your hands if you think this item is a good use of resources. What are your reasons?'

'Put up your hands if you think this item is not a good use of resources. What are your reasons?'

16. Ask: 'How can we increase the benefits of this item?' Then ask: 'How can we reduce the costs of this item?'

For example, for a mobile phone we might increase the benefits by sharing it within the family, and reduce the costs by buying a basic phone.

17. Ask: 'What have we learned from this activity?'

18. Invite participants to try to weigh up the immediate and future costs and benefits, and consider how to reduce costs and increase benefits, next time they are making a decision on whether to buy something.

19. Invite participants to form small groups, and to share ways they could spend less, use resources wisely, avoid waste, and save for the future.

20. Ask each group to share their best methods with the whole group.

 EXERCISE 29.8 HELPING EACH OTHER GET STARTED

AIMS: To build confidence in contributing to household income in a small way that can grow as we grow older. To see how children might start, or make progress on, an income-generating project in their community, using local skills, in addition to going to school. To look for ways of supporting children who are struggling with poverty.

DESCRIPTION: Participants hear a story, then draw or write what they want to do now to learn skills, earn money, or support their children in making steps towards a good future. Participants develop their plans, with those who have similar starting ideas working together. This includes identifying local resources such as loans or vocational training.

GROUPS: All the peer groups do this exercise together. If you have invited any local organizations to join you in this exercise, do introductions; invite the visitors to talk about what support they can offer and to work with the participants in developing their plans.

Directions[68]

1. Bring the children and caregivers together. Explain that we are going to work together to see how we might start, or make progress on, an income-generating project in our community, using local skills. We understand the importance of going to school and doing well, so we will talk about activities which we could do after school or at weekends. If some participants want to prioritize school at this time, they can think about a time in the future when they are ready to start income-generating activities.

2. Begin by reading, or inviting people to role play, the story of a child of their age / their child's age who started growing or making things in a small way, and gradually built up their skills and capital to become the owner of a good business. (Make up your own story to fit the context.)

3. Explain that we will now explore what we might do to gain skills and capital with the support of our caregivers.

4. Ask people to call out different kinds of income-generating activities in the community.

5. Ask caregivers and children to do this homework together:
- Select a way of making money that the child is interested in, and find out: i) the skills needed to do the work and how people learned these skills; ii) whether adults are passing these skills on to their children; and iii) what opportunities exist for the child to learn them, informally or through vocational training (in which case, how can someone become a student, and what does the training involve and cost?)
- Share what they learn with the group in their own time or at a future follow-up.

6. Ask: 'What economic support is available locally for children and their families in our community?'

You might want to arrange a meeting after the workshop, and invite someone from a relevant organization to talk to participants about their services, and answer questions.

7. Support pairs of children and their caregivers in deciding what actions they might want to take now to get skills or earn money. Give them paper and invite them to draw together what steps they might take along their road to a good future. If any participants feel that they or their children do not have the time or resources to get involved in income generation at this time, remind them that they can imagine a time in the future instead.

8. Ask everyone to hold up their paper and to form groups with other participants who have a similar idea for a first step.

9. Ask each group to make a start-up action plan.
- How will they learn the skills they need? How will they use them?
- How will they move along their path to their vision of a good future?
- How might they support each other in meeting their needs?

Add ideas from Box 29.k as appropriate.

Box 29.k Ideas for earning skills, earning money, and supporting each other

- Caregivers teach children to grow food and do household tasks, for example, maintaining the roof.
- Caregivers who have a skill (for example, sewing or carpentry) hold free classes to teach children.
- Caregivers train older children as apprentices, after school.
- Children participate in agricultural projects, benefiting from training and produce.
- Caregivers and children from the *Stepping Stones* group organize a revolving savings fund. When it is their turn to receive a lump sum, they use it for school or business expenses.
- Caregivers and children from the *Stepping Stones* groups hold fundraising activities to help those among them who struggle most. For example: a concert, a school fair, a play, the sale of healthy snacks to school children, the sale of old clothes, the creation and sale of toys and other items.
- Caregivers and children collect items, such as unwanted uniforms, school books, stationery, and soap, to share with the poorest children among them.

Closing circle

Ask each child and caregiver to draw a big flower, and write or draw in it something that has helped or is helping them / their child to achieve their vision of a good future. Bring all the flowers together to make a display of ideas on 'how to nurture our visions'. Ask each child and caregiver to explain aloud what they have drawn and written.

Praise the children for all their great ideas and encourage them in supporting one another. Explain that the flowers represent the changes they've made, or good things they have continued to do, to reach their dreams. And the flowers lead to their visions for the future!

REFERENCES

The material in this manual has been compiled from a large range of manuals, books, newsletters and websites. Below is a list of references to the sources used in developing exercises. See also Acknowledgements (p.vii) for list of permissions and acknowledgments.

Introduction

1. Welbourn, A. (2016) *Stepping Stones and Stepping Stones Plus: A training package on gender, generation, HIV, communication and relationship skills,* Practical Action Publishing, Rugby, UK, <www.steppingstonesfeedback.org> [last accessed 22 October 2015].

2. McAdam, E., Welbourn, A., Steinberg, C., Oljemark, K., and McAdam, K. (2011) *NAMWEZA Friends' Intervention Programme.*

3. Popov, L. K. (2000) *The Virtues Project Educator's Guide: Simple Ways to Create a Culture of Character,* Jalmar Press, and Pro.Ed USA, <www.virtuesproject.org> [last accessed 22 October 2015].

4. Keeping Children Safe (2014) *Child Safeguarding Standards and how to implement them,* Keeping Children Safe <www.keepingchildrensafe.org.uk/resources> [last accessed 22 October 2015].

5. International HIV/AIDS Alliance (2014) *Safeguarding the rights of children and young people: A guide to facilitating a workshop with Alliance Linking Organisations and partners working with vulnerable children and young people.* International HIV/AIDS Alliance. <http://www.aidsalliance.org/assets/000/001/694/LinkUp_safeguarding_manual_original. pdf?1433343519> [last accessed 22 October 2015].

6. Ibarra, K.; Miller, J.; Wagner, F., and the Teresa Group on behalf of the Coalition for Children Affected by AIDS (2014) *Difficult Decisions: A Tool for Care Workers* <www. careworkerethics.org> [last accessed 22 October 2015].

Session 1 Getting Started

7. Brakarsh, J. (2005) *The Journey of Life: A community workshop to support children. Section 3 The Journey of Life for children* REPSSI (Regional Psychosocial Support Initiative) <http:// childprotectionforum.org/wp/wp-content/uploads/downloads/2011/11/Journey-of-Life-1-Community-Workshop.pdf> [last accessed 22 October 2015].

Session 2 Using our Brains

8. Siegel, D. J., and Payne Bryson, T. (2012) *The Whole-Brain Child: 12 Revolutionary Strategies to Nurture Your Child's Developing Mind,* Bantam USA.

9. Siegel D. J., Payne Bryson, T. (2014) *No-Drama Discipline: The Whole-Brain Way to Calm the Chaos and Nurture Your Child's Developing Mind* Bantam, USA.

10. Gilbert, P. (2009) *The Compassionate Mind.* London, Constable and Robinson.

Session 3 Gender and Sex

11. International HIV/AIDS Alliance (2006) *Our Future: Sexuality and life skills education for young people, Grades 4–5* International HIV/AIDS Alliance <http://www.aidsalliance. org/resources/351-our-future-sexuality-and-lifeskills-education-for-young-people> [last accessed 22 October 2015].

12. International HIV/AIDS Alliance (2008) *Sexuality and Life-Skills: Participatory activities on sexual and reproductive health with young people* International HIV/AIDS Alliance <http://www.aidsalliance.org/assets/000/000/709/295-Sexuality-and-life-skills_original. pdf?1406297244> [last accessed 22 October 2015].

13. Popov, L. K. (2000) op. cit., page 151.

Session 4 Children's rights

14. Sr Mallmann, Silke-Andrea (2003) *Building Resilience in Children Affected by HIV/AIDS*. Maskew Miller Longman.

15. Popov, L.K. (2000) op. cit., pp.191–192.

16. International HIV/AIDS Alliance (2006) op. cit., Pages 19–21.

Session 5 The Tree of Life

17. Georgia, Jovia, Kenny, Lucy and Sandra (2009) 'The "Tree of Life" in a Community Context', *CONTEXT* number 105, October 2009, pp 50–54 <http://dulwichcentre.com. au/wp-content/uploads/2014/01/tree-of-life-community-context.pdf> [last accessed 22 October 2015].

Session 6 Assertiveness

18. Popov, L.K. (2000) op. cit. p.135.

19. International HIV/AIDS Alliance (2008) op. cit. pp.48–53.

Session 7 All About Virtues

20. Popov, L.K. (2000) op.cit.

Session 8 The power of love

21. Siegel, D. (2012) op.cit. page 129.

22. Popov, L.K. (2000) op.cit. page 195.

23. Moyo Fulata Lusungu (2011) *Parenting: A journey of Love Called to Care No.10* Strategies For Hope Trust. <http://www.stratshope.org/o-order.htm> [last accessed 22 October 2015].

24. Moyo Fulata Lusungu (2011) op.cit. pp.38–39.

Session 9 Bringing out the best in each other

25. Popov, L.K. (2000) op.cit. pp.143–144.

26. Neff, K. (2011) *Self-compassion The proven power of being kind to yourself* William Morrow <www.mindfulselfcompassion.org> [last accessed 22 October 2015].

27. Siegel, D. (2014) op.cit. pp.20–23.

28. Ibid., pp.226–227.

29. Moyo Fulata Lusungu (2011) op.cit. pp.45–46.

30. Neff, K. (2015) *Self-compassion Guided meditations and exercises. Exercise 4* <www.self-compassion.org/category/exercises> [last accessed 22 October 2015].

Session 10 Loss and the Tree of Life

31. Carnegie, R. (2006) *River of Hope: Child-centred approaches to HIV and AIDS. A resource manual for working with children and their communities* Healthlink Worldwide.

32. Brakarsh, J. with Project Concern International (2009) *Say and Play: Tulande no kwangala. A tool for young children and those who care for them.* Project Concern International, e-mail info@pcizambia.org.zm

33. REPSSI (2005) The Journey of Life. A community workshop to support children. *Action Workshop 2: Helping our children to understand Death* Pages 35–37.

34. Brakarsh, J. with Project Concern International (2009) Op.cit. page 32.

35. Crossley, G. Sheppard, K. (2000) *Muddles, Puddles and Sunshine: Your activity book to help when someone has died,* Hawthorn Press and Winston's Wish, UK.

Session 11 Coping with Loss and Death

36. Brakarsh, J. with Project Concern International (2009) op.cit. pp.32–34.

37. Crossley, G., Sheppard, K. (2000) op.cit. pp.18–19.

38. REPSSI (2005) *Action Workshop 2* op.cit. pp.38–42.

39. Carnegie, R. (2006) op.cit. p.75.

40. Crossley, G., Sheppard, K. (2000) op.cit. p.26.

Session 12 All About HIV

41. Winkler, G. and Bodenstein, M. (2005) *Teaching about HIV and AIDS,* Macmillan Education.

42. Clay, Sue; Chiiya, Chipo; Chonta, Mutale (2007) *Understanding and challenging HIV stigma : toolkit for action.* Module I: children and stigma. <http://www.icrw.org/files/images/ Understanding-and-challenging-HIV-stigma-Module-I.pdf>, [last accessed 22 October 2015].

43. International HIV/AIDS Alliance (2008) op.cit. p.137.

Session 13 Testing and talking about HIV

44. Carnegie, R. (2006) Op.cit Page 57.

45. Friends Intervention Programme (2011) Op.cit. Page 146.

46. Namiba, Angelina (2013) 'Telling you child you have HIV', Guest blog post on *Speaking Up! The Diary of an HIV+ Activist* <http://hivpolicyspeakup.wordpress.com/2013/04/11/telling-your-child-you-have-hiv> [last accessed 22 October 2015].

Session 14 Living well with HIV

47. Hejoaka, F. (2009) 'Care and Secrecy: Being a mother of children living with HIV in Burkina Faso', *Social Science & Medicine* 69: 869–876 http://www.deepdyve.com/lp/elsevier/ care-and-secrecy-being-a-mother-of-children-living-with-hiv-in-burkina-PSrBbo1pRU

48. Ramsden, N. and Vawda, C. (2007) *You and Your Child with HIV – Living positively,* Children's Rights Centre <http://botswanateenclub.files.wordpress.com/2009/03/you__ your_child_with_hiv_living_positively.pdf> [last accessed 22 October 2015].

Session 15 Partners in Health Care

49. International HIV/AIDS Alliance (2007) '*The Health Journey: Understanding the dimensions of care and treatment for people with HIV A community centred methodology*', International HIV/AIDS Alliance.

50. Siegel, D. (2012) op. cit. p.113.

Session 16 Friendship

51. Popov, L.K. (2000) op. cit. pp.171–172.

Session 17 Going to School

52. Harrison, K., International AIDS Alliance (2009) *Building Hope: Supporting work with children affected by HIV and AIDS by UK*: Macmillan Education. Order from Teaching-Aids at Low Cost: http://www.talcuk.org

Session 19 Growing Up

53. International HIV/AIDS Alliance (2006) *Our Future Grades 4–5* op. cit. pp.39–44.

54. Gordon, G (2007) *Choices: A guide for young people.* London: Macmillan Education, pp.28–29, order in English or French from: <http://www.talcuk.org>.

Session 20 Relationships, love and sex

55. International HIV/AIDS Alliance (2008) *Sexuality and Life-skills,* op. cit. pp.44.

Session 21 Our Sexual Feelings and Sexual Safety

56. International HIV/AIDS Alliance (2008) *Sexuality and Life-skills* op. cit. p.71.

Session 22 Pornography

57. Bish Training (2015) *Planet Porn Making it easier to talk about porn,* Bish Training <www.bishtraining.com/index-php/planet-porn> the exercises in this session draw on material from Bish Training.

Session 23 Delaying and stopping early sex

58. International HIV/AIDS Alliance (2008) op. cit. p.65.

Session 24 All about condoms

59. Garvey, M. (2003), *Dying to Learn, Young people, HIV and the churches,* Christian Aid, London, <http://www.christianaid.org.uk/images/dying_to_learn.pdf> [last accessed 22 October 2015].

Session 25 Children by Choice not Chance

60. International HIV/AIDS Alliance (2006) *Our Future Grades 4–5* op.cit. p.89.

61. Gordon, G. (2007) op. cit. p.111.

Session 26 Protecting each other from sexual abuse

62. International Save The Children Alliance (2008) *A Common Responsibility: The role of community-based child protection groups in protecting children from sexual abuse and exploitation.* UK: International Save The Children Alliance <http://www.savethechildren.org.uk/resources/online-library/a-common-responsibility-the-role-of-community-based-child-protection-groups-in-protecting-children-from-sexual-abuse-and-exploitation> [last accessed 22 October 2015].

Session 27 Supporting survivors of sexual abuse

63. Brakarsh, J. with Project Concern International (2009) op. cit. p.22–24.

64. McAdam, E., (2015) Personal communication.

Session 28 Learning and Contributing

65. Popov, L.K. (2000) op. cit. pp.161–2.

Session 29 Livelihoods

66. Bolles, Richard (2013) *What Colour is Your Parachute? A Practical manual for Job Hunters and Career Changers,* Ten Speed Press, USA.

67. United States Department of Labor's Bureau of International Labor Affairs (2011) *Findings on the worst forms of child labor* <http://web.archive.org/web/20131022050307/http://www.dol.gov/ilab/programs/ocft/2011TDA/Tanzania.pdf> [last accessed 22 October 2015].

68. Carnegie, R. (2006) op. cit. pp.65–67.

FURTHER READING

Kent, Ros; Iorpenda, Kate and Fay, Alice (2012) *Family-centred HIV programming for children: Good Practice Guide.* International HIV/AIDS alliance <http://www.savethechildren.org.uk/resources/online-library/family-centred-hiv-programming-children> [last accessed 22 October 2015].

Save The Children (2010) *The Essential Package Holistically Addressing the Needs of Young Vulnerable Children and Their Caregivers Affected by HIV and AIDS* http://resourcecentre.savethechildren.se/sites/default/files/documents/the_essential_package_holistically_addressing_the_needs_of_young_vulnerable_children_and_their_caregivers_affected_by_hiv_and_aids_11.pdf [last accessed 22 October 2015].

Save The Children (2012) *Child Protection in the Context of HIV and AIDS: Responses, Research, Recommendations,* Save The Children, <http://resourcecentre.savethechildren.se/sites/default/files/documents/6008.pdf> [last accessed 22 October 2015].

Appreciative Inquiry

McAdam, E. (1996) 'Tuning into the Voices of Influence: The Social Construction of Therapy with Children', *Human Systems* 6(3) https://drive.google.com/file/d/0B5TWuGoJVPe_NU1GOGJZM2xYVk0/edit [last accessed 22 October 2015].

McAdam, E. and Lang, P. (2003) 'Working in the worlds of children: Growing, schools, families, communities through imagining' *International Journal of Narrative Therapy & Community Work,* 2003(4): 48–57 <http://search.informit.com.au/documentSummary;dn=661365349642706;res=IELHEA> [last accessed 22 October 2015].

McAdam, E. and Mirza, K. (2009) 'Drugs, hopes and dreams: appreciative inquiry with marginalized young people using drugs and alcohol' *Journal of Family Therapy* 31(2):175–193 <http://onlinelibrary.wiley.com/doi/10.1111/j.1467-6427.2009.00461.x/abstract> [last accessed 22 October 2015].

Psycho-social Support

Berg, I.K. and Steiner, T. (2003) *Children's Solution Work,* W. W. Norton & Company.

Fontana, D. and Slack, I. (1997) *Teaching Meditation to Children: The Practical Guide to the Use and Benefits of Meditation Techniques.* London, Watkins Publishing.

Gilbert, P. (2005) *Compassion, Conceptualisations, Research and Use in Psychotherapy* London, Routledge.

Karkara, R., Fahmida, F.S. and Bhandari, Neha (2006) *Safe You and Safe Me,* Save the Children Sweden <http://srsg.violenceagainstchildren.org/sites/default/files/images/childrens_corner/Safe_You_and_Safe_Me.pdf> [last accessed 22 October 2015].

Morgan, J. (2007) *Making a Hero (Active Citizen) Book A Guide for Facilitators,* REPSSI, Johannesburg. <http://www.globalizationandhealth.com/content/5/1/8> [last accessed 22 October 2015].

Ranking, J., Cochrane, R. and Khulakahle Child Counselling Training Forum (2011) *The Child Within: Connecting with Children who have experience grief and loss.* UK: Strategies For Hope Trust.

Selekman, M.D. (1997) *Solution-focused therapy with children: Harnessing Family Strengths for systemic change.* New York, Guilford Press.

Siegel D.J. and Bryson, T.P. (2014) *Brainstorm: The Power and Purpose of the Teenage Brain*, New York, Penguin.

Siegel, D.J. (2015) *The Neurological Basis of Behavior, the Mind, the Brain and Human Relationships Part 1* https://www.youtube.com/watch?v=LleKn9BgSr0 [last accessed 22 October 2015].

Skovdal, Morten, Ogutu, Vincent O. (2009) '"I washed and fed my mother before going to school": Understanding the psychosocial well-being of children providing chronic care for adults affected by HIV/AIDS in Western Kenya', *Globalization and Health*, 5(8).

Skovdal, Morten (2011) 'Picturing the Coping Strategies of Caregiving Children in Western Kenya: From Images to Action' *Am J Public Health.*; 101(3): 452–453. <http://www.ncbi.nlm.nih.gov/pmc/articles/PMC3036692/> [last accessed 22 October 2015].

Stokes, J., Crossley, D. and Stubbs, D. (2007) *As big as it gets: Supporting a child when a parent is seriously ill.* UK: Winston's Wish.

HIV testing, Treatment and Care

Hejoaka, F. (2010)'"The Child Went Back to the Village!" Rethinking HIV Positive Child Care and Treatment through Mobility and Family Nomadism in Burkina Faso' <http://www.academia.edu/1706053/Hejoaka_F._2010_._The_Child_Went_Back_to_the_Village_Rethinking_HIV_Positive_Child_Care_and_Treatment_through_Mobility_and_Family_Nomadism_in_Burkina_Faso._Oral_Abstract_Session_AIDS_2010._Session_Lifecourse_Perspectives_on_Families_Affected_by_HIV_and_AIDS_._- XVIII_International_AIDS_Conference_21_July_2010._Vienna_Austria [last accessed 22 October 2015].

Neema S., Atuyambe, L., Otolok-Tanga, B., Twijukye, C., Kambugu, A., Thayer, L. and McAdam, K. (2012) 'Using a clinic based creativity initiative to reduce HIV related stigma at the Infectious Diseases Institute, Mulago National Referral Hospital, Uganda' *African Health Sciences* 12(2) *http://www.ncbi.nlm.nih.gov/pmc/articles/PMC3462528/* [last accessed 22 October 2015].

Teachers and Children

Badoe, A. (2005) *My Sister Julie*. Macmillan Education. Available from www.talcuk.org

Hanbury, C. and Carnegie, R. (2005) *Child-to-Child Approaches to HIV and AIDS: A manual for teachers, health workers and facilitators of children and young people.* UK: The Child-to-Child Trust. Available from www.talcuk.org

International HIV/AIDS Alliance (2008) *Our Future: Preparing to teach sexuality and life skills, an awareness training manual for teachers and community workers,* UK: International HIV/AIDS Alliance. <http://hivaidsclearinghouse.unesco.org/search/resources/Alliance_Preparing_to_Teach_554a_EN.pdf> [last accessed 22 October 2015].

International HIV/AIDS Alliance (2006) *Our Future: Sexuality and Life Skills education for young people, Grades 4–5, 6–7, 8–9* International HIV / AIDS Alliance. <http://www.aidsalliance.org/resources/351-our-future-sexuality-and-lifeskills-education-for-young-people> [last accessed 22 October 2015].

Steinitz, L.Y. (2010) *My Life – Starting Now: Knowledge and skills for young adolescents; Number 8 in the Called to Care Toolkit Series*. UK: Strategies For Hope Trust.

Winkler, G. (2009) *Understanding more about HIV and AIDS: Teacher's Guide and Student's Book.* Macmillan Education. Available from www.talcuk.org

Winkler, G. (2009) *Learning about HIV and AIDS: Teacher's Guide and Student's Book* Macmillan Education. Available from www.talcuk.org

UNESCO (2009) *International Technical Guidance on Sexuality Education: An evidence-informed approach for schools, teachers and health educators,* UNESCO <http://unesdoc.unesco.org/images/0018/001832/183281e.pdf> [last accessed 22 October 2015].

Sexuality, children and HIV

Edgework Consulting (2012) *The anatomy of a health seeking choice.* UNICEF Namibia. <http://assets.sportanddev.org/downloads/the_anatomy_of_a_health_seeking_choice_.pdf> [last accessed 22 October 2015].

International Planned Parenthood Federation (2010) *Healthy, Happy and Hot. A young people's guide to rights.* <http://www.ippf.org/resource/Healthy-Happy-and-Hot-young-peoples-guide-rights> [last accessed 22 October 2015].

Van Reeuwijk, M. (2010) *Because of Temptations: children, sex and HIV/AIDS in Tanzania.* Diemen: AMB Publications <http://hdl.handle.net/11245/1.313676> [last accessed 22 October 2015].

Websites

<http://www.cdc.gov/lgbthealth/youth.htm> Information on lesbian, gay, bisexual and transgender issues.

<www.memorybooks.org.uk> Guidance on making memory books or boxes.

<www.ovcsupport.net> A global hub for children and HIV.

ANNEX OF PICTURES

We have provided larger copies of certain pictures in this Annex, to use in Stepping Stones with Children workshops. If you can photocopy and enlarge them that would be best. If not, you can show participants pictures by holding up the manual.

We have not labelled the pictures, but in each case there is a small version of the picture in the session, so you just need to find the same picture in this Annex.

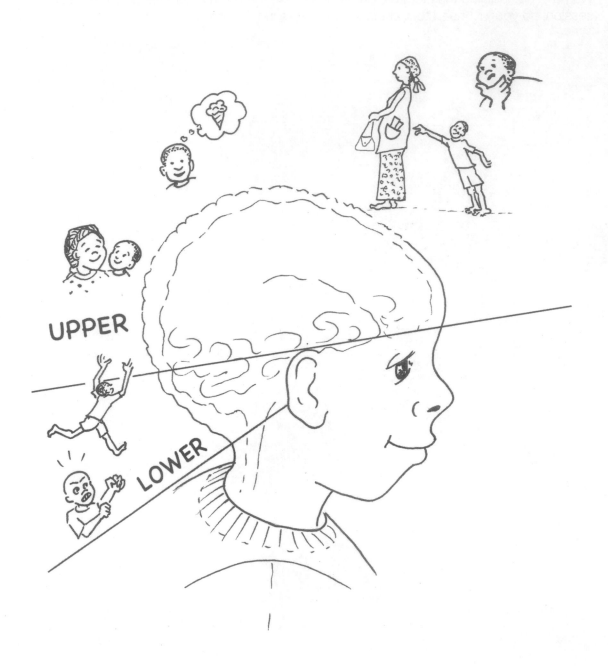

UPPER

LOWER

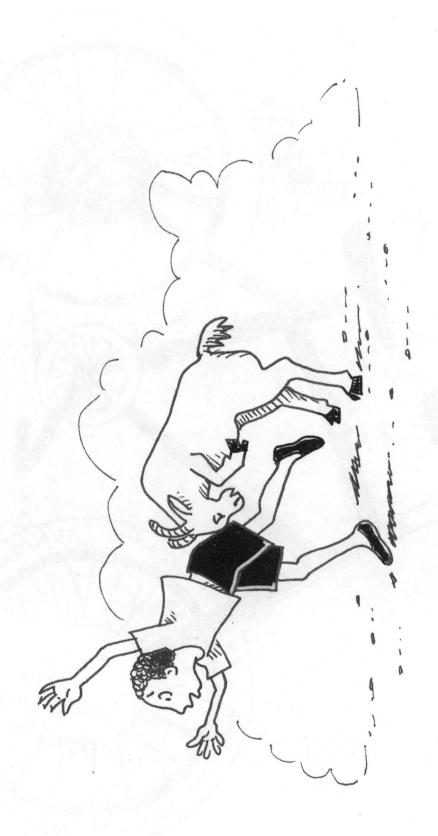

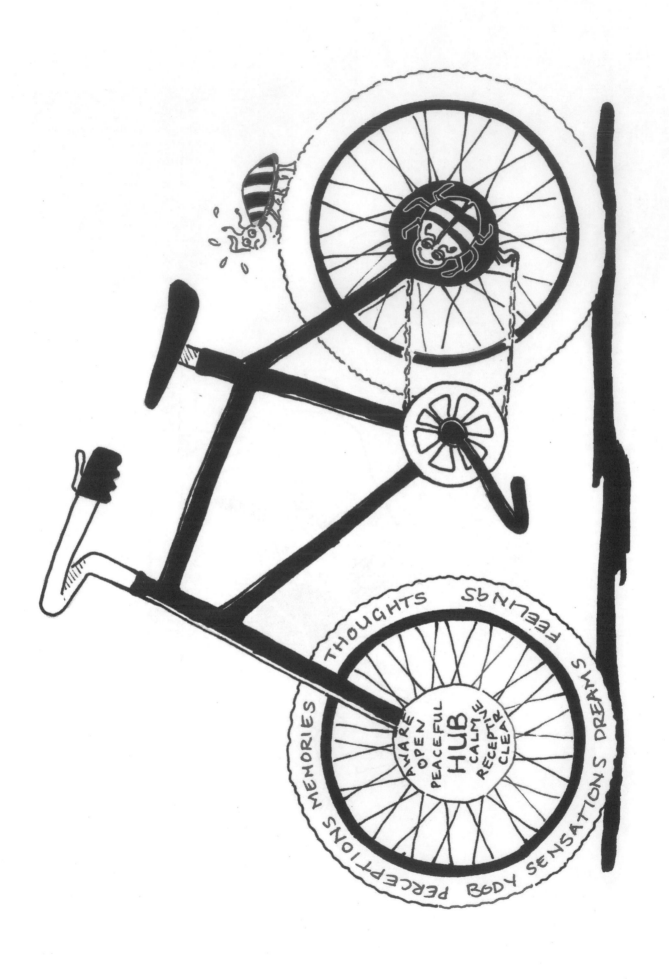

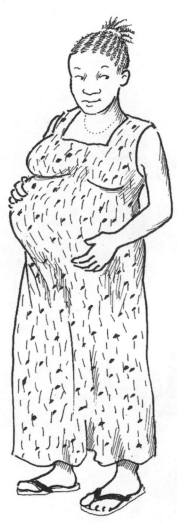

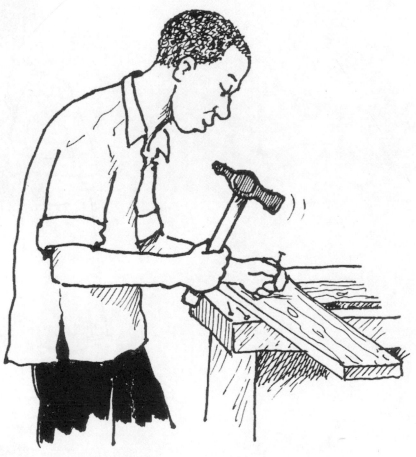

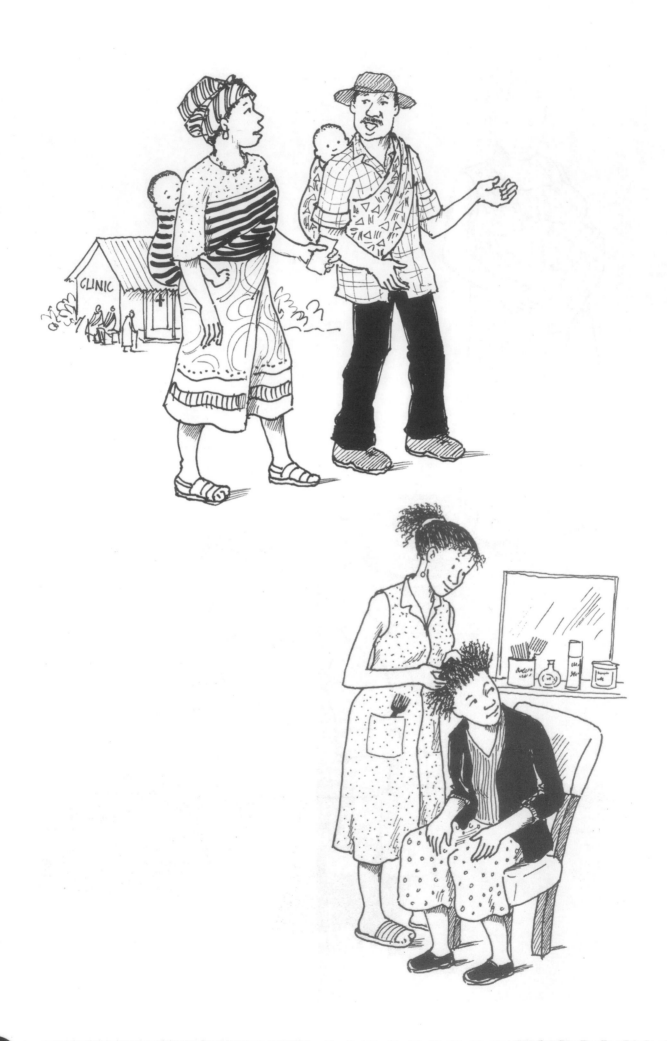

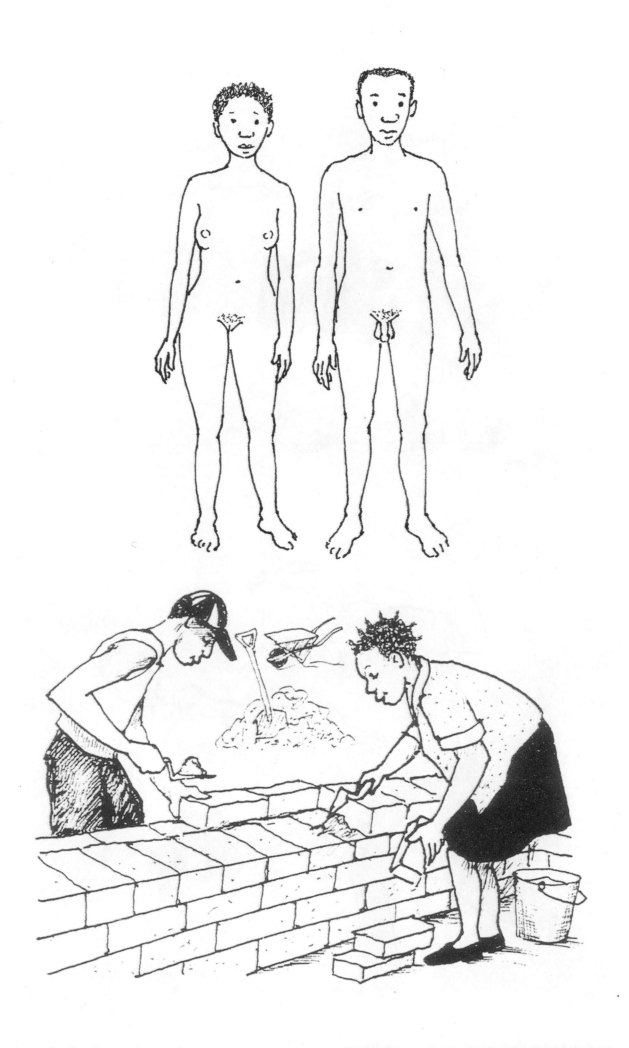

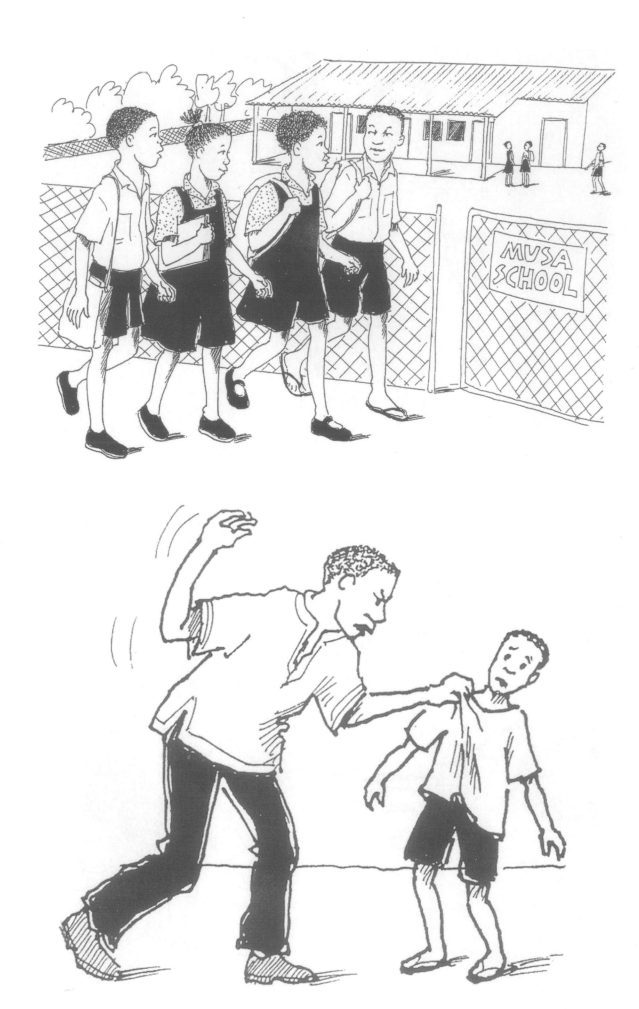

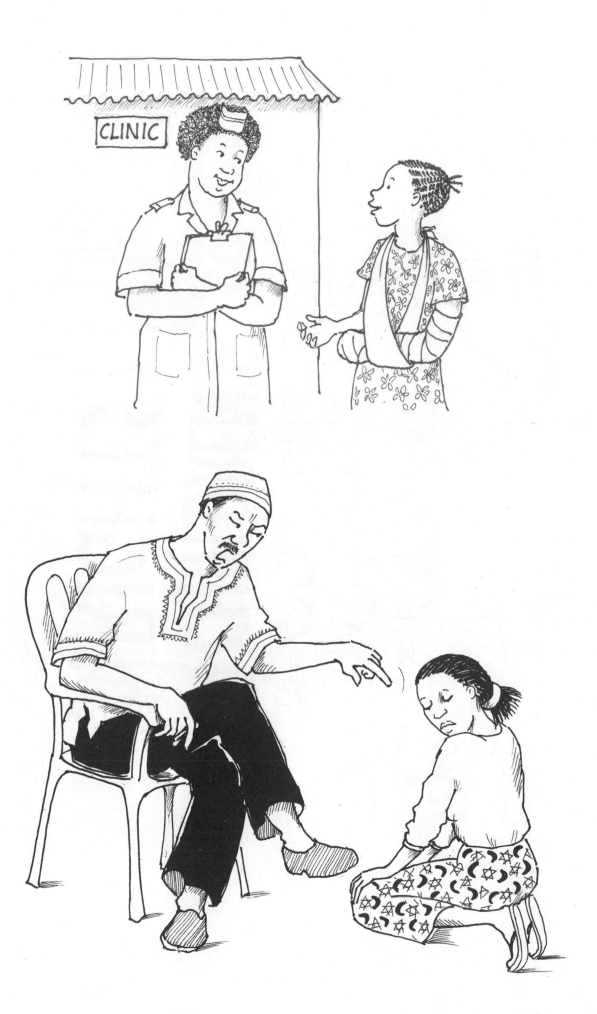

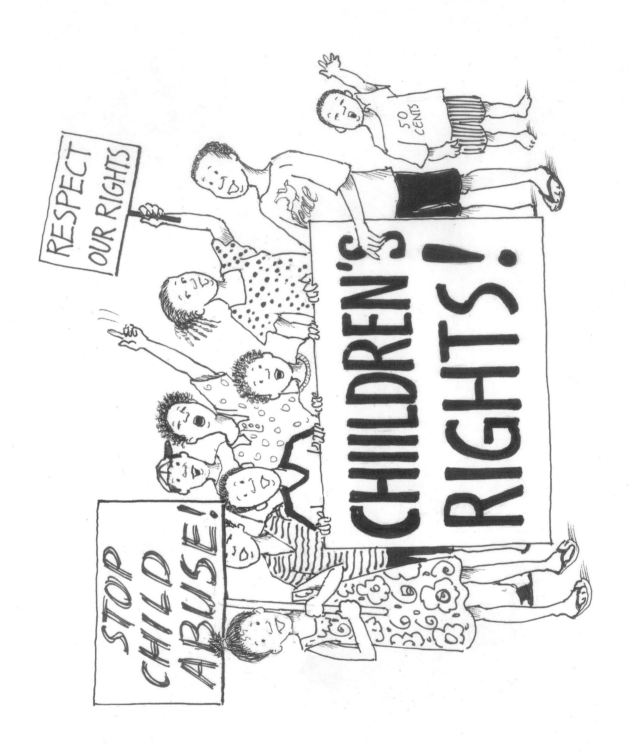

Assertiveness   Generosity   Reliability

Compassion   Honesty   Respect

Cooperation   Justice   Responsibility

Courage   Kindness   Self-discipline

Diligence   Love   Thankfulness

Enthusiasm   Moderation   Tolerance

Flexibility   Patience   Trustworthiness

Forgiveness   Peacefulness

Friendliness   Purposefulness

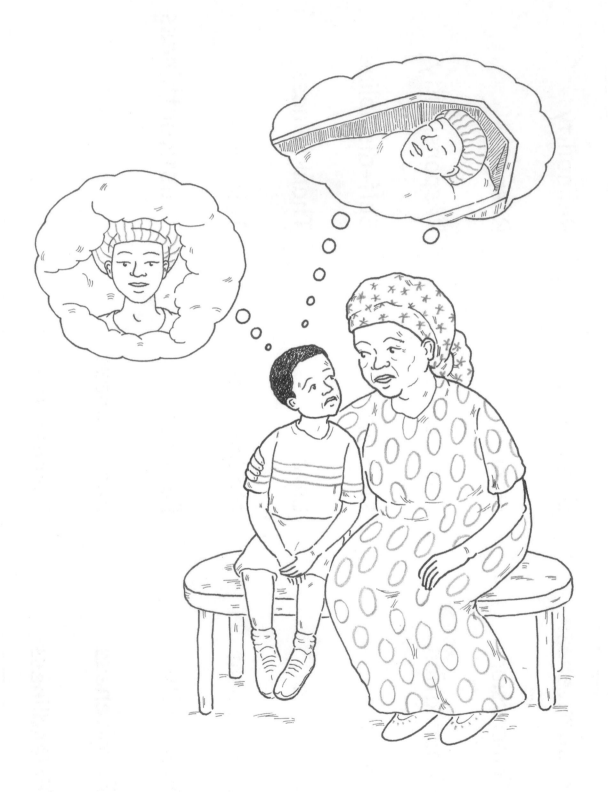

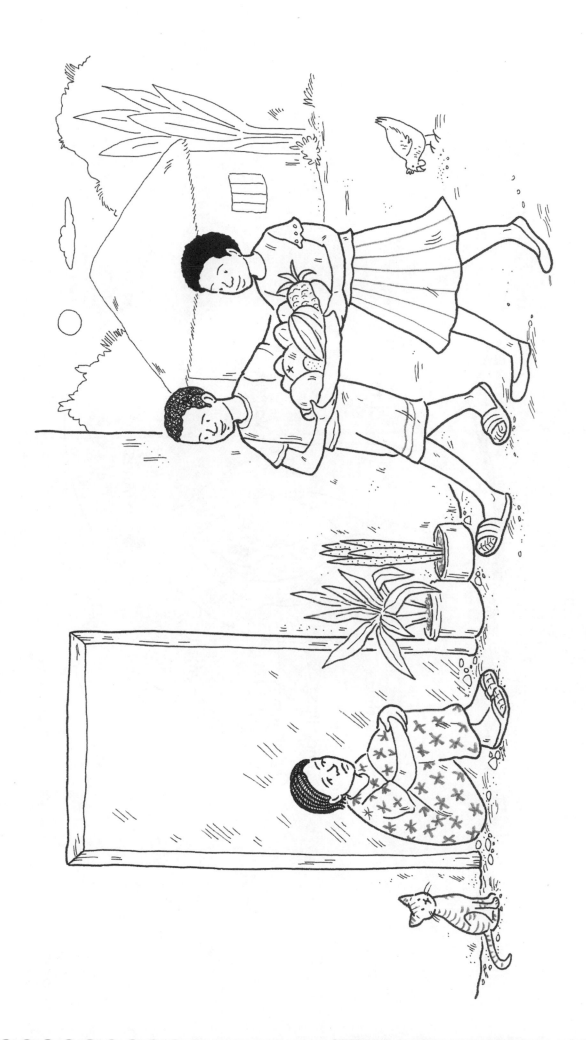

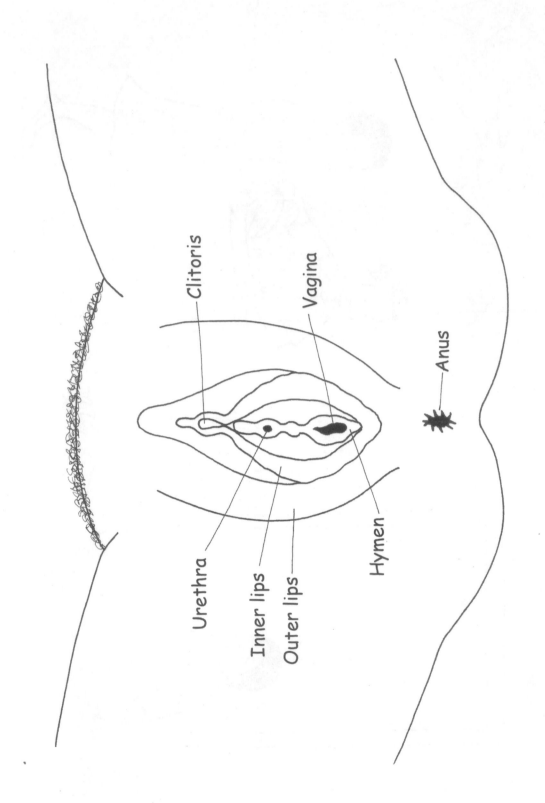

Clitoris

Vagina

Anus

Urethra

Inner lips

Outer lips

Hymen

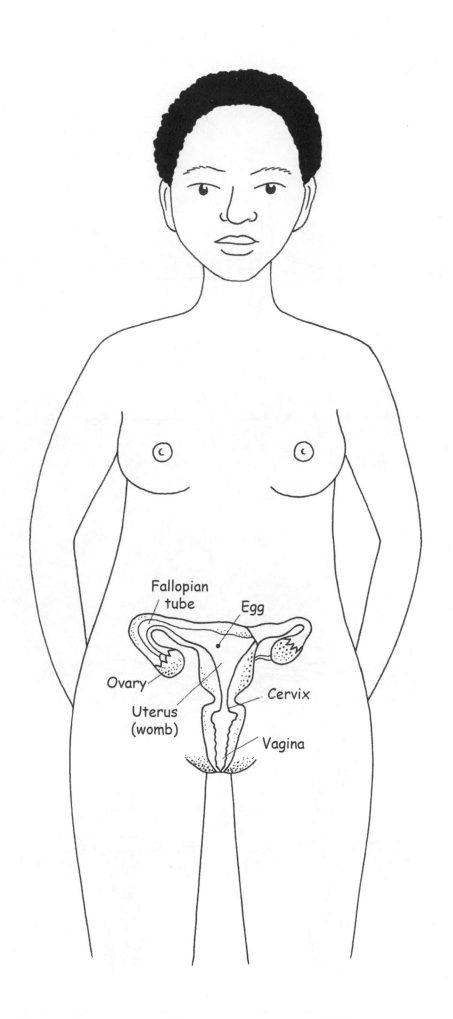

Fallopian
tube

Egg

Ovary

Cervix

Uterus
(womb)

Vagina

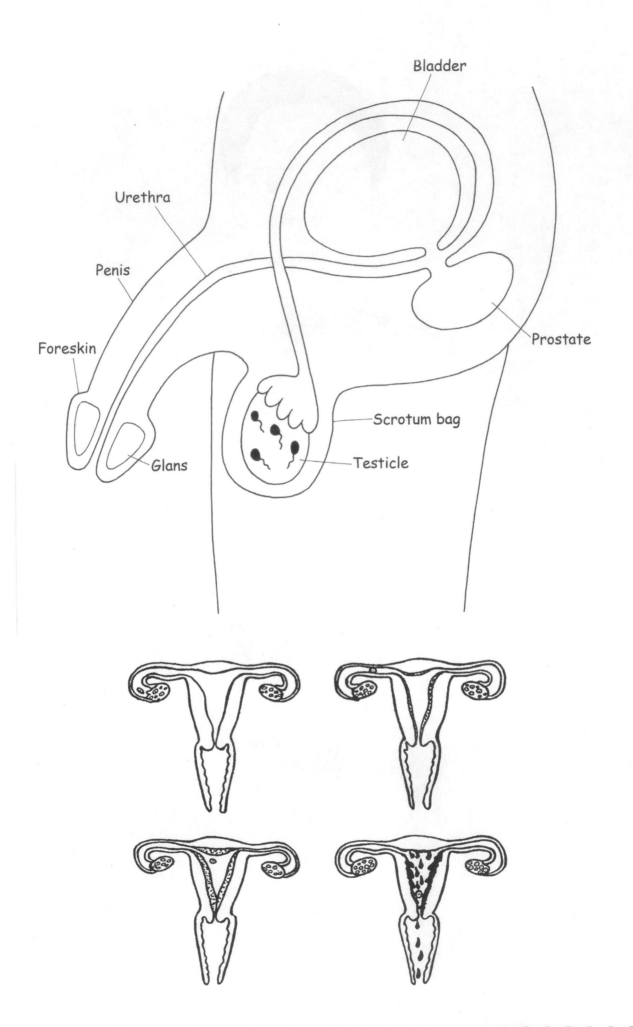

Bladder

Urethra

Penis

Foreskin

Glans

Scrotum bag

Testicle

Prostate

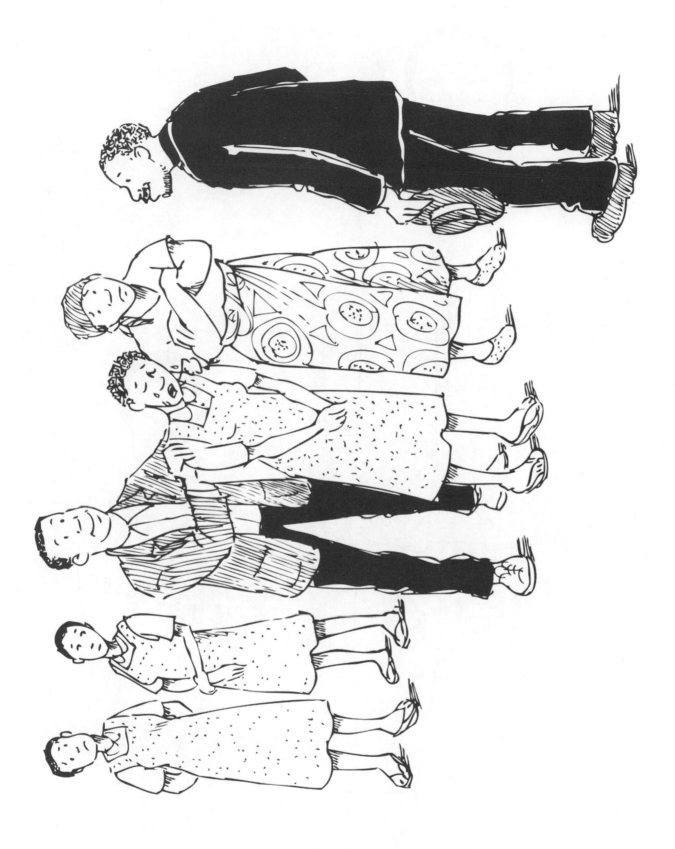

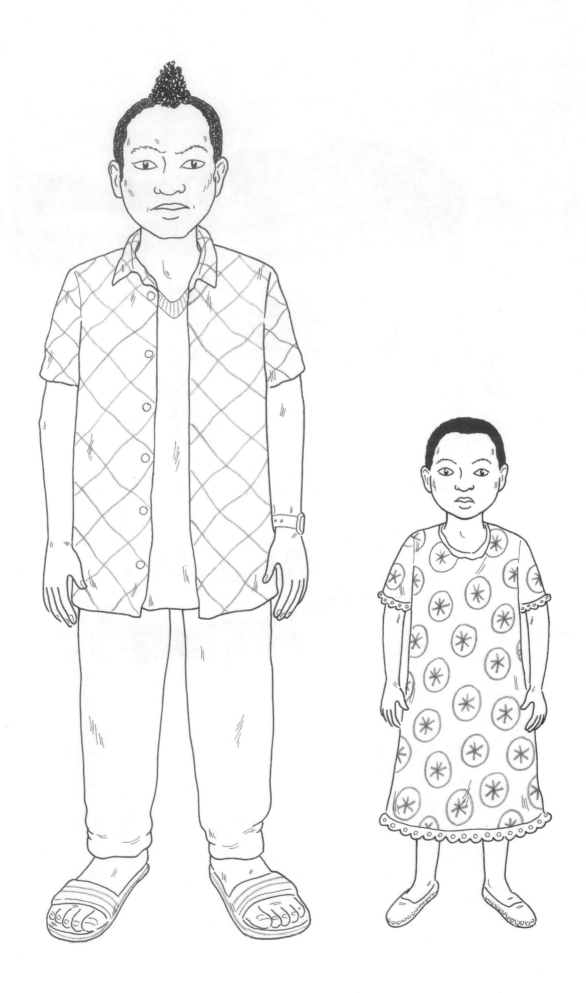